PROF. KERRYN PHELPS AM

FOREWORD BY *HIS ROYAL HIGHNESS PRINCE CHARLES*

THE
CANCER
RECOVERY
GUIDE

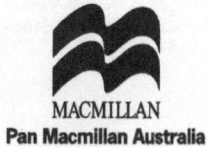

MACMILLAN
Pan Macmillan Australia

I dedicate this book to the patients whose personal cancer journeys have inspired me throughout my career and encouraged me to become a better doctor.

First published 2015 in Macmillan by Pan Macmillan Australia Pty Ltd
1 Market Street, Sydney, New South Wales, Australia, 2000

Cataloguing-in-Publication entry is available
from the National Library of Australia
http://catalogue.nla.gov.au

Typeset in 11.5/17 pt Sabon by Midland Typesetters, Australia
Printed by McPherson's Printing Group
Text design by Christa Moffat

Professor Kerryn Phelps AM is a doctor, public health and human rights advocate, past president of the Australian Medical Association, and past president of the Australasian Integrative Medicine Association.

She is an Adjunct Professor at Sydney Medical School, Conjoint Professor in the faculty of medicine at the University of New South Wales and Conjoint Professor in the National Institute of Complementary Medicine at the University of Western Sydney.

In 2001 she was awarded the Centenary Medal for services to Health and Medicine and in 2011 she was made a Member of the Order of Australia for service to medicine, particularly through leadership roles with the AMA, education and community health, and as a general practitioner.

In 2014 she was awarded an Honorary Doctorate of Letters by the University of Western Sydney.

She is a mother of three and lives in Sydney with her wife, Jackie, and youngest daughter, Gabi.

Also by Kerryn Phelps
Ultimate Wellness
General Practice: The Integrative Approach
Prostate Cancer for the General Practitioner

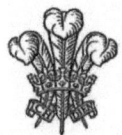

CLARENCE HOUSE

I greatly admire Professor Phelps' work in integrated health and care and I am delighted that she has produced this wonderful book for patients with cancer. It is a disease that is often accompanied by feelings of fear and helplessness but, with her integrated approach, Professor Phelps offers those with cancer both hope and some very practical information and advice on what they can do for themselves.

For very nearly thirty-five years, I have been a strong advocate of integrated healthcare. Conventional medicine has become effective in so many areas of medicine, and particularly with cancer. Nevertheless, it is not the whole story and changes in lifestyle and complementary treatments in combination with conventional medicine can, as we are often told, help symptoms and survival.

To some it may seem self-evident that what we eat may increase the benefits of the medicines that we take. Professor Phelps provides invaluable information on healthy eating and how this can be tailored to some specific conditions such as prostatic cancer. She also provides details of herbal and other complementary approaches, which can be used for different ailments and conditions as well as amplifying the effects or reducing the side effects of specific conventional remedies.

Crucially, proper integration is also about mind, body and spirit and I can only welcome a book that takes all three into account. I have always argued that when pursuing integrated approaches, safety and attention to evidence must be paramount. Professor Phelps has studiously attended to both in this book, often offering the reader the choice of whether a treatment or its given evidence makes it right for him or her. Facing cancer is a very personal thing and therefore, within the confines of safety and evidence, it is important that patients are helped to find the path that suits them best.

I have often described integrated medicine as "The best of both worlds", combining the conventional and the complementary. Professor Phelps has described how patients can ensure the best of both worlds for themselves in this book. She has combined her experience as a G.P. with a meticulous approach as an academic. On top of that, she has produced a clear and readable book which, I hope, will be of help to cancer patients everywhere...

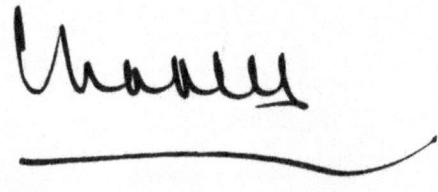

Contents

Prologue

A visit to my dermatologist is usually more a casual social affair than a serious medical consultation. And, like a lot of my patients who come to me for a general check-up, I had no particular concerns that day.

The dermatologist asked me to slip off my shirt and we began to chat about the start of the school year. What I was not expecting was to hear the words, 'Hmm, I don't like the look of that pigmented lesion on your back. I think I'd better take that off and send it for a biopsy.'

You know the old saying about your life flashing before your eyes? Well one of the problems for a doctor in the role of patient is that you see other people's lives flash before your eyes: the fifteen year old in my brother's old rugby team who had a melanoma and didn't make it to the next season; the friend with a massive scar on his back; the friend of my parents who had a mole removed from his chest and thought it was all over and done with, only to have it return and take his life years later; the patients with metastatic melanoma I have fought to get onto clinical trials because all other options have failed.

This might sound like an exercise in catastrophising, but while having the lesion removed I had to admit to myself that I felt confronted by fear and doubt. I knew the procedure itself was a simple one, yet it made me feel very apprehensive.

The biopsy results took a few days to come through, and during that time I thought about the possible outcomes. The result could go either way. If it was a melanoma I knew exactly what sort of decisions would need to be made about how to manage it. If it was small and contained then a wider excision might be all that would be needed. But it might be more serious with all the implications that may bring. I thought about my future, my family, my wife, my children and my dogs. The days ticked by as I worried and waited.

Luckily for me, pathology showed a dysplastic naevus, a benign mole. Not a cancer. I was relieved but I regarded the experience as a very personal reminder of the trauma that people go through when they are waiting for results or receiving the bad news that their test results show a cancer that may threaten their survival and need to be treated, casting them instantly into the role of 'cancer patient'.

I thought back thirty-something years, to when I was fresh out of medical school and working as a hospital resident. I was pregnant with my first child. Not the greatest timing, I admit. I knew I would have to take some time off during my training to look after my new baby, so I asked to be given the most medically difficult and challenging term to start, in a specialty where I would learn the most. I was assigned to the oncology team.

To say that starting my medical career on the cancer wards of a major teaching hospital was challenging is an understatement. Our team was responsible for looking after the sickest patients in the hospital. There were the technical aspects of the job, such as taking blood from veins that had no more blood to give, learning to perform a peritoneal tap or inserting a pleural drain, and there were the pompously named 'grand rounds', when a dozen or more doctors, nurses and medical students would crowd around a bed while a patient's latest test results were delivered or the next part of their treatment plan decided.

And, of course, there were the confronting emotional aspects of working on an oncology ward.

I remember discreetly dashing to the bathroom with horrible morning sickness to vomit, in between helping patients to cope with far worse nausea and vomiting from chemotherapy. This was years before we had effective medications or other tools to treat chemotherapy-related nausea.

The work was physically and emotionally exhausting. I was reminded daily of the irony of carrying a new life inside me while around me our patients were fighting for their lives or losing their struggle to survive.

I see that first term as a great gift, to have begun my career gaining the blinding insight of the impact that a serious and life-threatening disease can have on a person and their family. In my decades since then and as an integrative general practitioner, I have had the privilege of seeing the bigger picture. The cancers that are prevented, the cancers that are treated successfully, the long-term survivors, and the elements of successful living after a cancer diagnosis from a physical, emotional and spiritual perspective. And the reality that some people do not survive their cancer in the long term, and quality of life issues become the paramount issue.

A common theme that emerges when patients come to our clinic for help and advice is that they are looking for a plan of action, a template for the way forward. They want to be guided through the options for treatment and symptom relief, and provided information with clear, truthful explanations. They are looking for emotional support and practical solutions delivered with empathy and respect.

I am often asked when discussing options with a patient and their family, 'What would you do?'

I tell patients, and I teach my students this philosophy, 'I will only advise you to do what I would be prepared to do in your position.' The advice in this book comes with that philosophy.

Obviously every individual is different. We have different perspectives and different life stories, but there is much that is common about all of our experiences of health and illness.

This book is the result of many years of guiding patients through all aspects of cancer management in general practice. It is also the culmination of decades of learning from my patients about what they need at every stage in order to make their way through the often confusing and distressing maze they face when they are diagnosed with a cancer.

The field of cancer research is moving at a breathtakingly rapid pace. We know so much, yet there is still so much more we have yet to understand. In the process of writing this book, many areas of knowledge will have grown and changed.

If you have been diagnosed with cancer, you will need the concentrated and focused knowledge of your medical oncology specialists in the decision-making about your cancer-specific treatments. In this book I have attempted to distil the most practical and current information across the spectrum of other issues and decisions you may face throughout your individual cancer journey. This can be a confusing and stressful time and, for a while at least, it will take over your life.

I hope that with the advice in this book and the support of your healthcare team, family and friends, you will be able to navigate your way through it, recover and, literally, get your life back.

All my best,
Professor Kerryn Phelps AM

Introduction

Your doctor has told you that you have cancer. You might have had dozens of routine screening tests, never really expecting one to come back with bad news, or you might finally have an explanation for symptoms you have been experiencing.

No matter how positive or optimistic your usual nature might be, being told you have cancer turns your world upside down, at least for a while. Your first reaction is usually one of shock, or a sensation of surrealism that this couldn't really be happening to you.

Once you are told the likely diagnosis, you will initially have a million questions:

'Why me?'

'How did this happen?'

'What does this mean to me and my family?'

'What are my chances of recovery?'

'What specialists will I need to see and what treatments will they recommend?'

'What else can I do to improve my chances of a cure or remission?'

You may also feel many conflicting and intense emotions: fear, anxiety, anger, despair or hope.

You will be faced with a barrage of tests and information, which can be confusing and have you feeling scared and powerless. The advice you are given and the decisions you make will determine what treatment you have, and this will in turn help to determine your future. It is important for you to know that you are not powerless. The more information you have, the more confident you will feel to engage in the decision-making process. Obviously you will rely heavily on the experience and advice of your medical experts, but once you have that information, you are the one who will have to make the final decisions and give informed consent for any treatment.

Immediately after diagnosis, your doctors will guide you towards treatment options with a variety of goals:

- curing your cancer
- getting your cancer to a manageable state, or
- relieving discomfort caused by the cancer for as long as possible.

These 'cancer-specific treatments' will be recommended by your GP, surgeon, medical oncologist, radiation oncologist, or other cancer specialist.

It is possible you will also be offered treatments that fall outside the mainstream biomedical 'surgery, chemotherapy, radiotherapy, immunotherapy' set. More commonly though, in my experience, people find they have to proactively hunt around beyond established mainstream cancer services for advice on the additional treatments they can use to help make the cancer treatment process easier and, possibly, more effective.

Advice on whether a cancer-specific treatment is warranted, or which combination of chemotherapy is right for your particular cancer, or which radiotherapy or surgical procedure is best in a particular case is a matter for expert individual assessment. Oncology is a fast-moving field, where new treatments come along all the time and clinical trials are conducted to test them. If new treatments prove themselves in clinical trials to be superior to existing treatments, they will become part of the generally accepted treatment protocol.

Being diagnosed with cancer is undeniably scary. I want to show you how to be one of those people who turns a cancer diagnosis into a call to action; to do whatever you can to get through the treatment the best you can, and clean up your lifestyle to give yourself the best possible chance of survival and an optimal quality of life.

Many people find they feel very vulnerable and may try anything with the promise of curing cancer, regardless of the cost or the potential risk. I have seen people make all sorts of choices. Some of them I have agreed with, some I have not.

I believe the best thing I can do for you is to give you easy-to-understand information about the range of options you may want to consider, based on the best available evidence, as well as clinical experience. I will also steer you away from treatments that are likely to be ineffective, unsafe or excessively expensive without a high prospect of delivering on their promise.

Treating cancer is not only about procedures and drugs and supplements and therapies, although they all play a very important role. With cancer recovery, it is often a case of what old habits you can change to improve your chances of survival, and a sense that you can get your life back as good as, or maybe even better than, before.

USING THIS BOOK

The Cancer Recovery Guide is designed as a user-friendly guide for your cancer journey and beyond. You can read it through from start to finish, or you can jump into chapters that are relevant to you at a particular time. Where topics are referred to repeatedly or cross-referenced (such as dealing with fatigue), follow the cross-referencing and use the index to find the specific information useful to you. Use the information in this book to navigate your way through your journey, help you to reduce the side effects of cancer-specific treatments, consolidate your physical and emotional resources, and improve your ability to heal physically, emotionally and spiritually.

THE INTEGRATIVE APPROACH

In my experience, patients attend our integrative medicine clinic, Sydney Integrative Medicine, at a variety of stages along their cancer journey. There are those patients who see our doctors and other practitioners regularly for their usual health screening or disease management. We may have detected their cancer as part of their regular healthcare process. We may have arranged the investigation of symptoms such as a lump or pain or a change of bowel habit that led to a cancer diagnosis.

Where we are involved in a patient's care from the outset, we are able to guide that patient to oncology specialists and integrate and interweave adjunctive therapies throughout their cancer-specific treatment including preparation and support throughout treatment.

In many cases, patients seek us out because they have already been diagnosed with cancer and want a plan for getting through treatment. Some patients are able to work with their GP to put together an integrative plan with the cooperation of their oncology team. Unfortunately, however, patients can sometimes encounter resistance or hostility to the suggestion of treatments that are considered to be outside of the 'mainstream'. I have seen this reaction even when the suggestions for adjunctive treatments have a strong evidence base and low potential risk. Patients tell me they needed to find doctors who have special training or interest in integrative approaches, or who at the very least are open-minded and not hostile to discussions about different adjunctive treatment options.

Then there are the patients who have been through cancer-specific treatment without integrative support and find their way to us because they are struggling with their recovery. Treatment has left them feeling fatigued, drained, depressed and depleted.

With the right information and professional guidance, you can protect yourself from some of the negative impact of cancer treatment on your physical and emotional health, and optimise your potential for wellbeing.

I want to define the terms 'adjunctive' and 'integrative' because I use them a lot throughout this book and it is important that you know exactly what I am talking about. These terms are not the same as 'alternative'. 'Alternative' therapy implies a treatment that is intended to replace mainstream cancer-specific treatments.

Adjunctive therapies, on the other hand, are forms of treatment that are usually professionally guided or provided before, along-side, or following completion of mainstream cancer treatment. The aim of adjunctive therapies is to to reduce the side effects of cancer treatment – making the cancer-specific treatments more tolerable or cause less damage – and to enhance recovery. In the real world, the vast majority of people who choose to use adjunctive therapies do so alongside and in addition to their conventional cancer-specific treatments.

The term 'integrative' implies a plan to safely amalgamate various types of treatment, the 'cancer-specific' and the 'adjunctive' therapies in an individual or personalised way.

Even the term 'mainstream' is difficult to define, and the boundaries are shifting all the time. Your definition of mainstream will differ depending on your perspective, the available evidence, and the prevailing opinions of the medical profession at that time. I have been around long enough to see that even within 'mainstream' there is a wide range of opinions.

You may want to pursue adjunctive treatments that you hear about from friends or relatives, or read about in magazines or on the internet. But not all of the treatments you will read about or hear about are safe or effective.

In *The Cancer Recovery Guide* I will take you through many of the options and guide you to formulating a personalised, individual program to cancer recovery.

A HOLISTIC APPROACH

It should go without saying, but you are more than your cancer. At all stages of treatment and recovery you need to think of yourself in a holistic way, and consider all aspects of your physical, emotional and spiritual health. The incidence of chronic diseases such as diabetes, heart disease, arthritis, osteoporosis and kidney disease increases with age, so it is quite possible that you could be dealing with other health issues in parallel with your cancer. Chronic disease needs to be taken into consideration in any cancer treatment decision, and it also needs to be taken into account when you are planning your life ahead so that you can benefit in multiple ways from the decisions you make to live a healthier life.

Your GP needs to be aware of all of your health concerns and remind you to keep on track with all your health checks and screening along with your cancer specific checks.

PALLIATIVE CARE

This book is about managing your cancer, getting control and getting your life back after a cancer diagnosis. Even with the best care and treatment, for some people their cancer journey will be marked by recurrence or metastatic disease and for some this will require palliative care. The information in this book will continue to be relevant throughout any cancer journey but depending on the outcome, additional specialised information might be necessary when remission or cure is not considered possible, and quality of life and symptom management become the aim of treatment.

The following resources may prove useful when seeking additional information about palliative care:

- www.health.gov.au/palliativecare
- www.cancercouncil.com.au/87416/b1000/palliative-care-41/palliative-care-key-questions/
- Palliative Care Australia Multilingua: www.palliativecare.org.au/6Old/MultilingualResources.aspx
- Life Hope and Reality: www.caresearch.com.au/caresearch/WhatisPalliativeCare/tabid/63/Default.aspx
- End of Life Care: www.nhs.uk/Planners/end-of-life-care/Pages/what-it-involves-and-when-it-starts.aspx

· PART ONE ·

Diagnosis

Hearing the Word 'CANCER' is Scary

Being diagnosed with cancer can force you into a fog of fear for your future. What treatment do I need to have and what effect will it have on me? What are my chances of survival? How will it affect my family? Once it is treated, could the cancer come back? If you have been close to someone who has battled against cancer you may have a well-founded fear of the disease, its treatment and its possible outcome.

> For more information regarding coping with cancer emotionally, turn to page 63 for a full discussion and information regarding support and coping strategies.

We know the statistics about cancer. And they are scary.

According to the Cancer Council Australia, cancer is one of the leading causes of death in Australia, accounting for about three in 10 deaths. Cancer remains the second most common cause of death in the US, accounting for nearly one of every four deaths.

While these are the frightening numbers, it's important to realise that they're not the whole equation. Keep in mind that when you hear about 'cancer statistics', you often hear only the negatives.

In the early part of my career in the 1980s, a woman diagnosed with metastatic breast cancer would have been told there was nothing more to be done, and to make plans for the limited time she had left. Nowadays, it is a vastly different picture. That same woman would now be told about her options for the next phase of treatment which might include chemotherapy, hormonal therapy, radiotherapy or targeted therapy (sometimes called biological therapies) which are drugs that stop the growth of particular types of cancer cells. Even with metastatic disease, we are often able to plan for long-term survival.

The survival rate for many common cancers, such as breast cancer, has increased by 30 per cent in the past two decades as a result of earlier diagnosis and more effective treatments. Additionally, more than 60 per cent of people diagnosed with cancer in Australia will survive more than five years after diagnosis. So we have developed this relatively new concept of 'survivorship', how you live your life beyond a cancer diagnosis. At its most positive, a diagnosis of cancer is a signal to reassess your life goals, and to live as well as you can.

Unless you are told that there is 100 per cent chance that your cancer will be cured, you are going to experience a sense of uncertainty and anxiety. What can you do to reduce that level of fear? Arming yourself with information is the first step.

WHAT IS CANCER?

It is important to realise that cancer is not a single disease. The word 'cancer' refers to literally hundreds of diseases that have common features, but which can have very different outcomes.

Different cancers behave differently. There has been a great deal of debate recently in the medical profession about what we should even call 'cancer'. This has arisen out of decades of progress in screening and early detection, resulting in many cancers being found that might otherwise not have made themselves known, or ever needing to be treated at all.

A group from the National Cancer Institute in the United States recently called for an overhaul of the use of the word 'cancer', suggesting that we reserve the word for malignant disease with a reasonable likelihood of causing death if it were to be left untreated. This means there are some diseases in the cancer spectrum that will cause little or no harm in your lifetime, or which are low grade and very treatable. A low-grade prostate cancer might fall into this category.

Some cancers have been shown to respond well to changes in the way you live your life. On the other hand, a cancer diagnosis may mean you are in for the fight of your life . . . literally.

One of the most effective ways of reducing your level of fear after a diagnosis of cancer is to gather as much credible and useful knowledge as you can. You need clear and honest information from your cancer specialists about your situation and what lies ahead.

First and foremost, you need accurate information on your type of cancer and its apparent level of aggressiveness. Then you need a plan of action with estimated time frames.

Make sure you do some homework and gather a support team around you. This will include your special people: family and friends. Your medical and allied health team will be essential, of course. I will explain later about how to do this.

Make sure the cancer specialists you see are experienced with your particular type of cancer. For the less common cancers, this may mean referral to a larger cancer treatment centre.

It is important to talk about your fears and anxieties about your cancer and its treatment. Your doctors or other health professionals can help by giving you the time to ask all your questions and provide you with honest answers to the extent that they are able to predict what is likely to happen.

Connect with support groups or telephone help-lines that can give you information and share experiences with you at times when you need to talk to people who have been through the same experiences of cancer treatment.

Signs that fear is getting in the way include:

- you are having trouble sleeping at night
- you feel anxious most of the time
- you feel hopeless about the outcome of your cancer
- you have trouble concentrating
- you don't look forward to the activities you usually enjoy
- you lose your appetite.

Long-term remissions and 'cures' are not achieved without struggle and change. Surgery, radiotherapy and chemotherapy can be very harsh physically and emotionally. If you explore adjunctive treatments and activities alongside your conventional cancer treatment, it is important to ask yourself questions about why you are seeking these complementary approaches.

- Is it to reduce the side effects of treatment?
- Is it to help you recover from surgery or chemotherapy?
- Is it to improve your chances of survival?

If you choose to add some adjunctive treatments, be clear about what you are trying to achieve and make sure the health professionals you see are well qualified and experienced in working with people undergoing cancer treatment. Warning bells should start to ring if a practitioner tells you to abandon your conventional medical treatment, or to conceal any treatment they recommend from your medical team.

DON'T GET CAUGHT UP IN THE WEB

Informing yourself is a vital part of engaging in the decision-making process at every stage. To avoid confusion, I would caution you to focus only on the websites of recognised organisations or institutions. Some websites are not well researched or credible and may steer you in the wrong direction.

Your doctors will be able to direct you to some of the more credible and useful websites. Throughout the book I will also provide you with some resources and references.

Speaking the Language

In preparation for any discussion you might have with your medical specialists, you need to be clear about how much you want to know and what you want to know, and communicate that to your significant family members or support people. It is also necessary for you to have a clear understanding of the terms that will be used in that discussion. Nobody expects you to understand all of the medical jargon.

If your doctors use any terminology that you do not understand, ask them to explain the meaning to you. It is easy to misunderstand the words that are used in discussing the outcome of your cancer and what it means for your future, so it is important to get the terminology clear.

PROGNOSIS AND SURVIVAL

Prognosis is not definite. It is not a certainty. Prognosis is a prediction of the likely chances of surviving a disease based on your age, the type of cancer, where it is located in your body, its stage at the time of diagnosis and treatment, and the current experience of the success rate of the treatment protocols that can be offered.

The statistics are gathered over many years and involve analysis of many thousands of similar cases. I say similar, because no two people will be exactly the same.

Factoring in your past general health, or your individual current state of health, the uniqueness of your cancer, your diet (past, present and future), your genetic make-up, your attitudes and mental state into your prognosis can be difficult. Predicting with any accuracy how you, as an individual, will respond to a particular treatment can also be impossible. As the study of cancer genetics expands and treatments become more refined and personalised, many of these uncertainties will become clearer in the future.

The probability of a particular outcome for you as an individual is based on the collection of data from many thousands of patients with the same type of cancer over many years and matching it up your particular situation as closely as possible. Given the number of variables, it is amazing how accurate these assessments can be. But you can see that working out a prognosis can be complex and it is not always possible to be accurate.

Cancer survival statistics are usually given in terms of the percentage of people who survive a particular length of time. If you are given a survival prediction, it will usually be the likelihood of surviving for the next five years or ten years.

There are a number of terms you might hear and it is important to understand what your doctor means when you are having these conversations.

'CANCER-SPECIFIC SURVIVAL'

This term refers to the number of people in a treatment group who have not died as a result of the specific cancer in a defined period of time. The time period usually starts from the time of diagnosis or the start of treatment and ends at the time of death. This calculation excludes people who die from a cause other than the cancer. For example, this calculation would not include a man with prostate cancer who dies as a result of a heart attack.

'RELATIVE SURVIVAL'

This is a measure of the number of people with a cancer who survive, compared with the life expectancy of a similar group of people who do not have the cancer, usually calculated over five years from the date of diagnosis or the start of treatment. This is a way of finding out whether a particular cancer shortens life.

'OVERALL SURVIVAL'

Overall survival is the length of time that patients diagnosed with a particular cancer are still alive, from either the date of diagnosis or the start of treatment.

'DISEASE-FREE SURVIVAL'

This term refers to the length of time someone survives without any signs or symptoms of cancer once they have completed their primary cancer-specific treatment. This measure is often used in research to work out the success of a new treatment. This might also be referred to as 'recurrence-free survival'.

WHAT DO YOU WANT TO KNOW?

Given that prognosis is not an accurate or individual prediction, do you want to know how long you are likely to live? What difference would knowing that make to you?

You may want to know what the diagnosis means for your immediate future, but also what it means in terms of your long-term quality of life, and length of life.

Let's look at the situation where decisions need to be made about the best treatment approach for you. If the treatment is likely to significantly prolong your life, and without treatment there is a high likelihood that you will not survive, then you would be more inclined to decide to have the treatment, even if the treatment process itself was likely to be very difficult to go through.

On the other hand, if the treatment is not likely to give you a great deal of benefit in terms of survival or quality of life, then you might consider other options.

I remember when a friend's father was in the terminal phase of pancreatic cancer. He was told he could have chemotherapy, which would have kept him in hospital. When his oncologist was questioned about how effective the treatment was likely to be, she told the family that statistically, the chemotherapy would give him maybe another 10 days. Reasonably, the patient and his family decided against having it. He went home and, with palliative care support, died peacefully in his familiar surroundings.

On the other hand, I have also seen people resist recommendations for treatment because of the fear of adverse effects, when the potential benefits seemed to me to be obvious. I remember having an animated conversation with a patient who, without treatment, would inevitably die within months as a result of her cancer. With treatment, there was a good chance of remission. To me it was a no-brainer. She was determined to press on with alternative therapies, convinced that she could defeat it without medical intervention. I asked her a simple question: 'If you were standing in the middle of the road and there was a bus speeding towards you, would you jump out of the way?' She said of course she would. 'The bus is coming,' I said. 'You need to jump out of the way.' She reluctantly agreed to treatment and survived another four years with a good quality of life to see her children graduate from university.

Some people say they just want their doctors to make the decision and let them know what is best for them. But if your preference is to have a very active role in the decisions about your treatment, then you will need accurate and detailed information on which to base your decisions.

I find some people don't want to know every detail, or have personal, cultural or religious reasons for not wanting to discuss prognosis, so it is important that you have that discussion up front with your significant others and your medical oncologist and other team members.

I have to declare my hand at this point, because my view is that to make informed decisions, you need information. Most of my colleagues in Western medicine share this belief these days.

CULTURAL DIFFERENCES

The custom in many cultures, including Mexican, Filipino, Chinese and Iranian, is for a patient's family to be the first to hear about a poor prognosis, after which the family decides whether and how much to tell the patient. Members of such cultural groups may believe that it would be insensitive for a patient to be told bad news and doing so would only cause the patient great stress and even hasten their death by destroying hope.

But this is a generalisation, and not every member of a cultural or religious group would share the same beliefs. Doctors need to be careful not to make assumptions about our patients' views based on culture, religion or ethnicity, and it is important for you as a patient that you not assume your doctor will automatically know what you want to know. If you have cultural or religious beliefs that may influence your decision about the information you want to know about your fate, or prognosis, then this needs to be explained to your doctor, nursing staff and other healthcare team members.

If you have never faced this situation, you may not have thought about whether you would want to know 'everything'. In a 2012 study of older disabled adults (with an average age of 78 years), 65 per cent of participants said they would want to discuss the prognosis if their doctor estimated they had less than five years to live and 75 per cent said they would want to know if the estimate of their survival was under one year.

Among the people who said they would want to discuss prognosis, there were three prominent reasons given: to prepare themselves, to make the most of the life they had left, and to make medical or health-related decisions.

Those people who said they would prefer not to discuss prognosis gave these reasons: emotional difficulty, the uncertainty of prognosis, or they felt it would not be useful.

CURE, REMISSION, AND RELAPSE

Other terms you may hear from your doctor are 'cure', 'remission' and 'partial remission'.

A 'cure' is a situation where a cancer has been detected and treatment has been completed so that the treating doctors are confident that all traces of the cancer have been eliminated, and it will not ever come back. This is a big call. Doctors almost never use the word 'cure' because it calls on us to give a 100 per cent guarantee that there are no cancer cells remaining that could ever, under any circumstances, develop into a significant disease again.

Having said that, there are some examples of where using this word is appropriate. We would confidently apply the word 'cure' to a localised basal cell carcinoma of the skin that has been completely removed surgically and where there is no microscopic evidence of any cancer cells at the margin of the excision. The same could be said of a very localised focus of cervical or endometrial cancer, which is treated surgically.

Some other cancers are also so successfully treatable that they can be considered 'cured', but your doctor may still be reluctant to use the word and give you that 100 per cent guarantee if there is even a remote possibility of later recurrence. In this situation your doctor may use the term 'complete remission'.

A 'complete remission' is a situation where any signs of cancer have disappeared. You have no residual symptoms of cancer and there are no signs of the cancer on scans or in blood tumour markers or on physical medical examination. Tiny but undetectable amounts of cancer could still be present in your body. It is still possible that there could be a recurrence, but the longer the remission lasts, the less likely it is that the cancer will recur.

A 'partial remission' is when most of the signs and symptoms of the cancer have diminished or gone as a result of treatment, but the cancer is still demonstrably present. The possibility of recurrence is higher than with a complete remission.

'RELAPSE' OR 'RECURRENCE'

'Relapse' refers to a return of signs or symptoms of cancer after a period of remission. The cancer may recur at the same site or at a different site to where it started or was first detected. For example, breast cancer may recur in bones and is still referred to as a relapse or recurrence of breast cancer.

QUESTIONS FOR YOUR MEDICAL TEAM

The discussion about your prognosis is a two-way conversation. So that you have all the information you need, there are questions you may have for your medical team, particularly your oncologist. One of the ways you can prepare for the visit with your oncologist is to have a list of questions, such as:

- What are my chances of surviving without treatment compared with having the treatment you are recommending?
- What are my chances of surviving with this particular treatment compared with other treatments?
- Is there a realistic prospect of cure or long-term remission?
- Is there any risk in delaying treatment?
- What can I do to improve my state of health physically and psychologically before treatment starts?
- What are the potential adverse effects, in the short term and the long term, of the treatments being proposed?
- Are there clinical trials showing promise for new or future treatments for this cancer?

Prevention and Screening after a Diagnosis of Cancer

———————————————•———————————————

I want to explain the inclusion of this chapter on prevention and screening, in case you think that it is a case of shutting the gate of the paddock after the horse has bolted. After you have been diagnosed with a cancer, it becomes your main focus of medical attention for some time. There are important reasons to continue to screen for other medical problems and you will need to discuss with your general practitioner a plan to reinstate your regular health checks, which are often interrupted during cancer treatment.

PREVENTION

There are three levels of prevention: primary, secondary and tertiary.

The aim of primary prevention is to literally take action to prevent an illness or injury before it happens. Primary prevention involves identifying and changing any personal features or lifestyle habits that are known or suspected of increasing your risk of a particular disease or injury. It is at this level that the side benefits of lifestyle change will have the most impact. If you have already been diagnosed with a cancer, primary prevention still applies to other conditions that can be prevented by introducing a healthier way of living. An example might be stopping smoking, increasing activity, and improving nutrition to prevent heart disease. Another simple example is immunisation against infectious diseases.

The aim of secondary prevention is to identify an illness early in its development before it has caused significant symptoms and while it is still reversible, such as the early detection of precancerous polyps or an early stage bowel cancer with faecal occult blood testing or colonoscopy.

Once you have been diagnosed with cancer, you are in tertiary prevention territory for that particular cancer. Here the condition is well underway and causing you symptoms, or it has been detected and the treatment process is underway or completed. The aim of tertiary prevention is to reduce the impact of the disease by restoring function, and preventing recurrence and complications.

SCREENING

Health screening is a test or investigation that is done to detect a disease before there are any symptoms. These tests can be offered to whole populations where they are usually funded by a government program, or can be done on an individual basis.

For a screening test to be worth the effort and expense, the test needs to fulfil a number of criteria:

- It needs to be able to detect a condition that is common, disabling, or life threatening.
- The test also needs to be simple, safe, accurate and cost-effective.
- Treatment should be available and accessible.

- Intervention needs to have a reasonable chance of resulting in longer life and greater quality of life than if the disease was left to run its natural course.

Screening programs that are subsidised by governments also have to pass a cost–benefit test. Those that are not subsidised by governments or other organisations can still be offered to you as an individual, but similar criteria usually apply and you have to make a personal decision about having the test, including its cost. But there is room for a more personalised approach. For example, if you are concerned about a family history of ovarian cancer, you might want to talk to your doctor about a yearly pelvic ultrasound and blood test for the CA 125 tumour marker. This approach is commonplace in the US, but not recommended in Australia because it does not satisfy the whole-of-population economics test for a publicly funded program.

Debates within the medical community about different screening protocols range back and forth depending on the latest evidence and how different professional subgroups interpret that evidence. Screening for prostate cancer has been a particularly heated debate in recent years because of the controversy about which cancers would never have needed treating and which ones were likely to cause disability and death if left untreated. This controversy will settle as we are developing better ways of working out which prostate cancers are likely to be aggressive and significant.

The most common screening programs across populations include:

- Pap smear for cervical cancer in women
- mammography for breast cancer in women
- Prostate Specific Antigen (PSA testing) for prostate cancer in men

- faecal occult blood testing and/or colonoscopy for bowel cancer
- specialised ultrasound scans in early pregnancy to detect foetal abnormalities.

It is important to have a carefully coordinated plan of action for health screening. I usually find that routine screening goes on hold while people are going through cancer treatment, but once the treatments are completed, and with the help of your GP, it is important to get back on track and have a plan for maintaining your future health. The plan will involve monitoring for any sign of the cancer that has been diagnosed, as well as screening for other diseases according to your gender and your particular health concerns.

Health Audit

After you have been diagnosed with cancer, one of the most important things you can do to help you persevere with treatment and to optimise your chances of recovery is to audit your entire lifestyle. While doing the audit, it is important to be as accurate and honest with yourself as possible. The idea is to identify those habits that have a positive effect on your health, as well as the areas where you need to focus your attention and make changes.

There will be a lot of demands on your time and attention during the early phases after diagnosis, but I need to stress the importance of taking stock at any and every stage, and making changes that are within your capability to improve. As you move through the different stages of cancer treatment and recovery, I encourage you to repeat the audit to see how you are going.

HEALTH AUDIT

ENERGY

Rate your energy level on a scale of 1 to 5, 1 being very low energy, 5 being peak energy.

	1	2	3	4	5
On waking					
Around midday					
Mid afternoon					
In the evening					

The value of this self-assessment is to give you and your health advisers a guide to the reasons you might be experiencing low energy at some times of the day. The reasons may not be obvious and could relate to your sleep patterns, diet, activity or work situation, stage of treatment, side effects of medication or other factors. The assessment also gives you a comparison to assess your degree of wellness as you progress through treatment or make changes to some of your habits.

WHAT ARE YOUR MAIN CANCER-RELATED PROBLEMS RIGHT NOW?

1. ....

2. ....

3. ....

4. ....

5. ....

Your cancer and its treatment may be your current number-one priority, but you quite possibly have other health challenges too. Think broadly about these and list them in order of the most important priority for you right now:

1. ....

2. ....

3. ....

4. ....

5. ....

WHAT OTHER MEDICAL PROBLEMS HAVE YOU BEEN DIAGNOSED WITH IN THE PAST?

YEAR	DIAGNOSIS	TREATMENT	OUTCOME

HOSPITAL ADMISSIONS

Have you had any admissions to hospital in the past five years? YES/NO

DATE	REASON	PROCEDURE	OUTCOME	PROBLEMS

Outpatients visits:

DATE	REASON	INVEST-IGATIONS	PROCEDURE	OUTCOME

YOUR HEALTHCARE TEAM

Who are the healthcare professionals you have consulted since your cancer diagnosis? ....

Do you have copies of their reports, opinions or advice?

PRACTITIONER	
DISCIPLINE OR SPECIALITY	
REASON FOR CONSULTATION	
OUTCOME	

WHAT INVESTIGATIONS HAVE YOU HAD?

TEST	DATE	SITE	RESULT
Blood tests			
Biopsy reports			
X-rays			
CT scans			
MRI			
PET scans			
Ultrasound			
Special investigations (e.g. colonoscopy, mammogram)			

Obtain and file copies of your results in chronological order.

For X-rays, CT scans, MRI scans and PET scans: keep the original images as a CD, DVD or film copies, and make sure there is a result included with the images. If you do not have the images, the radiology practice should be able to provide you with a copy on a disc or USB stick. If you do not have copies of the results, contact the radiology practice or radiology department in the treating hospital. If that proves difficult, ask your cancer specialist. Your GP may have also been copied in on results.

For biopsy and surgical pathology reports: the surgeon will have copies of the original biopsy and pathology reports. Your GP should also have been copied in on these results. Ask for copies for your records.

SYMPTOMS OF CANCER AND SIDE EFFECTS OF TREATMENT

Think about the symptoms of cancer and its treatment that you are experiencing:

- pain (location, severity, quality, timing) ....
- nausea and vomiting ....
- anxiety ....
- depression ....
- fatigue ....
- poor appetite ....
- weight loss ....
- mouth ulcers ....
- constipation ....
- diarrhoea ....
- swollen limb(s) ....
- hot flushes ....
- hair loss ....
- skin problems (from radiation) ....
- frequent infections ....
- breathlessness ....
- reduced exercise tolerance ....
- other symptoms ....

Do you experience other symptoms that have not been investigated or diagnosed? Examples include headaches, loss of libido, erectile dysfunction, incontinence, irregular menstrual cycle, excess gas, abdominal cramps, period pains, rashes.

Record all symptoms and include features such as timing, severity, duration, what makes it better, what makes it worse:

....

....

....

....

....

....

....

....

DIGESTION

Describe your bowel function:

- Has there been any recent sustained change in your bowel habit? ....
- What is the consistency? ....
- Are your stools well-formed/watery/hard/variable? ....
- How often do you open your bowels? ....
- Is there any blood? If so, is it bright or dark? ....
- Do you suffer abdominal bloating? ....
- Do you pass excessive gas? ....
- Do you suffer from heartburn, indigestion or dyspepsia? .....
  ....
- Other specific symptoms and signs ....
  ....

There are literally hundreds of different symptoms to describe unpleasant physical sensations. Examples include pain, cough, wheeze, trouble breathing, swelling, lump, palpitations, loss of appetite and nausea, frequent urination, urinary incontinence, abnormal bleeding (including vaginal bleeding), swollen ankles, dizziness and many more. List any symptoms and report them to your doctor who is trained to make sense of them.

HOW DO YOU MEASURE UP?

Height H (in metres) ....

Weight W (in kilograms) ....

Body Mass Index (BMI) W(kg)/H(m) × H(m) ....

This calculation can be confusing. There are online tools that can calculate it for you. To calculate it yourself, take your weight in kilos and divide it by your height in metres. Then divide that number by your height in metres.

Depending on this number – your BMI – you will get an indication of how your body weight relates to your health risk.

Ideal BMI: 18.5–25
Too light: under 18.5
Overweight: over 25
Obese: over 30

WAIST MEASUREMENT

Hold a tape measure against your skin and breathe out normally. Measure around your waist halfway between your lowest rib and the top of your hipbone, roughly in line with your belly button.

Your waist measurement (centimetres)..

'Safe' zone (meaning there is no evidence of increased risk of cancer associated with waist circumference):

Men: under 94 cm

Women: under 80 cm

Moderately or significantly increased risk for some cancers:

Men: more than 100 cm

Women: more than 85 cm

SLEEP AUDIT

Keep a sleep diary like the one below.

	MON	TUES	WED	THUR	FRI	SAT	SUN
What time did you go to bed?							
Time you spent reading/watching TV in bed before sleep?							
Time taken to go to sleep?							
How many times did you wake in the night? At what times? Why?							
How many hours did you sleep?							
Did you have any dreams/ nightmares or other night-time events?							
Did you nap in the day?							

SLEEP DIARY

Your sleep diary will reveal your sleep behaviours and patterns that will help to identify whether sleep is a problem for you, and act as a guide to solve your sleep problems.

- After a week, look at the patterns in your sleep diary.
- How many hours do you sleep at night on average?
- How long does it take you to get to sleep on average?
- Is your sleep disturbed during the night? Why?
- Do you wake refreshed, feeling as though you have had enough quality sleep?

See the chapter on sleep (page 360).

DIET

For this section, keep an accurate food diary and record everything (yes, everything) you eat and drink (including alcohol) over a seven-day period.

As a result of your cancer or its treatment, you may have difficulties with appetite, or digestion, and you may have special nutritional needs. Also, these will vary over time.

	MON	TUES	WED	THUR	FRI	SAT	SUN
Breakfast							
Other food/drink consumed in the morning							
Lunch							
Other food/drink consumed in the afternoon							
Dinner							
Other food/drink consumed in the evening							

This information should be recorded during a period of time when you are in a normal schedule of daily activities, work and socialising. If your schedule is interrupted – for example, during a treatment cycle or if you go on a business trip or a family holiday – then you need to keep a separate record of those meals and transfer them to your diary to get an accurate assessment of potential problem areas.

If you are going through an unusual period, such as a loss of appetite or a distaste for certain foods, where you are unable to keep up your food intake, it is important to document this too so that adjustments to your food intake can be made or supplements recommended to maintain your nutritional status.

MEDICATIONS AND SUPPLEMENTS

Do an audit of all medicines and supplements. On this list note down any:

- prescribed medications
- cancer-specific treatments including chemotherapy protocols
- over-the-counter drugs
- supplements
- herbal medicines and combinations

Include brand names and generic names, doses and how often you take them. Note whether the strength is in mg (milligrams), μg (micrograms) or IU (international units).

You will need to go through your medicine cabinet, first-aid kit, bedside tables, kitchen and pantry, handbags and briefcase to see what is in your house, car and office. While you are doing that, discard any medications that are out of date or that you do not expect to take.

If you are taking a combination herbal product, particularly one dispensed by a naturopath, herbalist, or Traditional Chinese Medicine practitioner, you will need a list of all ingredients. If you have a smartphone, it can be helpful to take photos of labels and keep them as a reference. If the ingredients are not in English, ask the prescribing or dispensing practitioner to translate them for you.

- Include all medications, whether you take them regularly or only occasionally.
- Do you ever take more than the prescribed or recommended amounts? If yes, why?
- Do all members of your healthcare team have the details of these lists?

DO YOU HAVE ANY KNOWN DRUG OR HERB ALLERGIES?

DRUG(S)/HERB(S)	TYPE OF REACTION(S)

GENERAL MEDICAL CHECK-UP

It is common for the detection and treatment of cancer to take over your medical consultations and all other medical check-ups to go on the backburner. But it is important to treat the 'whole you'.

PREVENTION

Are your preventive health checks up to date?

Discuss with your doctor what preventive health checks you need that are specific to your cancer and its treatment, but remember all of the other health checks even though your cancer treatment takes priority.

DATE AND RESULT OF LAST

- Pap smear (women)...
- Mammogram (women) ....
- Prostate cancer check (men) ....
- Bone density..
- Blood sugar ....
- Cholesterol and other blood lipids ....
- Blood pressure...
- Bowel cancer check ....

IMMUNISATIONS

Keep a record of all of your immunisations, including the type of immunisation and date, as well as a note of when any boosters are due. If necessary, discuss with your doctor a program for updating your immunisations. This is particularly important if your immune system has been compromised or is likely to be affected by cancer treatment or you plan to travel internationally. See the chapter on travel plans, page 396.

DATE	DISEASE TARGETED	VACCINE AND DOSE	BOOSTER DUE

EXERCISE

Like your food diary, keep a diary of the amount of exercise you do. This might include walking the dog, a game of tennis or golf, gardening, a dance class, tai chi, yoga, special exercise classes, gym sessions.

EXERCISE DIARY

DAY	TYPE	TIME	INTENSITY
MONDAY			
TUESDAY			
WEDNESDAY			
THURSDAY			
FRIDAY			
SATURDAY			
SUNDAY			

How much time do you spend outdoors each week?......................

TOBACCO SMOKING

Do you currently smoke? YES/NO

If YES, do you intend to quit?

When?

If YES:

- Do you consider yourself a 'social' or 'occasional' smoker?
  ....

- Are you a regular (most days) smoker? ....
- Have you attempted to quit? YES/NO
- How many times have you tried to quit and using what methods? ....
- If you are an ex-smoker, when did you quit? ....

See the chapter on smoking page 385.

ALCOHOL

Over an average week, and referring to your food diary, record the number of standard drinks you consume. Remember that a bottle of wine contains seven to eight standard drinks. A single nip of spirits is equivalent to one standard drink. A cocktail might contain two or three standard drinks.

How much is a standard drink?	
Can/Stubbie low-strength beer	= 0.8 standard drink
Can/Stubbie mid-strength beer	= 1 standard drink
Can/Stubbie full-strength beer	= 1.4 standard drinks
100ml wine (13.5% alcohol)	= 1 standard drink
30ml nip spirits	= 1 standard drink
Can spirits (approx 5% alcohol)	= 1.2 to 1.7 standard drinks
Can spirits (approx 7% alcohol)	= 1.6 to 2.4 standard drinks

ALCOHOL DIARY

DAY	No. of STANDARD alcoholic drinks over a 24-hour period
MON	
TUES	
WED	
THUR	
FRI	
SAT	
SUN	

Do you average 1–5 drinks per week? You are low risk

Do you average 5–10 drinks per week? You are medium risk.

Did you average more than 10 drinks per week? You are high risk.

Did you have more than 4 drinks in any 24-hour period? This is classified as binge-drinking.

Has alcohol ever caused any problems in your work, social or family life?

Do you consider alcohol a problem for you now?

See the chapter on alcohol page 295.

WHEN WAS YOUR LAST DENTAL CHECK-UP?

Sound dental and oral health is important for general well-being, particularly for making sure you are getting high-quality nutrition. Some types of chemotherapy and radiotherapy will necessitate oral and dental preventive strategies as part of your cancer prehabilitation workup.

When was your last visit to the dentist for a check-up and maintenance?

Within 12 months or over 12 months?

Before some cancer treatments, I recommend the patient has a dental check-up and oral health treatment. See pages 157, 273 and 278 for information on dental and oral health.

EMOTIONAL WELLBEING

There are a number of self-assessment questionnaires for emotional wellbeing. One of the best known assessment tools is the Kessler Psychological Distress Scale, or K10.

The maximum score of 50 indicates severe distress. The minimum score is 10, which indicates no distress.

Lower scores mean a higher degree of emotional health. Higher scores mean you need to pay attention to aspects of your emotional health. Talk to your doctor if you score over 20.

You can rate your general level of emotional wellbeing, but it is also important to look more closely at some of the influences that impact on your emotional world.

	None of the time (1 point)	A little of the time (2 point)	Some of the time (3 point)	Most of the time (4 point)	All of the time (5 point)
In the past 4 weeks how often did you feel tired out for no good reason?					
In the past 4 weeks how often did you feel that everything was an effort?					

	None of the time (1 point)	A little of the time (2 point)	Some of the time (3 point)	Most of the time (4 point)	All of the time (5 point)
In the past 4 weeks how often did you feel nervous?					
In the past 4 weeks how often did you feel so nervous that nothing could calm you down?					
In the past 4 weeks how often did you feel hopeless?					
In the past 4 weeks how often did you feel worthless?					
In the past 4 weeks how often did you feel fidgety?					
In the past 4 weeks how often did you feel so restless you couldn't be still?					
In the past 4 weeks how often did you feel depressed?					

	None of the time (1 point)	A little of the time (2 point)	Some of the time (3 point)	Most of the time (4 point)	All of the time (5 point)
In the past 4 weeks how often did you feel so sad nothing could cheer you up?					
Total					

SPIRITUALITY

Consider the following questions about your spirituality. Is faith (religion, spirituality) important to you?

- Has faith been important to you at other times in your life?
- Do you use religion or spirituality to help cope with illness or is it a source of stress, and how?
- Do you have any religious or spiritual beliefs that might influence decisions about your medical care?
- Are you a member of a supportive spiritual community?
- Do you have any troubling spiritual questions or concerns?
- Do you have someone to talk to about matters of faith or religion?
- Would you like to explore religious or spiritual matters with someone? If so, who would that be?
- Do you have any spiritual beliefs that might influence decisions about your medical care?

See part two, 'Dealing with cancer emotionally' on page 63 for more information.

Your Healthcare Team

When you are diagnosed with cancer, you will find that a team, or a 'virtual team' springs up around you surprisingly quickly. If your GP has been conducting screening or diagnostic testing for you, then he or she will initially arrange referral to appropriate specialists. That may involve a medical oncologist for further investigation and a cancer-specific treatment plan, or you might be referred to a surgeon who will then advise you on which other cancer specialists from their team need to be involved.

Depending on where you live and the extent of the cancer services and other health services around you, there may or may not be much choice in this decision-making. If you are living in a major city with a variety of large cancer treatment centres, then you may be able to choose a centre that has particular experience and expertise in the treatment of your particular type of cancer, and with a comprehensive service providing a range of different types of health care to respond to your needs at each stage of treatment. This will be especially important for the less common types of cancer.

Unfortunately this type of well-planned and -resourced cancer treatment service is not always available. It is also quite possible there will be some assistance or interventions you need or want to access that are not provided by your cancer service.

You may need to draw together a 'virtual team' of health professionals to provide all of the assistance that you need. This means a group of practitioners who are not a formal team working together all the time in one location, but your own team of practitioners who provide the services you need in different locations and at different times. For example, you may want to see an acupuncturist who helps you manage pain and nausea and a dietitian near your home who helps you with a nutrition plan. They are not working in the cancer centre, but they are part of your virtual team.

The best place to start your treatment plan is with your general practitioner, who will have a network of local practitioners for referral.

WHY YOU NEED A GP

I can't emphasise enough how important it is for you to have a primary care physician, or GP, you like and trust. If you don't have one, now is the time to find one.

I mention GPs first, not out of bias but because we have pivotal roles to play in your cancer care at all stages. The vast majority of cancer screening and investigations for early detection of cancer are arranged by GPs. This would include screening activities such as performing Pap smears, prostate checks, or skin cancer checks, or arranging for your mammograms or colonoscopies, and so on. It is likely that your GP ordered the initial screening test or arranged the initial investigations that led to the diagnosis of your cancer.

The first presentation of any symptoms of cancer is likely

to be to a GP, who will take your medical history and examine you for signs that are suspicious for cancer. The initial diagnostic investigations are ordered by your GP and the results come back to your GP who then needs to coordinate the appropriate referrals for further investigation and treatment with the right cancer specialists.

Your GP has a crucial role in advising you about your options and advocating on your behalf within the specialist cancer treatment system, which can be a confusing maze. The so-called 'cancer journey' can be a very bumpy ride and the familiar face of your own GP can provide a much greater sense of security for you and your family at times when you are trying to make sense of the diagnosis and its implications for your lives in the short and long term.

Sure, your surgeon and oncologist and radiation oncologist all play their roles in the cancer-specific treatment and follow-up, but there has to be a central, professional navigator who helps you to coordinate all aspects of your cancer care, and who is also there for you during your rehabilitation and recovery.

In the spirit of 'whole person care', your GP will also monitor your general health and manage any other healthcare issues that might arise now and into the future.

In an ideal world, the specialists working in the tertiary (hospital) sector will keep your GP informed of any results, progress and setbacks you experience. But, sometimes from our perspective in general practice, once a patient is diagnosed with a cancer, they are then seemingly swallowed up into the tertiary sector's cancer services for surgery, and/or chemotherapy, and/or radiotherapy, and then eventually turn up back in our offices somewhat the worse for wear.

A good GP will help to troubleshoot problems you have along the way. Then it is the GP's task to organise rehabilitation and monitoring of your recovery and remission. Sadly, in some cases it is palliative and terminal care which we need to coordinate.

YOUR CANCER-SPECIFIC SPECIALISTS

In larger cancer centres, specialists from a range of disciplines – pathology, radiology, nuclear medicine, surgery, oncology, radiation oncology – will hold multidisciplinary meetings to discuss your case prior to treatment and assess, on the basis of best available evidence and experience, what is the most appropriate cancer-specific treatment for you. They will also discuss your progress during treatment and advise each other on the treatment plan as you progress through the various stages of treatment. In this section I will describe some of the health professionals you may see along the way and what their roles should be.

SURGEON

The cancer surgeon is responsible for removing body organs or cancer tissue. If a screening test or other investigation has discovered an area suspicious for cancer, a surgeon may be needed to take a small sample of tissue (biopsy) to help in getting a definitive diagnosis so that treatment can be accurately planned. If a cancer mass needs to be removed or an organ removed or repaired, that will be the surgeon's job.

Surgeons in major centres usually subspecialise and treat specific body parts or tumour types. It is important for you to check that the surgeon you are seeing has training and experience with your particular type of cancer. Your GP will usually know or can help you find the right surgeon.

MEDICAL ONCOLOGIST

Your medical oncologist is the cancer-specific specialist who is usually most responsible for your overall cancer treatment plan.

He or she will confirm your diagnosis, including staging, and then liaise with the other cancer specialists involved in your case to develop a treatment plan. They plan the chemotherapy part of your treatment and monitor your progress.

Some medical oncologists have a special interest in particular types of cancer such as breast cancer. There are some oncology subspecialties such as haematology-oncology that concentrate on the diagnosis and treatment of cancers of the blood, such as leukaemias, lymphomas and myeloma. Your initial referral will consider which oncologist is most appropriate to treat your cancer.

The medical oncologist will also anticipate possible treatment side effects and work out an action plan to manage these medically, as well as your cancer-related symptoms.

RADIATION ONCOLOGIST

The radiation oncologist is a cancer specialist who uses ionising radiation (also called radiotherapy) targeted at primary cancers or metastases to shrink the size of tumours and kill cancer cells. The radiation oncologist has to carefully plan and target treatment to minimise side effects, knowing that radiation damages healthy cells as well as cancer cells.

CANCER (ONCOLOGY) NURSE

A cancer nurse or oncology nurse is a registered nurse specialising in the care, monitoring and education of people with cancer. These nurses work in multidisciplinary teams in a variety of settings. You might see them in the chemotherapy suite administering prescribed chemotherapy drugs, on the wards, in the outpatients department, working with your surgeon or medical oncologist in their private rooms or doing home visits where they might help with symptom management and coordinating supportive or palliative care.

ONCOLOGY SOCIAL WORKER

Cancer and its treatment are likely to change your day-to-day life, at least for a while. Cancer centres will usually have an oncology social worker whose job it is to provide you with information services, organise any home-based care you need after discharge from hospital, and put you in contact with community resources such as home nursing or accessing welfare payments for you and your family. You will usually have contact with the social worker while you are in hospital before discharge home, but this can also be arranged as an outpatient through your cancer nurse, GP, or oncologist.

OTHER HEALTHCARE PRACTITIONERS

A range of allied health practitioners will be involved in your care from time to time, depending on your needs. Your GP or oncologist will advise you on which health professional to see, such as a dietitian to ensure you are getting optimal nutrition, an exercise physiologist to plan your return to physical activity, a physiotherapist, speech therapist, lymphoedema therapist, occupational therapist or psychologist. The selection of health professional will depend on the stage of your treatment and an assessment of your needs. It will also depend on where you live and the availability of suitable local services.

Other health professionals include acupuncturist, audiologist, chiropractor, counsellor, dentist, dietitian, exercise physiologist, herbalist, massage therapist, naturopath, nurse/nurse practitioner, occupational therapist, optometrist, osteopath, personal trainer, pharmacist, physiotherapist, podiatrist, psychologist, social worker, speech pathologist and Traditional Chinese Medicine practitioner.

ADJUNCTIVE THERAPIES

If you are like most people diagnosed with cancer, you will be thinking about or actively seeking out complementary or adjunctive therapies to help you get through treatment or assist your recovery. In fact, experts estimate that at least 80 per cent of cancer patients use some form of complementary therapies during the course of their treatments and rehabilitation, almost always as an 'adjunct' or added extra.

There is an out-dated argument you will hear that 'non-conventional' treatments are synonymous with 'unproven', but the growth in evidence for treatments that fall outside the basic training and expertise of most Western-trained medical practitioners makes that argument unsustainable and plain wrong.

The delivery of so-called 'complementary' or adjunctive treatments is almost exclusively in the community rather than in the hospital environment and it is often not connected with general practice or oncology services. Yet they are so common that they should now be considered usual practice, if not yet mainstream, and carefully integrated into your treatment plan at every stage if that is your choice.

Many major cancer services are responding to patient demand and starting to integrate cancer treatments within their service. Your GP may be able to refer you to some or all of the extra services you need, but in reality you may have to seek out and arrange some of the services yourself.

It is important that any adjunctive therapies are well planned for their effectiveness and safety and for timing, and that you ask for professional advice.

The types of complementary or adjunctive treatment combinations are as varied as the options available.

If you refer to the chapters on chemotherapy (page 129), radiotherapy (page 154), and part five 'Symptoms and side effects of cancer treatment', (page 245), you will see that a number of the evidence-supported therapies are delivered within some comprehensive cancer services. Commonly these might include counselling, meditation, lymphoedema therapy and exercise classes. To access the full range of services you might require, you will probably need to find health professionals who work outside conventional cancer services. Examples would be oncology massage therapists, naturopaths and acupuncturists.

Many people who seek complementary therapies or are taking supplements are not disclosing that information to their GP or oncologist, and the problem is that if you do not inform your practitioners there could be problems coordinating your care. This raises potential safety issues. Lack of coordination means you might be missing out on the health benefits you could get through detailed professional advice on the best possible combinations and doses and timing. It can also mean the potential detrimental interactions between drug, herbs and other supplements are not anticipated and avoided.

Throughout the book I will look at the best adjunctive treatments at different stages, and precautions you need to take, including coordinating their timing with your chemotherapy or radiotherapy.

ATTITUDES OF DOCTORS

In recent years I have seen a major shift in attitude within medical circles to embrace the type of care that patients are saying they want. This shift has led to the development of integrative cancer centres, which aim to deliver many of the complementary/adjunctive treatments patients are seeking.

Sometimes resistance to adjunctive treatments is based on a lack of evidence of effectiveness and safety of a therapy if it is used in a patient who has cancer.

In other cases the doctor may not be familiar with the evidence for a therapy so he or she may believe it is safer to say, 'Don't take anything I don't prescribe'. Unfortunately, following this advice could mean you miss out on safe and effective treatments that could relieve your symptoms or side effects and improve your quality of life. Sometimes, the resistance is based on cultural bias or lack of exposure to information about these therapies.

If you want to explore adjunctive treatments in conjunction with your medical treatment, you will probably test your doctors for their openness and competence in discussing the options with you. Ideally you will be able find doctors who are well informed, balanced in their views and encouraging of safe and effective treatments while warning you appropriately of unsafe or ineffective treatments.

Most Australian GPs believe the risks of complementary therapies mainly arise from incorrect, inadequate or delayed diagnoses, and potential interactions between complementary medications and pharmaceuticals, rather than concerns about any specific risks of the therapies themselves. Where we start running into difficulty with consensus on the safety of treatments is in the 'ingestibles and injectables', or therapeutic substances that are swallowed or injected, particularly the types, combinations and doses of nutritional supplementation, herbal products and other biological agents.

We do need to be particularly cautious about potential interactions when these therapies are considered alongside or interspersed with courses of chemotherapy. But this should not be to the point of excluding you, without good cause, from treatments that can safely reduce the toxicity of cancer treatments and improve your recovery.

Case study

A young mother in her thirties was diagnosed with breast cancer. She undertook surgery, radiotherapy and chemotherapy. She also explored and adopted a range of adjunctive treatments throughout her conventional treatment schedule. I remarked to her that she seemed to tolerate treatment extremely well compared with some other patients I had watched going through similar treatment without adjunctive therapies.

I asked her for details of what she had been doing.

Her reply was thought provoking. She said that her oncologist had made a similar remark about how well she seemed to have tolerated the chemotherapy compared with other patients, but that the oncologist had not asked the next question, 'What did you do differently that other patients did not do?' She never did tell her oncologist about the adjunctive therapies which helped her and distinguished her cancer journey from those who had suffered far more through the treatment process.

YOUR INTEGRATIVE HEALTHCARE TEAM

What do you need to look for in a health professional?

First and foremost, any practitioner you see needs to be well trained in their professional discipline. When you see a doctor, you know they have attained a minimal specific level of education and that they have compulsory continuing professional development. Doctors who define themselves as 'integrative medicine practitioners' generally have a wider frame of reference for providing treatment advice. They may or may not have had formal postgraduate training but many have gathered knowledge through courses, conferences, clinical experience and wider reading.

With other types of practitioners, it is important to check whether there is a system of professional registration and regulation. That means that the profession has agreed on minimum standards

for training, education and continuing professional development, and that an independent regulatory body is responsible
for upholding those professional standards. This administration
of standards applies to most healthcare professions you will find
in a hospital environment, including medicine, nursing, physiotherapy, podiatry, audiology, dietetics, psychology and so on.

Some practitioners will have special post-graduate training in a
particularly specialised area of their profession. For example, some
massage therapists have completed specialised training in oncology
massage and oncology nurses will have had post-graduate training
in cancer care.

In the field of natural therapies there is a wide variation in
training and knowledge. Traditional Chinese Medicine in Australia
took many years to gain recognition, but registration went national
in 2012. However some professions or philosophies of health care
do not fall under any scheme of professional registration and
regulation, which makes it difficult to choose a practitioner. This
also makes it difficult for the registered professions to interact
with those that are not registered, for safety reasons as well as for
medico–legal reasons.

This situation will change with time because professional
groups such as naturopaths and herbalists have recognised this
as a problem for consumers and for the standing of responsible
practitioners, and they are actively seeking a system of registration. There are professional membership groups but these are not
the same as formally recognised registration.

WHO ARE THE RIGHT PRACTITIONERS
FOR YOU TO SEE?

If you want to combine a number of different healthcare philosophies in your cancer recovery, you will need to carefully select
the right practitioners.

If you would like to see a particular practitioner, you may be able to discuss their suitability with your GP or oncologist. Or your GP may be able to point you in the right direction and refer you directly to a practitioner because he or she will have assessed their training and skills and be aware of their areas of special interest and expertise.

Self-referral to complementary medicine practitioners is also common among cancer patients. Sometimes you will be relying on the recommendation of friends or relatives or some other source to see a practitioner. If you are doing your own research on a practitioner, check whether that health profession has a system of registration, then you can check that the practitioner is registered to practice in that discipline.

To check qualifications, you will need to ask the practitioner directly or check their website for their qualifications. If necessary, track down the institution that granted the qualification and find out what the course entails in terms of length of study and content, and whether it is a certificate, diploma or degree course.

But be aware that even this is not a guarantee of the right skills to suit your needs. For example, a practitioner might have a science degree or a nursing degree from a university – or no degree at all – and practice as a naturopath without having trained as one.

Whichever non-medical practitioner you see, alarm bells should immediately ring if they discourage you in any way from continuing care with your GP or cancer specialists. Discuss any planned treatments with your cancer-specific specialists (preferably one with an integrative mindset or expertise) to make sure there are no potential interactions with your cancer treatment.

ACCESS AND AFFORDABILITY

One important point about the use of evidence-based complementary medicines in cancer care is that most patients need to pay for them out of pocket, with limited subsidies coming from private health insurance for those who have insurance. The specialist hospital sector is making noises that it is interested in integrative cancer centres but realistically, it is unlikely that a comprehensive range of subsidised services will be available when and for as long as you need those services. Public funding doesn't stretch that far and private cancer centres need to charge for their services, so even if a therapy is likely to help you, affordability can be an issue.

The scope of therapies is also limited in cancer centres. In the foreseeable future it is highly unlikely that conventional hospitals and cancer centres will venture beyond therapies like massage, acupuncture, exercise, meditation and nutrition.

Some integrative medicine advice or interventions cost very little. These might include support groups, meditation classes, walking regularly or adopting sound nutrition. Other interventions are more therapist-intensive or expensive, such as massage therapy or herb/vitamin therapies. Unfortunately this places some complementary therapies in the luxury category for many people.

It is essential for you to be able to turn to your GP as a filter for reliable information at a time when you are likely to be emotionally vulnerable and looking for answers, and to direct you away from potentially harmful or expensive therapies with little or no likelihood of benefit. It is equally important for your GP and oncologists to be able to give you accurate and unbiased information about the full range of evidence-based medical and adjunctive treatments that may help relieve your symptoms, prevent or mitigate the side effects of cancer treatments, accelerate your recovery, and help you live longer.

COMMUNICATION BETWEEN YOUR PRACTITIONERS

The protocols for doctors to communicate with each other are well established. Your GP writes a letter to the specialist covering all your relevant information, including your medications and medical history. The specialist sees you and writes back to your GP with the results of any investigations or treatments and their opinion. If a specialist does not communicate efficiently back to the GP, they tend to get fewer referrals and their reputation suffers, so there is an incentive to make sure they do.

Hospitals ideally, but not always, send a discharge summary to the GP so that your GP knows if you have been admitted to hospital, and they also provide your GP with any changes to your medical treatment and requests for follow-up. Patients will often be provided with a copy of the discharge summary. Increasingly, this communication is done via secure electronic transmission to computerised records held by the doctors and hospitals. It is very frustrating for a GP if a patient has been in hospital and been told to follow up in a few days or weeks with their GP, but the GP has not been informed of exactly what happened in that admission or what changes have been made to treatment plans.

Other health practitioners tend to be less consistent with their communication. For example, the GP might or might not hear about your visit to the physiotherapist. I always let allied health professionals know that I want a written report about their assessment with recommendations so that I have complete documentation in my patients' files.

Keeping track

I encourage every one of my patients to consolidate their medical records and keep them up to date. This is particularly important in cases that are complex or deal with serious medical conditions such as cancer. All it takes is a ring folder that can hold trans-parent plastic sleeves, a little assertiveness and a tiny bit of organisational skill.

Here's what you need to record:

- to start with, ask your GP to provide you with a health summary, which is usually just one or two sheets of paper with a summary of relevant details, such as your past medical history, current medications and supplements, allergies and immunisations
- ask your surgeon for copies of your original operation report and results of the pathology reports of biopsies or surgically removed tissues
- the original pathology report so that we know exactly what cancer we are dealing with, including documentation of staging of your cancer
- what investigations have already been done
- when and what exact treatment combinations have been tried
- who recommended and supervised the treatments
- how effective they were – or were not
- what side effects were encountered and how they were managed
- what the follow-up care plan is once cancer-specific treatment has been concluded
- the names, addresses and other contact details of all the health professionals you have consulted in the past, and those who you are currently seeing
- the written details of the chemotherapy treatment protocol you had or plan to have
- an information sheet from your oncologist with the exact chemotherapy drugs and their doses and a treatment plan, including a list of possible side effects

- information about any adjunctive therapies that have been recommended, and other advice – examples of this might be hormone therapy for breast cancer or prostate cancer, or medication for chemotherapy-associated nausea
- a schedule of dates and a precise description of the type of radiotherapy you had or plan to have.

Ask for you and your primary care doctor, your GP, to be copied in to any blood results, and make sure you file copies of any investigation reports into your record. Even the normal results can be relevant. Then ask your specialists if you can be provided with copies of their reports, including investigations, procedures and opinions. The same goes for any allied health practitioners and complementary medicine practitioners. It is not possible for your GP to work out a comprehensive summary with you if they do not know what supplements or herbal treatments or other treatment modalities you have tried, whether successfully or unsuccessfully, or you are currently using.

With supplements, if your GP can see a precise list of ingredients, he or she can work out what doses and combinations you are taking and whether there are any potential interactions or risks of adverse events. You can take the bottles of herbs or supplements to the appointment so your GP can see the labels with ingredients or use your smartphone to take photos of the labels of your medications and supplements showing the ingredients and doses.

· PART TWO ·

Dealing with cancer emotionally

Mental Health

The initial reaction to a diagnosis of cancer is usually one of extreme shock. At that moment you know your life has changed inexorably and your future is, at least for the time being, determined by the cancer, the results of medical investigations, the treatments you need to deal with the cancer, and the implications of the cancer on your future health and wellbeing.

I am not a psychologist, but as a GP I am in the position of seeing the psychological influences and the emotional fallout of cancer in all its forms and stages. Many people fear that a cancer diagnosis is the end of their life as they have known it and in some respects that is true, but not as you may think. A word you will hear often applied to your ability to cope with cancer is 'resilience'. There is no question that any serious medical condition tests your ability to cope, your resilience. Fortunately, most of the studies into the psychological dimensions of cancer show that the majority of people, sooner or later, manage very well psychologically.

The study of the psychological impact of cancer and how to manage it is a very big subject and is collectively known as psycho-oncology. At every stage, your emotions and your mental state have a bearing on the cancer disease process and its outcome and the decisions you make along the way.

It is beyond the scope of this book to cover the entire field of psycho-oncology, but I can point you to some areas to think about, and also to some further resources if you think they may be useful to you. I also want to discuss some of the issues you are likely to confront, and give guidance on how to deal with them and when and where to get help.

SCREENING FOR CANCER

Fear may motivate most people to have cancer screening, but it can work in the opposite direction too. I was told of one case of a woman in her early forties who had noticed some blood in her bowel motions. She thought it was 'just haemorrhoids' but it persisted for months. She was so scared of needles and hospitals that she refused to go to her doctor until she started to get pain in her abdomen and terrible constipation. It was then that her doctor discovered what was by then an extensive and inoperable rectal cancer.

After you have a screening test, most people think that 'no news is good news', and in the vast majority of cases that is true. If your doctor receives an abnormal test result that may indicate a cancer, they will make every effort to contact you. But in the real world, results can go astray or follow-up systems slip up for all sorts of reasons. So you have a responsibility to yourself to make sure that after you have a cancer screening test, regardless of whether you think it is going to be normal or not, you call to check the result has returned and that it is negative.

You may get a call that a screening test has come back with a positive result. This is not a trigger for panic, because a positive initial screening test does not necessarily mean you have a cancer.

If you are called back because of a positive test, it will be to arrange further investigation to work out whether the positive test really does indicate a cancer.

RECEIVING BAD NEWS

Obviously the type of diagnosis you receive will have a huge impact on your emotional response, but the way your diagnosis is delivered can make all the difference to the way you cope initially.

Most medical and nursing staff show great skill and empathy when they are delivering bad news to a patient. Unfortunately, however, some of the stories I hear from patients about the way they found out about their cancer tell me that there is room for improvement.

Case study

Rachel was in hospital waiting for the results of investigations. She told me that a registrar she had never met picked up the chart at the end of her bed and said, 'So you're the lymphoma?' That was the first time she had heard the diagnosis and, as you can imagine, it came as a terrible shock. Not to mention that she is a person, not a 'lymphoma', a detail that should never be overlooked.

Doctors have individual personalities and styles of practice and this will influence how they communicate with you. From my perspective of having to deliver bad news from time to time, I am direct and clear about the results. I deliver the results in person and not on the phone where I possibly can. Before the patient comes in for their appointment, I have all the information I need and I have already organised referrals and appointment times for specialists so there is a plan of action. I give patients time to respond and ask questions.

Initial reactions differ, of course. Some people are distraught. Some are numb and uncomprehending. Some retreat into denial. Some are really angry.

There is no right or wrong way to react and no way to plan or prepare for it. Your reaction will be whatever it was. It will be automatic and visceral.

Sometimes your doctor will have the answers to all or some of your initial questions, but there are times when we need to wait for more information to be clear about questions on your prognosis.

Everybody experiences a cancer diagnosis uniquely because each person has a unique history, different family and friendship structure, and different pre-existing physical and psychological health and wellbeing. These conditions will all frame how you react emotionally to a cancer diagnosis and the treatment that follows. They will also be the influences on the way you live your life beyond diagnosis and treatment.

Your emotional responses will also depend on your particular life stage. For example, if you are a younger woman and you need to have your uterus or ovaries removed and you desperately wanted to have children, your reaction will be different from an older woman who has adult children. In the case of a man being diagnosed with prostate cancer, the implications of the diagnosis for a man in his forties may be very different from a man in his eighties.

Sometimes a cancer diagnosis is a kind of strange relief. A woman in her fifties had been feeling exhausted, lethargic, and had uncontrollable night sweats for months. Her doctors did not seem to be able to work out what was wrong or what to do to help her. She felt as if she was dying and didn't know why. Then a lump came up in her armpit and a biopsy showed lymphoma. She understood that treatment would be a challenge on many levels, but at least she knew what was making her feel so unwell and that there was a prospect of long-term remission after treatment.

Whatever your initial reaction, a cancer diagnosis is emotionally traumatic and you may have to dig deep to find ways of coping and getting through each phase of treatment. If you or your family have been through tough times before, then you will be able to use the lessons of the past to inform you about how to get through this current challenge. But if you have never had to face a major trauma, then you are likely to need some extra guidance. It is a common reaction at this time to review your life, to look back fondly or critically at decisions and actions you and others have taken. You may or may not intend to review your past, present and future life, but it will almost certainly happen.

GETTING THROUGH TREATMENT

You will hear the term 'cancer journey'. Anyone who has been through diagnosis, treatment and recovery from cancer may come out of it older and wiser and a bit worse for wear, but this journey is no vacation.

PSYCHOLOGICAL PREPARATION FOR CANCER TREATMENT

It is important for you to prepare yourself emotionally for what lies ahead.

Information – Be as knowledgeable about the process as you can, but be wary of Dr Google or scary anecdotes from friends or well-meaning strangers, as you will always find conflicting information, information not relevant to you, and stories that often show the worst-case scenarios.

Bring someone with you – When you are in shock or overwhelmed, your capacity for information processing is greatly reduced. A trusted friend or family member can help fill in the gaps post-appointment. Ask your doctor for notes of the major points of information and advice.

Ask questions – Bring a list of questions with you to your appointments so that all of your concerns are answered.

Keeping daily routines – Keeping connections with your normal life as much as possible is better than allowing excessive time to ruminate over the uncertainty of your experience with cancer.

Cull your diary – If there are events or responsibilities that are too demanding or unpleasant, delegate them or cull them.

Enjoy the small moments – Put rewards into your day and have a laugh where possible.

Bring distractions – Every appointment will leave you stuck in a waiting room for minutes or hours. Really think how you want to spend this time – with emails, books, crosswords, sudoku, movies already downloaded, music loaded onto a device with earphones for quiet listening. That way you are not just ruminating while you wait for them to call your name at the appointment.

It is important to point out that building resilience does not mean you have to be upbeat, positive and perky the whole time. Nor does it mean you sail through the process unchanged or untouched. Quarantining yourself from the emotional conse-quences of cancer diagnosis, treatment and what it all means for your life beyond your role as a 'patient' is virtually impossible.

You might feel angry at times. If your default emotion is anger, you may find you are angry at the cancer and the situation you have been thrust into. You may not necessarily be angry at someone specific, but it can be easy to take anger out on the people close to you, the ones who don't have cancer while you do, and pick faults with the people who are there to manage your treatment. This is understandable but unproductive. Acknowledging the situation and turning the anger into a determination to get through the treat-ment process and focus on your recovery is far more constructive.

WHO DO YOU TELL?

Different people have different ideas about disclosing their cancer. Some of my patients adopt a need-to-know basis. That is, they tell their close family members and a few friends what they are going through, but prefer to maintain a veneer of normality to the rest of the world. Others prefer complete openness and let everyone around them know what is going on. Who you choose to tell about your cancer, and how much you choose to disclose to them, is entirely up to you. You need to communicate clearly about your wishes for confidentiality with the people who you do choose to tell.

I would always recommend that, as a minimum, you tell enough people around you to make sure you have a strong support network. That may mean someone you can call on to drive you to and from chemotherapy, someone to pick the children up for school on days when you can't make it, and someone to attend medical appointments with you.

It is vital to surround yourself with people who are genuinely caring, supportive and loving at a time you need it most. If you feel you need support that cannot be accommodated within your community of friends and family, then looking further afield is the next option. Broader cancer care networks and support groups can help to fulfil this function.

One of the conversations I always have with patients who are about to go into treatment is about reducing your commitments and pacing yourself. You may think you have amazing coping skills and reserves of energy, but even people who seemingly sail through treatment find that they have needed to modify their usual activities, if only temporarily.

If you are anxious about medical treatments, take a buddy along for consultations and treatments, and let the cancer nurses know you are anxious and that you need to have every step of the treatment explained to you along the way.

A professional counsellor or psychologist experienced in working with people who have been diagnosed with cancer may be necessary if your emotional distress is interfering with your life or your ability to function. Meditation, mindfulness and cognitive behaviour therapy can help you manage treatment-related anxiety. You will need professional advice to develop these skills.

Some patients will talk to me about seeking so-called 'alternative' cancer treatments because they fear the side effects of conventional chemotherapy or radiotherapy. This can be a difficult conversation. Because I have a special interest in integrative medicine they have an expectation that I will support their decision to abandon recommended medical treatments and construct an alternative treatment protocol, whereas this is not the role of an integrative doctor. An integrative doctor will work synchronously with your oncologist to help you through your cancer treatment. It is important for you to know which treatment is most likely to give you the best possible outcome in terms of achieving remission and survival. If your cancer team has told you that there is no available medical treatment that will give you a remision (for example, advanced mesothelioma which has failed conventional treatments), a program of integrative management can help to support your general health but cannot promise a long-term remission or 'cure'.

I often find that fear of the unknown is more potent than the fear of the actual disease or its treatment. Finding out as much as you can so that you understand the medical terms being used and what you can expect along your journey will help with this.

For many people the first thought they have when they are diagnosed with cancer is: 'I am going to die'. This is a terrifying thought. You may also experience a type of grief that, even in the short term, your life will not be the same. Depending on the type and seriousness of your cancer, there may be short-term or long-term disabilities such as reduced fitness, less strength in your limbs, sexual dysfunction, or chemo brain, which affects your memory. It is also possible that your cancer may shorten your life.

Case study

Shelley was 67 and had lived alone for many years since her divorce. She had two sons and several grandchildren who were the light of her life. Four years ago she was diagnosed with metastatic cancer and was told she had maybe six months to live. 'Obviously that was a profound shock,' she said. Standard cancer treatment failed to have any effect on her tumours. She took some time to think through her options and decided to accept her oncologist's offer to take part in a clinical trial of a new drug. 'I was determined to stay alive for my grandchildren,' she said. So with a focused and positive outlook, Shelley started the trial. Initially she felt very tired but she persisted. After a few months she got the wonderful news that she had responded to the treatment and the cancer metastases had shrunk. 'I was over the moon. I went back to work and carried on with life as if nothing had happened. Then at one of my routine check-ups about a year later they found some metastases in my brain. That was when I felt the battle was lost. I wanted to give up but my sons encouraged me to keep trying. The radiation oncologist said that he could treat the metastases, so I decided to have the gamma knife treatment he suggested. I was terrified that I had gone through it for nothing . . . until I got back the result that the treatment had made the brain metastases almost disappear. I don't know what the future will bring, but I will keep fighting this until I have no option left.'

DEPRESSION

Depression is common after a cancer diagnosis. Sadness, depression, uncertainty, and anticipatory grief – grieving a loss before it occurs – are some of the natural responses to the thought that life could end sooner than you anticipated. Suicidal thoughts are also possible. These feelings can also appear during your treatment or recovery, or when you are trying to adjust to life following treatment.

SYMPTOMS AND SIGNS OF DEPRESSION

In your thoughts

Have you been thinking, 'life is not worth living', 'I hate myself', 'only bad things happen to me', 'I'm worthless', 'the world would be better off without me'?

In your behaviour

Have you stopped going out to social events, not been getting things done at work or school, been relying on alcohol and sedatives to feel better, stopped doing the things you previously enjoyed, had trouble making decisions, found it hard to concentrate?

Feelings caused by depression

A person with depression may feel sad, angry, frustrated, irritable, overwhelmed, despondent, hopeless. If this sounds like the way you are feeling, you need to talk to someone in your family about it, and ask for professional help from your GP, a psychologist or psychiatrist or your cancer treatment team.

Physical symptoms of depression

Depression can have physical manifestations such as fatigue, lacking energy, feeling sick and 'run down', headaches, muscle pains, churning gut, trouble sleeping, loss or change of appetite resulting in weight loss or gain.

As you can see, it can be difficult to determine if some of these symptoms are related to your cancer or your cancer treatment or separately caused by depression, so we need to address possible underlying physical or medical causes before we attribute symptoms to a diagnosis of depression.

You need to be able to recognise the symptoms of depression:

- a deep feeling of sadness or a marked loss of interest or pleasure in activities
- changes in appetite that result in weight loss or gain
- insomnia or oversleeping
- loss of energy or increased fatigue
- restlessness or irritability
- feelings of worthlessness or inappropriate guilt
- difficulty thinking, concentrating, or making decisions
- thoughts of death or suicide or attempts at suicide.

If you experience some of these symptoms of depression, it is important to ask your doctor for help.

SYMPTOMS OF ANXIETY

There is lot of crossover between anxiety and depression, and the two conditions often coexist. Symptoms of anxiety may include a sense of impending doom, uneasiness or panic, jitteriness or agitation, trouble concentrating, sweaty palms, racing heartbeat, dry mouth, trouble sleeping (particularly in getting to sleep).

COMBATING DEPRESSION

I recommend an integrative approach to combating depression that involves incorporating the lifestyle measures in this book, plus the following:

Get organised – Make a plan of action for each day and across the week. This will include getting all your documentation in order, timetabling appointments and treatments, meeting other commitments, and taking time for relaxation.

Optimise the management of any other illness you have – As you get older it is increasingly likely that you will have chronic diseases other than the cancer that is the current focus of your attention. Remember always that you are more than the cancer, and this includes doing all you can to manage your health as best you can.

Correct any nutritional inadequacy – Some types of nutritional deficiency such as iron and vitamin B_{12} can mimic depression. I refer you to the chapter on nutrition (see page 323). If you have any issues with appetite or nutrition, I advise you to see a dietitian to analyse your diet and advise you on nutrition.

Exercise – Exercise elevates your mood and relieves symptoms of anxiety and depression. It also helps to improve the quality of your sleep. (See the chapter on exercise, page 307.)

Learn and practise mindfulness activities – The Black Dog Institute has some suggestions for mindfulness techniques to practise: www.blackdoginstitute.org.au

Maintain adequate vitamin D – Make sure to have your vitamin D level checked and if it is low, increase your skin sun exposure and supplement with vitamin D if necessary.

Ensure light exposure, especially in the morning

Reduce stressors in your life and make time in your day to relax

Arrange counselling and professional advice on psychological techniques

Look after your sleep routine. (See the chapter on sleep, page 360.)

Strengthen your social connections – Family relationships, friendships and support networks help you to get through the hard days and weeks. It can be tempting to take out your frustrations, anger or distress on the people who are closest to you, but try not to take out your stress on loved ones. Instead, tell them about your problems and ask for their support and suggestions.

Consider spirituality as an important part of your emotional wellbeing (see page 101).

Avoid mood-altering substances – This includes tobacco, alcohol and caffeine.

Ask for advice on herbal medicines – St John's wort has a number of significant drug interactions, including with some chemotherapy agents, so it is important to get professional advice on this herb rather than self-prescribe.

Talk to your doctor about pharmaceuticals that may be appropriate if your depression is persistent or severe.

WHEN TO GET PROFESSIONAL HELP

There will be some people around you who will be able to monitor your psychological health and give you feedback about whether they have noticed any personality change or signs of distress or depression. The people closest to you will be the first to notice. Ideally, you will have regular contact with your GP and/or cancer nurse. You will need the help of a psychologist if your emotions are disabling, distressing, limiting your quality of life, or keeping you from accessing your recommended treatments. Your GP may offer you counselling, or refer you to a psychologist for further help. If you are diagnosed with anxiety or depression, you will qualify for a mental healthcare plan. Under these plans, Medicare in Australia provides some subsidy for counselling with a qualified psychologist.

If you do not have the resources to get the psychological help you need in the private sector, most publicly funded cancer units have psychologists and social workers who can work through the emotional issues with you. Organisations such as the Cancer Council have advice lines with trained counsellors, and suitable support groups are also available.

You may not think you need professional help with the emotional aspects of your cancer but having cancer is a major and traumatic life event. If you or the people close to you are concerned about how you are coping or you want some preventive strategies, reach out for help.

TAKING CONTROL

You may feel you have absolutely no control over the cancer or its outcome, and in some senses that is true. Yet there are many ways you can exert some control, particularly in how you live your life and the health-affecting habits you can change.

If you have already been diagnosed with cancer, is it too late to change your lifestyle? Absolutely not. In the chapter on prevention and screening after diagnosis of cancer (see page 24), I discuss secondary prevention. That means that even though you have been diagnosed with cancer there are things you can do to help yourself to recover from the rigours of treatment, get yourself into a state of remission, and stay there.

There will be times during your treatment when you feel you do not have control over what is happening to you, but there will be aspects of your self-care where you can take control. In fact, this is at the core of the purpose of this book – to take control of those things you can change.

The way you think can influence your actions and your quality of life. From the moment you are told you have cancer, you will experience a high degree of stress and there will be emotional issues that will need to be addressed. It is likely that you and your significant others will experience shock, fear, anxiety, anger and depression. Sometimes you can deal with these feelings through your support network of friends and family, but there will be times that you need to talk to a skilled counsellor or psychologist.

THERAPY AND SUPPORT

Each person's experience of cancer is unique. What cancer means to you will be different from its meaning for others. For instance, some people feel they have been unlucky, others feel they have failed themselves or their loved ones, while others think they may be being punished for something they have done in the past. When you talk to people who have been through similar experiences, you will find you have many feelings in common with them.

Cancer does not occur in a vacuum. Your response to a cancer diagnosis is affected by your previous life experiences, your current relationships, and your dreams for the future. Your relationships with some of the people in your life will be enhanced as they move closer to offer you support, but others may distance themselves as a protective mechanism for themselves. It's not always possible to predict which people will fall into either of these categories.

Many people think they have to pretend to be happy and positive for others around them and to generate the impression that they are coping well, almost as a badge of honour. You don't have to be up and positive all the time to be coping well. And if you are not coping well, you need to find help and support to get back on track.

Therapy can help you to express exactly what you feel in a protected, private space. It will help you to share those fears you may not be able to express elsewhere, and that sharing will help you to understand the fears and put them in perspective.

I want to say a few words to you if you are one of those people who thinks, 'Well, there's nothing I can do about the fact that I have cancer. I'm not going to be able to talk it away. What's the point of therapy?' If the people around you are suggesting you have therapy, it could be that you cannot see yourself realistically right now. The people close to you will notice concerning changes in behaviour. Some examples would be withdrawing from social interactions, flying off the handle at minor provocations, irritability, or drinking too much alcohol. Try not to be defensive or angry if they do suggest you see a therapist. I recommend that you take their advice, even if just for a couple of sessions. Nobody can make you talk about your emotions or feelings, but you may find there are issues you need to work through that you do not want to tell a friend or a partner or one of your children.

It is not a sign of emotional weakness to think you can benefit from therapy during a significant and traumatic life event. You can also view therapy as an investment in your emotional future, giving you strategies for coping with challenges to come. If you do not have a space to reflect and think about yourself and what the cancer means to you individually, you can be left with a nameless dread that will have a detrimental effect on your psychological and physical health.

Support groups provide a forum for people at various stages of cancer treatment and recovery to get together and share their feelings and support each other. Depending on the cancer unit where you are being treated, you may or may not be linked to a psycho-oncologist in the healthcare system, so it is up to you to find the help and support you need. Due to a lack of resources, it may not be offered in a routine way within the healthcare system. You may not have someone in your usual support network you can confide in, and you may even need to be the 'strong one' holding those around you up.

You can start with your GP, who will be able to refer you to an appropriately qualified professional.

COGNITIVE BEHAVIOUR THERAPY (CBT)

One popular form of therapy is called cognitive behaviour therapy. CBT shows you how to adjust your thinking about yourself and your circumstances and change negative thought patterns and damaging behaviours. In a nutshell, the aim is to gain control of your reactions to stress. This is achieved by teaching you to recognise the thought patterns that produce anxiety, and change your behavioural responses to avoid the anxiety reaction.

Psychotherapy is different as CBT generally won't be able to address existential issues and 'nameless dread'. A therapist's job is to respond in a calm and non-anxious manner, guiding you and enabling you to think clearly.

Issues you might want or need to discuss with a therapist include:

- the consequences of your illness on practical issues such as your work and finances
- facing more abstract issues such as your mortality; for example, 'I am not going to live forever'
- coping with the uncertainty of the progression of your disease
- concerns about the consequences of your illness on your friends and family
- existential concerns, such as what do you believe happens to you after death (see the chapter on spirituality, page 101). An unexpected diagnosis of cancer may be a time of psychological growth and deepening of your relationships with the people you love and an enhanced sense of who you are and what you really value in life
- preparing yourself for the reactions of others
- if at other times in your life your body has been out of your control, whether from psychological or physiological reasons, then a cancer diagnosis can reactivate all those longstanding feelings and affect your mental wellbeing.

You will need to speak to your GP or find a therapist who is able to address the overwhelming feelings when dealing with existential issues, or the depression or trauma that has been activated by the cancer diagnosis.

REMEMBER THE BASICS

Anxiety and depression can dominate your life, and take your attention away from the basics of good health such as nutrition, sleep routines and exercise. Healthy lifestyle habits also work as therapy.

If you are anxious, you need to avoid caffeine completely. Alcohol is best avoided too, as are illicit substances such as amphetamines, cocaine and ecstasy.

The right diet is essential. The *Medical Journal of Australia* reviewed the evidence on the direct effects of food on mood and concluded the following:

- Eating breakfast regularly leads to improved mood, better memory, more energy and feelings of calmness.
- Eating regular meals and nutritious afternoon snacks may improve cognitive performance.
- Slow weight reduction in overweight women can help to elevate mood.
- Consuming high levels of refined sugar was found to be linked to a greater prevalence of depression.

Make sure you are eating the recommended five vegetables and two pieces of fresh fruit a day as well as daily sources of protein including seafood. High levels of saturated fat consumption may be linked to a greater prevalence of depression so a low-fat diet is helpful. And eat regular meals throughout the day to avoid hypoglycaemia (low blood sugar).

Regular moderate exercise elevates your mood and can

improve your energy and concentration. Make sure you get exposure to sunlight during the day because lack of sunlight can depress your mood.

It is important to look at sources of stress that you can reasonably avoid. Get organised and cull things that are not important for you to deal with. Make space in your life for activities that will help you manage your anxiety and depression.

Allow enough time for a good night's sleep and provide a calm quiet sleeping environment.

Supplements

If your diet is deficient or you have medical problems that make it difficult for you to absorb nutrients from food, you may benefit from a balanced multivitamin and mineral supplement, at least in the short term. Avoid excessive B vitamins as they can cause jitteriness that exacerbates anxiety. Calcium and magnesium work together and can help with anxiety.

HERBAL MEDICINES

Traditional herbal treatments for depression and anxiety have been used for many hundreds of years. If you are planning to try herbal medicines in conjunction with your lifestyle changes, you need to see an expert to prescribe them correctly and to make sure there are no interactions with your other prescribed medicines.

St John's wort (*Hypericum perforatum*) may be useful for treating depression following cancer treatment, but don't self-prescribe this herb or take it during chemotherapy as it can interfere with the action of some chemotherapy drugs. It must not be taken at the same time as SSRI antidepressants as the additive effect can cause serotonin syndrome, a toxic state caused mainly by excess serotonin within the central nervous system (confusion, agitation, racing or irregular heartbeat, nausea, tremor, loss of muscle coordination, sweating).

Particular care needs to be taken to check for potential herb–drug interactions during cancer treatment. Significant interactions include decreased effectiveness of cyclosporin, tacrolimus, irinotecan, and other chemotherapeutic agents. Your GP, oncologist, naturopath, or pharmacist can check these interactions for you.

St John's wort has also been shown to have some anti-cancer properties.

Other herbal and nutritional anti-anxiety and antidepressant supplements include kava kava (*Piper methysticum*), passionflower (*Passiflora incarnata*), lemon balm (*Melissa officinalis*), lavender (*Lavandula angustifolia*), withania and skullcap (*Scutellaria lateriflora*), GABA, and 5-HTP. These all require professional prescription and dosage advice.

ANTIDEPRESSANT MEDICATION

The symptoms of anxiety and depression can be very difficult to tolerate and there is a temptation to reach for a pharmaceutical solution to ease the emotional pain and the physical symptoms. It can be a struggle to have the patience to persist with a non-pharmaceutical strategy for anxiety or depression, but the effort is worth it.

Over recent decades there has been a dominant philosophy of prescribing medication for these problems. Antidepressants, sedatives, sleeping pills, and 'benzos' like Xanax or Serepax have become common ways of patching over mental health problems without providing skills that can help you to deal with the underlying issues.

In recent years a number of pieces of evidence have emerged to fundamentally change the way we approach the management of anxiety and depression. Scientific reviews have shown that antidepressant medications are ineffective in treating all but the most severe cases of depression, and the side effects of these medications often mimic anxiety disorder. Additionally, continuing or increasing medication can exacerbate the problem.

We have come to realise the disturbing impact of over-reliance or addiction to medication for anxiety. That being said, there is an important place for prescribing temporary anxiety-relieving medications and sedatives to help with sleep problems and traumatic situations provided there is a comprehensive plan of psychological support and monitoring of medication, and a plan for withdrawal when the stressful situation passes.

Where anxiety and/or depression is more severe or does not respond to other measures, you may need to consider pharmaceutical antidepressant medication. There are times when antidepressant medication is absolutely necessary.

I have seen many people who are reluctant to take anti-depressant medication when it was clearly indicated, and some who have taken medication and suffered adverse effects. However, I believe in balancing benefit against risk. Severe depression is disabling and can be life-threatening, and has to be treated seriously. The right medication can be extremely effective. The medication will probably be a temporary measure in most cases while your physical health is recovering, and works best if you have concurrent counselling.

MIND–BODY TECHNIQUES

Counselling and support groups and conversations with the people close to you all provide a form of emotional scaffolding. Most of the time, however, you are left with your thoughts. There are some effective techniques you can learn to help you contain and guide those thoughts.

MEDITATION

Possibly the most powerful and effective method of managing stress is to regularly practise meditation. You will find some form of meditation in most of the major religions and spiritual traditions, and meditation is now commonly recommended as an activity that will help your health and wellbeing.

In meditation, the aim is to create a wakeful but relaxed state of mental and physical calm. While there are different forms of meditation, most of them have common elements. They generally require:

- a quiet environment
- a comfortable posture, whether sitting, lying or standing
- a focus of attention which may be a mantra, your senses, or your breathing
- an ability to observe without judgement.

The most common types of meditation are transcendental meditation and mindfulness meditation. Transcendental meditation is a part of Ayurvedic tradition. In this meditation a repeated sound or mantra is used as the focus of attention. It emphasises positive emotions and the need to be in tune with your body's natural rhythms.

Mindfulness practice involves bringing your focus to the here and now. In a nutshell, it involves you giving deliberate and non-judgemental attention to the present moment, where you acknowledge and accept every thought, feeling and sensation in and around you at that given moment.

Mindfulness-based techniques have been found to be very useful in dealing with the distress of cancer. One study looked at mindfulness-based cancer recovery (MBCR) involving mindfulness meditation and gentle yoga and compared it with supportive-expressive group therapy (SET) in a group of women with stages I to III breast cancer. It found the mindfulness approach was more effective than the group therapy approach for improving quality of life and stress levels. Both approaches are useful and some people prefer one over the other, so my suggestion would be to try both and see which one benefits you most. You may choose to do both mindfulness and group therapy.

If you are planning to practise transcendental meditation or mindfulness mediation, then you will need to be taught by an expert. There is now extensive research on the effects of mindfulness practices to show that it is helpful in the treatment of pain, stress, anxiety, addictions, preventing relapse of depression, and other situations relevant to a cancer diagnosis.

We know that meditation changes brain activity, which results in an improvement in mood. One study measured brain electrical activity before and immediately after meditation, and then four months after an eight-week training program in mindfulness meditation. It found significant increases in left-sided frontal brain activation, a pattern known to be associated with positive mood, in meditators compared with non-meditators. The study also found significant increases in the antibody response to influenza vaccine among people in the meditation compared with those in the wait-list control group.

Long-term meditation is now thought to affect not only the electrical activity in the brain but the actual structure of the brain, and to slow age-related loss of brain cells, particularly in brain regions associated with attention and sensory processing.

There is also a measurable increase in immune function and changes in other parts of the body.

Meditation can be used to maintain your general wellbeing or it can be used as a part of integrative therapy for a range of illnesses. You can also use it to enhance your spiritual development.

The physiological and psychological benefits of meditation accumulate over time and with experience, resulting in:

- improved physical health
- enhanced immunity
- improved mental and emotional health
- faster rehabilitation after illness
- clearer thinking
- greater self-awareness
- reduced feelings of stress
- greater resilience to pressure
- improved sense of spiritual fulfilment
- improved quality of life.

YOGA

Yoga can help to improve your quality of life during and after cancer treatment. Studies have shown that yoga practice results in large reductions in distress, anxiety and depression; with moderate reductions in fatigue; moderate increases in general quality of life, emotional function, and social function; and a small increase in functional wellbeing.

Check with your doctor and yoga teacher about what form and level of yoga practice is suitable for you and what limitations you might need to apply. There are some yoga teachers who specially plan and supervise classes for people with medical problems. (See the section on yoga, page 239.)

TAI CHI AND QI GONG

Tai chi and qi gong are popular forms of combined exercise and mind–body practice for people who are looking for a safe, gentle, and effective activity. (See page 253.)

RELAXATION THERAPY

Relaxation therapy with breathing techniques and progressive muscle relaxation can help reduce anxiety during cancer treatment. The physiological relaxation response slows your heart rate, lowers your blood pressure, decreases oxygen consumption, and decreases your levels of stress hormones.

There are a number of relaxation techniques you can learn including controlled breathing, progressive muscle relaxation, visualisation, and various meditation techniques. Some of these techniques are taught in yoga schools, in private or group classes, or in private sessions with a psychologist.

CONTROLLED BREATHING

When you are stressed you tend to take shallow breaths with a rapid breathing rate. Controlled breathing is a method of focusing on deep slow breathing patterns to combat the effects of stress and to promote relaxation.

- Play some peaceful, 'smooth' instrumental music without a defined beat.
- Lie down or sit comfortably in a quiet place and close your eyes.
- Breathe in deeply and slowly through your nose but do not overfill your lungs.
- Pause briefly, then breathe out slowly and steadily.
- Gradually increase the duration of the breathing-out phase so that is about twice as long as the breathing-in phase.
- Slow down the cycle of breaths, but make sure it feels comfortable and not strained for you.
- Continue for ten to fifteen minutes.
- Repeat daily.

Once you have practised controlled breathing a few times, you can use it when you are feeling very stressed as a way of restoring your balance.

PROGRESSIVE MUSCLE RELAXATION

Progressive muscle relaxation is, as the name suggests, a methodical way of consciously tensing a muscle group then releasing it progressively, usually starting at your toes and finishing at your neck and head, or vice versa. It can be taught in groups or private lessons with a psychologist, other healthcare practitioner or yoga teacher, or with a self-help DVD. Once you have been instructed in the technique you can practise it yourself.

GUIDED IMAGERY

Guided imagery uses your imagination along with controlled breathing exercises to reduce unpleasant sensations. You might use mental images of sights, sounds, smells, tastes, physical sensations, or experiences to help you manage pain, discomfort, nausea, anxiety and distress.

You will need to be taught the techniques by an experienced professional.

MUSIC THERAPY

Music therapy has a long history in cancer recovery. You don't have to have any musical talent or experience to benefit. Music therapists may provide one-on-one sessions or group sessions based on your preferences.

The session of music therapy might include making music, listening to music, writing songs and discussing lyrics. It can be effective in reducing pain, nausea, depression and anxiety.

RECURRENCE

If there is one thing that is as difficult to handle emotionally as an initial diagnosis of cancer, it is a recurrence.

There is no way to sugar-coat the news of a cancer recurrence. It means that after initial treatment and remission the cancer has returned, either at the original site but more likely at a distant site. Most people embark on their initial treatment with the intention of a long-term, if not permanent remission, but a recurrence flings you back into the cancer 'system', and decisions about treatment or symptom management have to be faced again.

Case Study

Janette was diagnosed with breast cancer eight years ago. Then one day she developed a backache that kept her awake at night and just wouldn't go away. A bone scan showed metastases in her lumbar spine.

'I had just got to the point of feeling confident that the cancer was gone for good,' she said. 'I was fine with the initial breast cancer diagnosis. I felt positive. I convinced myself that I could beat this thing. I had my troops rallied around me and I read everything I could about getting through breast cancer. Then this. It was like being punched in the chest. I had much more trouble feeling positive about the cancer coming back and I really didn't know if I could face it all again.'

News of a recurrence can be frightening and demoralising. You will need accurate information about the meaning of the recurrence to your inmmediate future and your prognosis.

The level of stress at the time of finding out about a recurrence is similar to the time of initial diagnosis. Interestingly, you may find that you have a better idea of how to cope because at the time of initial diagnosis you had to learn new coping mechanisms.

Many patients find that the situation is familiar and they slip back into helpful habits such as meditation and taking care of sleep routines, nutrition and exercise, and connecting with known support people. How you cope will depend on how you learned to cope with your initial diagnosis and treatment.

A study by the Ohio State University supports this idea of learned resilience. Following a group of women in the first year after a recurrence diagnosis, and comparing them with patients who were coping with their first diagnosis, patients with recurrence had significantly lower anxiety and confusion. Breast cancer recurrence is currently managed as a chronic disease, so the way you adjust to a recurrence of your cancer will depend on the type of cancer and the meaning of its recurrence in terms of your prognosis.

It is crucial to take control of as much of this process as possible. Collect as much information as you can about your treatment process. Follow advice on what to prepare for each visit and what to bring to hospital. Keep an ongoing list of questions to ask your doctors and make sure that your sources of information are credible and reliable. If at any time you feel you are not coping emotionally, ask for help. It is crucial to remember during this process that you are the expert on you and you know best what your psychological needs are.

THE CONFIDENCE TO LIVE

Once your treatment is over you might expect to feel relieved, even elated. This may be true for you, but you may also feel insecure, cut off from the support structures of the cancer treatment centre and uncertain about your future. Don't be surprised if this turns out to be the most challenging phase for you.

Some treatment side effects, such as hair loss or nausea, pass quickly after treatment ends, but some occur months or even years later. These 'late effects' include serious conditions such as cancer recurrence, development of a second cancer, cardiotoxicity (damage to the heart), diabetes and other metabolic disorders, neurotoxicity (damage to sensory or motor function, learning and/or memory processes), osteoporosis, and premature menopause and fertility issues. There will likely be ongoing health challenges to manage over time.

Many cancer survivors experience fatigue, changes in their brain function, changed appearance (which may affect body image and self-esteem), and reduced mobility. Cancer and cancer treatments may also have a persistent psychological impact, such as the fear of the cancer returning and uncertainty about the future. There are also the practical considerations, such as loss of work or a reduction in your usual income, changed roles within your home relationship, discrimination in employment and insurance issues.

It is helpful to remember that this is a time of major life transition. You need to form new relationships with your body, yourself, your family and your friends. You will need to do a lot of thinking and reflecting on what you have been through and what lies ahead for you in order to regain some sense of familiarity with this new situation and to lay a new foundation to live your life confidently, both physically and emotionally. This is where support groups can be very beneficial. Simply knowing others have similar feelings can normalise your experience.

For a time, your cancer and its treatment govern most of your thoughts and occupy much of your time. As your remission time grows longer, the cancer will occupy less and less of your thoughts and energy.

You may think differently about yourself. Others may see you differently. You may have had to change many aspects of the way you lived before your diagnosis. Unexpected physical and psychological effects of the cancer and its treatment may have affected your ability to work, to care for your family, to be active, and to do the other 'normal' things of life. Take the time to think about how you can optimise the opportunities that life presents you and how your 'new normal' looks and feels.

I have seen many people go through cancer treatment and recover to long-term remission. Ideally, the internal chaos or depression you might experience along the way resolve, leaving you with a renewed passion for the preciousness of life and your connection to others.

Thanks to Lissy Abrahams, psychotherapist, and Jace Cannon-Brookes, clinical psychologist, Heath Group Practice, Sydney.

RESOURCES
See the following websites for more information:
Cancer Council NSW: www.cancercouncil.com.au/
Macmillan Cancer Support in the UK: www.macmillan.org.uk/
Cancerinformation/Cancerinformation.aspx
Stanford Medicine Cancer Institute: cancer.stanford.edu/
information/coping/

Conneƈtedness

In any health crisis you need a support structure, and this is a time when the support you need comes in the form of those connections to the people who matter to you.

During times of stress, as you will inevitably have experienced and may continue to experience through your recovery, your body produces hormones in the adrenal glands which are necessary to the body to face day-to-day challenges. But when these hormones are present in large amounts over time, they can impair the immune system and slow down healing, increase blood pressure, and affect blood glucose levels and bone density.

The act of connecting with someone releases the hormone oxytocin, which can impact on stress levels, depression, and perhaps is even the reason why women with good friends often have lower blood pressure, heart rate and cholesterol.

The Harvard Nurses' Study began in 1976 and has followed the health of 238000 women since then. In 2001 the study found that not having a good friend is as bad for your health as smoking or being overweight. According to a study conducted at the University of California, women tend to naturally seek out social contact and support from close friends as a way of coping with stress. In this way, women respond differently to stress than men, and that may help to explain why men are more likely to suffer the harmful effects of stress.

People feel much better when they talk about their worries or share their joys. Having a friend who will listen to you is sometimes all we need to feel better. In times of illness and emotional trauma, supportive and encouraging friends increase hope. And increased hope improves the functioning of the immune system.

Managing cancer is a team effort. This is not just in terms of the medical treatment, nursing care, and adjunctive therapies you need to directly treat the cancer. Your support team will also ideally include people who are willing to help you with the emotional and physical challenges of the treatment and recovery process. They might be the ones who help you shop and prepare food, listen to your worries, call you to see how you are feeling, help transport you to appointments, visit you in hospital and at home, arrange social events for you, or just be there for you when you need a friend.

I always encourage patients to take a trusted person with them to all their medical consultations to help them remember the details of the consultation, and also to reach out to friends and family for emotional and practical support.

AUDIT YOUR CONNECTEDNESS

A health crisis can be a catalyst for you to reflect on your connectedness. You can do a simple audit, which involves some fundamental questions. Most of the questions are very straightforward while others will need more reflection and perhaps be more challenging.

- Do you have a primary relationship? How would you describe this relationship?

- Who lives at home with you?
- Describe your extended family.
- Have there been any stresses or difficulties with any of your relationships recently? Can these difficulties be fixed?
- In general, does contact with the important people in your life make you feel better or worse about yourself?
- What is your cultural/ethnic background and what effect does this have on your life?
- How do you contact people who are important to you and how much time do you spend each week interacting with them?
- Who are your 3 am people? (See page 98.)
- Who do you trust to talk to about your concerns or problems?
- Do the people you spend time with make you feel valued and loved?
- Describe your workplace and the interactions with colleagues. Are there any conflicts or stresses with the people there?
- Do you love your job and do you look forward to going to work each day?
- How closely do you identify with your place of work? Is it 'just a job', or is it something you feel proud to be associated with?
- What social activities do you have and how often do you attend them?
- What non-work-related interests and hobbies do you have?
- What memberships do you have to clubs or organisations? What time do you spend there and what sort of activities do you do?
- What is your financial situation?
- What part, if any, does religion or spirituality play in your life?

You don't need to 'tick all the boxes', but thinking about all of these aspects of connectedness will give you an idea of the breadth of connection you might have and the impact that will have on your life now and into the future. Hopefully the exercise will get you thinking about some of the areas you can plan to address.

Then once you have conducted the audit of your own connectedness, you will have some clues about what to do to improve your sense of connectedness.

WHO ARE YOUR 3 AM PEOPLE?

Your 3 am people are your closest and strongest relationships and that connection is mutual. You would call them in a crisis at 3 am. This is particularly important when you are undergoing cancer treatment.

Your 3 am people might be family or friends. They may or may not be biological family members. They may be people you see only occasionally, but you have a strong connection to them.

They are the ones you need to have on speed dial during the intense parts of your cancer journey in case you have a medical emergency or an emotional crisis. You may never need to call at 3 am, but knowing they are there can have a very calming effect.

LAYERS OF CONNECTEDNESS

Think of your relationships with other people as a series of layers inside other layers, like an onion.

Your 'inner circle' is inhabited by your most intimate relationship. Ideally this will be your partner. It may be a parent or an adult child, your closest friend, or more than one of these.

Outside of that is another layer with your 3 am friends.

Next are the friends and family you like spending time with but are a little more emotionally distant from you.

Outside of that group are the acquaintances you spend time

with, but who do not share your personal details or your confidential health information.

Beyond that are your work colleagues, contacts, hairdresser, shopkeepers, people you say hello to while you are walking the dog.

There are the special purpose connections too, like cancer support groups. In healthcare we harness the power of connectedness in helping you to manage through difficult times or to recover from illness, with support groups, group therapy, and community-based activities. If you get involved in a cancer support group, you may find you meet people who become close friends because of your shared experience.

CONNECTING THROUGH SOCIAL MEDIA

Technologies such as FaceTime and Skype can allow a type of direct personal communication. If you cannot be in the same place at the same time with someone, at least you can see each other's faces and have a form of personal contact with voice and vision. You can join social media support groups set up for people who are going through similar cancer journeys.

There is huge potential for social media to improve connectedness for people with cancer and in the future I am sure that we will see much more exploration of how we can increase the use of technology to connect people.

ASK FOR HELP

There will be times when you need help. Don't be afraid to ask, or accept offers of help. I try to help my patients work out who they can ask for help, and if they say they feel uncomfortable stepping outside their usual support people, my advice is, 'If you are offered help and you need it, please accept the assistance'.

Another advantage of gathering a support team is that you are less likely to exhaust the people closest to you.

One helpful hint is to give your support people some guidance about what is useful to you. For example, if you need someone to pick up the children from school for a few weeks, let them know.

Maybe you are living alone, widowed, estranged from your family, or you have recently moved to your neighbourhood and you cannot realistically put together the support you need in the short term. Let your doctor or other members of your cancer team know and they will put you in touch with a social worker. This is the member of the cancer team who can gather any available community support for you.

MEND OR END DAMAGING RELATIONSHIPS

A cancer diagnosis will highlight the strengths and weaknesses in your primary relationship also. Living in an unhappy relationship, or one that is not bad enough to leave and not good enough to stay in, is a significant risk factor for death from a whole range of different causes. If you are living in an abusive, unhappy or unfulfilling relationship, consider relationship counselling as an essential part of your integrative cancer management and try to sort out your differences.

Spirituality and Cancer

Your concept of spirituality will be as unique and individual as you are, and quite different from someone with a different upbringing, life experience, culture or environment. To you it might mean your religion, your philosophy of life, or the sum total of the things that matter to you and give your life meaning.

Spirituality can and usually does come into focus when you face a health crisis, especially a potentially life-threatening situation. When I speak to patients who have been diagnosed with cancer, they are often looking for answers to questions, which, while not strictly medical, certainly have an essential place in an integrative approach to cancer care. Patients can experience the gamut of emotions from shock, grief, and anger to loss, depression, and hopelessness. Their questions can range from the metaphysical meaning of the disease to beliefs about God, death, and the prospect of an afterlife.

The question of spirituality and an afterlife came up for our family when my wife Jackie's mother was very ill with metastatic bowel cancer. Knowing she had limited time, probably only weeks to live, she told us that she had no belief in an existence beyond the present and known. She said that if there were, surely there would have been a sign. Soon after this conversation there were a number of events observed by many around her that were inexplicable other than being by some 'other-worldly' communication. These events fundamentally transformed her view of life and death, and she moved into a far more peaceful and accepting mindset. They certainly convinced me and other cynical and scientifically trained members of our family that, to quote Shakespeare's *Hamlet*: 'There are more things in heaven and earth, Horatio, Than are dreamt of in your philosophy'.

Spirituality is not the same thing as religion, although organised religion may be the framework for your own personal expression of spirituality. Separate from religious spirituality are the secular concepts of humanitarianism, love, compassion, tolerance, contentment and altruism. Your brand of spirituality may express itself in your appreciation of nature, your pursuit of social justice, your relationships, your belief in a universal force, or your appreciation of art or music. It might be a combination of all the influences on your personal philosophy.

There are spiritual practices such as prayer, meditation, appreciation of nature and altruistic voluntary work that increase your understanding of yourself and your place in the universe. However you express your spirituality, the things that give your life meaning, hope, comfort, and peace of mind make up very important elements of emotional health and resilience as you face the challenges of cancer treatment and recovery. There is growing research showing how important spirituality is in cancer survivorship. Spiritual beliefs will influence factors as diverse as treatment decisions, coping strategies, choice of complementary therapies and end-of-life care.

As cancer survivorship increases with more effective treatments, there has been more focus on issues of quality of life, including the spiritual dimension of recovery and the pursuit of wellness.

DEVELOPING YOUR SPIRITUAL SELF

In the Health Audit (see page 28), I asked you to consider spiritual aspects of your life – past and present – and how this might influence you as you face the future. It is important to give some thought to spirituality and its meaningfulness for you.

Developing your spiritual self is not just going to be a bolt from the blue. It will need contemplation and planning, and it may also mean you look for spiritual guidance. While on the one hand you might rely on your sense of spirituality to get you through the tough times with your illness, on the other hand your faith can also be seriously challenged after a serious diagnosis or if your prognosis is not optimistic. This can precipitate what we might call a spiritual crisis. You may find yourself questioning your previous beliefs, your religious upbringing, and your beliefs about God. If your prognosis is poor you may, literally, 'lose faith'. Revisit the audit on page 28 for a list of questions to reengage your spirituality.

YOUR BUCKET LIST

The definition of 'bucket list' is a list of experiences or achievements that a person hopes to have or accomplish during their lifetime. It goes hand in hand with spirituality, in that the exercise of formulating a bucket list is an opportunity to reflect on those things that have had meaning for you, and to make a plan for instilling purpose into your future.

Think back to when you were a child, a teenager, a young adult. Think of all the things you said you would like to do 'one day'. Backpack across Europe? Study Italian in Rome? A cancer diagnosis is a reminder that life is finite. For all sorts of reasons, prognosis is not always accurate, but it will give you some idea of your immediate future and how much time you may have to achieve some of your dreams.

A bucket list is not meant to be a fixed, immutable contract with the universe. It is a wish list of goals and dreams that may change from time to time. Your bucket list will depend on your current state of health and the prognostic prediction of whether you will be physically able to do the things you would like to have on your bucket list . . . and you may need to modify it to take into account any physical limitations you have as a result of your cancer or its treatment.

YOUR PERSONAL SPIRITUALITY

Whatever your definition or expression of spirituality, it is likely to have an impact on your experience of cancer, and on how cancer affects your life now and into the future. Many people with cancer draw on their spiritual or religious beliefs to help them cope with the disease and its treatment. Spiritual wellbeing is relevant to your cancer recovery because it has a direct impact on your mental health, lifestyle choices, current and future relationships, and coping strategies. It may also affect your survival. There are actions you can take to develop your spiritual self.

- Incorporate spiritual elements into all parts of your life.
- Think about what gives you positive feelings such as joy, comfort, hope, connectedness and strength.
- Develop a portfolio of achievable dreams and goals.
- Think about whether your work contributes in some positive way to others.
- Spend time in nature.
- Find time to do some of the things that are important to you every day.

- Consider some altruistic work such as community volunteering.
- Find someone who will listen to your hopes, fears, and dreams, and be there for others to express theirs.
- Think about the place of religion in your life and whether this might be incorporated in some way into your framework of spirituality.
- Consider art and music appreciation in your daily life.

Intimacy, Sexuality and Cancer Recovery

When you face a medical crisis such as the diagnosis of a significant cancer, it can make you take a long and critical look at yourself, the choices you have made in how you live your life and particularly your relationships with the most significant people in your life. You may ask yourself questions like, 'How important is my partner to me?', 'Have I truly appreciated this person?', 'Could we have spent more time together?'. You could even ask yourself the very challenging questions like, 'Am I truly happy in my life?' or 'Am I with the right partner?'.

Some cancers are more likely than others to raise issues of sexual function early in the course of treatment and recovery. Obviously this is particularly the case for breast cancer, prostate cancer, and some gynaecological cancers such as vulval cancer or ovarian cancer. Or sexual function may be a secondary issue that needs to be addressed later on. For example, when a change in libido is an unanticipated side effect of chemotherapy or hormone therapy.

Your sexual function after cancer treatment and how much of an issue it will be for you depend on a lot of factors:

- your sexual function and attitudes before you had cancer treatment
- the type of cancer
- the cancer-specific treatments you need to have and how much those treatments will affect your general health, energy, and libido
- the nature of your current relationship (if you are in a relationship)
- your plans for a future relationship (if you are currently single).

There are several ways that cancer and cancer treatment can impact on you sexually:

- the effect on your body image
- the direct impact of cancer treatment on your physical functioning: specifically, erectile function in men or sexual arousal in women, the presence of any physical discomfort or pain or restriction of movement, exertion tolerance and your ability to reach orgasm
- the psychological effect of cancer and cancer treatment on your thoughts and attitudes about yourself and your partner sexually
- your general emotional wellbeing.

The emotional and physical aspects of sexuality and intimacy are very much interconnected and one cannot be considered without considering the other.

BODY IMAGE

Many types of cancer treatment can change your body image and affect the way you feel about yourself sexually.

HAIR LOSS

One of the most immediately obvious visual effects of chemotherapy is hair loss. (See page 133 for more information on hair loss.) If you have a partner, it is important to involve him or her in discussions about how you will deal with hair loss and provide them with the opportunity to hear all the information and ask any questions, as hair loss can be distressing and confronting for both of you.

With chemotherapy you can lose all the hair on your body. I always warn people to expect to lose their eyelashes and eyebrows and to plan for that as well.

You can also expect to temporarily lose your pubic hair.

SCARRING

Surgery can aesthetically affect parts of your body that are important to your sexual identity. Apart from the pain of the healing process, both men and women can feel physically violated after an operation, and it is common to be embarrassed and self-conscious about scarring. Minimally invasive surgical techniques have progressed dramatically in the past decades so we don't see the extensive scarring of previous eras quite as often, but there are some conditions where the treatment necessarily has to involve surgery that is invasive and disfiguring, such as radical mastectomy or amputation of a limb.

There is no doubt that most cultures see the breast as a symbol of femininity, and the loss of a breast is frequently mourned because of this. Surgeons try to be as conservative as possible, but where the priority is long-term survival, and hopefully a cure, the aesthetics almost invariably have to take a back seat to the medical outcome. Losing a breast can cause a massive psychological reaction affecting sexual functioning, so it is now a relatively common practice for the cancer surgeon to work with a plastic surgeon to begin the process of reconstructing the breast at the time of the mastectomy if that is possible. Nonetheless, many women notice a change in their sexual attitudes or behaviour after a mastectomy. This seems to be particularly true of women who rely a lot on breast and nipple stimulation for arousal or orgasm. An exercise called 'sensate focus' is useful to helping with this problem. It involves using different touching techniques on other areas of your body which stimulate the erotic feelings that build towards orgasm. In the case of a mastectomy, it takes the emphasis away from the breasts by discovering other parts of the skin that may give you a similar response.

The loss of a breast can also mean a loss of self-confidence and a reluctance to initiate sex, in particular a new relationship.

Case history
Laura was 58 and divorced when her breast cancer was diagnosed and she was told she would have to have a mastectomy.

'I had been divorced for over five years and I'd been on a few dates but I just didn't feel ready to go into another serious relationship. Then this. At first my main priority was surviving the cancer, of course. My children and my friends were fantastic when I was going through the surgery and then the radiotherapy and the chemo but the nights could be very long and lonely. Once I was given the all clear, it was such a relief. The hormone treatment they put me on just killed off any libido that was left by then. I would love to meet someone special but I have resisted even thinking about it too much because I just don't know how I would cope with a new relationship with someone looking at the scar where my breast used to be.'

The situation is different for people who are in established relationships, but the potential impact on your sexual relationship needs to be discussed at each stage of treatment planning. Any surgery that involves the genital area, for instance, will obviously have sexual implications.

One of the most common genital operations in women is a hysterectomy, or removal of the uterus. This is done for a variety of reasons including cancer, uncontrollable menstrual bleeding, or benign conditions such as fibroids. There is still a lot we don't know about the effects of hysterectomy on sexual function, but it probably depends on the woman's sexual responses before the operation. Some women find that contractions of the uterus heighten their orgasm, and others depend on deep vaginal and cervical stimulation to trigger their orgasm. These women may notice a change in the quality of that orgasm after the operation. Other women say their sex life improved afterwards because they weren't tired all the time from heavy bleeding, and they no longer had to worry about contraception.

To a large extent, the reason for the operation determines the individual reaction to it. If the uterus is being removed because of cancer, then survival and getting through treatment will be the overwhelming issues, and the same is true for most malignancies.

In the case of prostate cancer surgery, the potential effect on erectile function can be one of the main factors in a decision about whether and how to treat the cancer, or wait and watch it. (See the chapter on prostate cancer, page 442.)

VAGINAL DISCOMFORT

After breast cancer treatment with surgery, chemotherapy and/ or radiotherapy, women with hormone-sensitive cancers will be advised to take hormone-blocking medications to improve their chances of survival. There are some predictable side effects of these medications, including vaginal dryness and a condition we call vulval atrophy, where the skin around the vagina becomes thin and can split easily if it is traumatised. This obviously can make sexual penetration extremely uncomfortable, painful, or impossible.

I don't mean to sound brutal, but along the lines of 'if you don't use it you lose it', unless the vagina is regularly stretched, it can become extremely tight and eventually penetration can become physically impossible. If you have a partner, regular sexual interaction increases blood flow to the genital area which helps to maintain the tissues, and also regularly stretches the opening of the vagina so that it maintains its openness. If you do not have a partner or if penetrative intercourse is not a part of your relationship, there are vaginal dilators that can perform this function. Vaginal moisturisers and lubricants can help.

For women on hormone-blocking medication, vaginal symptoms and sexual dysfunction can be a deal-breaker; the difference between being able to continue with the medication or not. A few years ago there was a zero tolerance attitude of oncologists to the use of topical vaginal oestrogen creams by women who had a history of breast cancer. Recognising what a big problem this is, in more recent years this attitude has relaxed. There is a balance between quality of life and assessment of risk, and while each case has to be assessed individually, oncologists are now more comfortable with women using vaginal oestrogen sparingly a couple of times a week.

ERECTILE DYSFUNCTION

One example of a cancer that can affect erectile function in men is prostate cancer. The surgery can sometimes damage the nerves responsible for erections. Hormone therapy for advanced cancers can also cause loss of libido and impotence.

The overall incidence of impotence (erectile dysfunction) from surgery is extremely variable depending upon the expertise of your surgeon. Generally, if you are potent preoperatively and you are under the age of 65 and both nerves are spared, you should expect at least a 70–80 per cent chance of sexual recovery over an 18-month period. This is the result from the best units in the world currently. It is quite common for the erectile recovery to be incomplete but adequate for intercourse, and often requiring medication with PDE5 inhibitors (such as the medications sildenafil, vardenafil or tadanafil) as well. It is also mandatory that sexual rehabilitation be arranged as part of your recovery process if future sexual function is important to you. Your surgeon or GP will be able to refer you to a suitable health professional for this.

If recovery after surgery or indeed after any form of therapy such as brachytherapy or radiotherapy is incomplete, then your first option is to try PDE5 inhibitors. If these medications do not work, then the next options would be a vacuum device and penile injection therapy, and the final option would be a penile implant. Generally, penile implants are reserved for those patients who do not respond to more conservative therapies.

Hormone therapies for treating advanced prostate cancers will severely affect sexual functioning. Prostate cancer is a hormone-dependent cancer, so the idea is to prevent any of the hormone reaching the cancer. You will not be able to get an erection if you are taking luteinising hormone (LH) blockers, such as goserelin (Zoladex), leuprorelin (Prostap), or buserelin (Suprefact). This is because the drugs stop you producing any of the male hormone testosterone. It is possible that erectile function could return if you stop taking the hormone treatment, but this could take some time. You need to be aware that the erectile dysfunction could be permanent.

About half the men treated for metastatic prostate cancer with an anti-androgen such as bicalutamide (Casodex) on its own maintain their previous sex drive and can get workable erections.

This is also true for high dose treatment with Casodex. But about four out of five men may still become impotent with long-term treatment.

BOWEL CANCER AND SEXUALITY

Bowel cancer surgery can also affect sexuality, particularly if there is an extensive scar, if the condition results in a degree of faecal incontinence, or if there is a colostomy bag.

After treatment for rectal cancer, some women feel their orgasm is less intense than before. It may also take them longer to reach orgasm. This is thought to be due to changes in the blood flow and nerves in the pelvic and genital area. You might need to experiment with different sexual positions, use placement of cushions, and control the speed and depth of penetration to find a more comfortable technique. Vaginal lubricants can also help.

If you have a stoma it can make you feel more self-conscious or anxious about sexual activity. The stoma nurse will anticipate the questions or areas of difficulty you might have with sexuality after a stoma and provide you with advice about how to manage this. If you are in a relationship it will be important to discuss this with your partner and you may need to ask for further professional advice if you are having difficulties.

YOUR RELATIONSHIP

There may be physical, or anatomical, or biochemical/hormonal reasons for sexual dysfunction after cancer treatment. Some of these problems are permanent but others are temporary or fixable. While it might take some effort and perhaps some professional help, it is possible to continue to enjoy your sex life during and after cancer treatment if it is physically possible.

The answer to, 'Will I have a great sex life after my cancer treatment?' depends largely on how things were before. Any major problems in a relationship are not going to suddenly resolve because there is a crisis. They may be put on the backburner for a while as priorities are reassessed, but they are not going to just disappear. That's where specialised counselling can help.

If a relationship is stable and supportive and there is good communication between the partners, then there's a very good chance of things getting back to normal, or even better than before. Your sexual routine may need to change, at least for a while, and the key to success in this is communication. Initially, that means communicating with health advisers so that you know what disruptions to your sexuality there are likely to be and you can plan ways of dealing with them. The next step is communicating with each other. Sometimes that communication has to be more detailed than ever before.

Some people worry that they will cause their partner harm or pain. Taking it slowly and telling your partner where and how to touch or moving their hand or body weight to avoid pain and finding the most pleasurable positions will help to get around this anxiety.

During and after cancer treatment it is common to feel weak and tired. If this is the case, it may help to ask your partner to take a more active role in lovemaking than they have before.

No matter what kind of cancer treatment, the ability to feel pleasure from touching almost always remains. Some couples will need to learn new techniques or, in the case of gynaecological surgery, may even need to relearn how to have orgasms. Keeping your options open means maintaining an open mind about ways to feel sexual pleasure. Many people have a narrow definition of 'normal' sexual activity. As an example, some people think 'sex equals penis-in-vagina intercourse in the missionary (what do you mean there's more than one?) position'. This restricted attitude stands in the way of sensual fulfilment.

Some forms of sexual activity are more strenuous than others, and a crisis like cancer and its treatment can be an incentive to explore new ways of sexual expression, such as massage, oral sex, sensate focus, or manual stimulation of yourself or your partner.

Using fantasies of happy memories or special places can distract you from the fears and unpleasantness of the realities. Taking time to explore sensitive parts of your body or playing around with a vibrator will increase stimulation. Trying out different positions to avoid pain, and using lubricating jelly to get around vaginal dryness will help to overcome some of the discomforts.

DO YOU HAVE ANY QUESTIONS?

It can be difficult to ask for professional advice about sex in the best of circumstances, and even if the question of resuming sex after your cancer treatment did occur to you, it's hard to get the opportunity to ask. Ward rounds before your discharge from hospital are definitely not the ideal time for a private conversation. You might have the surgeon, the registrar, a resident or two, the physiotherapist, dietitian, occupational therapist, ward pharmacist, nurses, spouse and assorted relatives crowded around the bed discussing anything from your latest scan result to working out your chemotherapy schedule.

'Any questions, Mrs Jones?'

'Well Doctor, my husband and I were actually wondering whether a big orgasm might burst my stitches or give me a stroke?' is probably not something you feel like asking out loud under the circumstances.

This is a conversation you need to have, ideally, in the prehabilitation stage. You can speak privately to your surgeon, radiation oncologist or medical oncologist. Your GP or cancer specialist can also arrange a referral to a sexual health practitioner who can assist with counselling and practical advice.

· PART THREE ·

Cancer-specific treatments

Prehabilitation

Cancer prehabilitation is a part of the process of cancer treatment that occurs ideally between the time you are diagnosed and the beginning of acute treatment. The process includes physical and psychological assessments to establish your baseline functional level, identifies any impairments you might have, and provides targeted interventions to improve your before, during and after cancer treatment.

The aim of cancer prehabilitation is to reduce the complications of medical treatment and to speed and enhance your recovery, and there is a growing body of scientific evidence that supports the benefits of preparing a newly diagnosed cancer patient for treatment and optimising their health before starting acute treatments. Most prehabilitation processes focus on nutrition, physical strength and fitness, and stress management techniques. Ideally, you will be living an optimal lifestyle at the time of diagnosis. Unless your treatment must start urgently, you may have time to undertake cancer prehabilitation for several weeks . . . even two to four weeks will show a difference.

Go back to the health audit (page 28) and identify the areas where you need to make improvements to your current wellbeing and lifestyle. That is a start. Then you will need specific advice on exercise, nutrition, supplements, and mind–body strategies to prepare you.

Your individual prehabilitation program will depend on your particular physical and emotional needs as well as the type of treatment plan and your current state of health. For example, if you have lung cancer and lung surgery is planned, stopping smoking and learning breathing and coughing exercises will be integral to your plan.

During the prehabilitation process you will also have the opportunity to plan your management of treatment side effects and your post-treatment rehabilitation and recovery.

Cancer prehabilitation will most likely be multidisciplinary and a plan might include:

- nutritional correction by improving the quality and content of your diet, such as increasing vegetable and protein content, and restricting sugar and fat intake
- supplementation with appropriate vitamins and trace elements before and after surgery
- supplementation with vitamin D to address deficiency
- ensuring adequate omega-3 fatty acids from fatty fish, nuts, ground flaxseeds or supplements
- an individualised aerobic and resistance training program to increase your strength and fitness
- relaxation and meditation techniques to relieve anxiety
- stopping smoking if you are a smoker
- stopping alcohol
- reviewing all of your medications and supplements
- looking after your oral and dental health.

A trip to the dentist might be the last thing on your mind when you are facing a cancer diagnosis, but it is an essential part of your prehabilitation. Cancer treatment can affect your gums, oral tissues, teeth and jaw, and anything that damages your mouth can affect your ability to eat. This can have a knock-on effect on your ability to maintain adequate nutrition.

You need to ask your medical oncologist and radiotherapy oncologist if the treatment is likely to have any side effects on your mouth and teeth, and ask for a letter explaining the details to your dentist, so that he or she can plan your preventive oral health advice and treatment.

Surgery

There are a number of aims of cancer surgery. A surgeon might remove healthy tissue to prevent future cancer. Examples of this would be bilateral mastectomy (breast tissue removal) and/or removal of ovaries and tubes in women who have the BRCA1 and BRCA2 gene mutations and are at high risk of a future cancer in those organs.

Surgery is also used in diagnosing and staging a tumour that has been discovered. For example, a small amount of tissue might be removed for examination under a microscope and other testing to work out the type of cancer so that treatment can be targeted. Cancer surgery might be potentially curative in cases where the tumour is localised and has not spread to the lymph nodes or other organs.

In cases where the cancer cannot be completely removed with surgery, a 'debulking' procedure might be undertaken. As the name suggests, debulking means reducing the bulk of the tumour with the aim of making chemotherapy or radiotherapy work more effectively because there is less tumour bulk to treat.

There are also situations where a tumour is causing symptoms such as pain or obstruction and removing some or all of a tumour will relieve pressure and help with symptom management.

PREPARING FOR SURGERY

Surgery is physically and emotionally challenging, so it is important to prepare yourself with information on what to expect, and with measures to build your strength and resilience.

Remember also that along with surgery goes anaesthesia. If you have had any adverse reactions to anaesthetics in the past, these need to be discussed with your anaesthetist in advance.

Unless you are having an urgent procedure, you may have time before your surgery to make some changes that will ease your recovery afterwards.

Your plan for prehabilitation before surgery would include:

- find out as much as you can about your cancer and the procedure that is planned for you, including the type of anaesthetic
- see your GP for a full medical check-up including heart and lung function
- ask your GP to test you for anaemia and for vitamin D, iron and vitamin B_{12} levels so that you can identify and correct any deficiencies as nutritional depletion increases the risk of complications after surgery. Also have a blood test for diabetes
- if you have some time to plan and you are overweight, pay attention to your kilojoule intake and the quality of the food you eat with the aim of achieving a healthy weight.

- if you are underweight, see a dietitian for detailed advice on nutritional support
- make sure you have an eating plan that includes adequate dietary iron, vitamin C, protein and omega-3
- stop smoking
- stop drinking alcohol
- seek advice on appropriate activity levels and an exercise program that you can reasonably do before surgery, and a plan for the rehabilitation phase after surgery
- learn some relaxation techniques such as deep breathing, meditation, or imagery
- talk to family and close friends about your planned surgery and accept offers of assistance
- make sure your home and work are in order
- on the day before surgery, shower with antibacterial soap or lotion to reduce the risk of infection.

QUESTIONS TO ASK YOUR ANAESTHETIST

- Will the procedure involve a general or regional/local anaesthetic or both?
- Are there any special risks for this type of anaesthesia?
- Do I have any special risks because of my medical condition(s)?
- Are any of my medications or supplements likely to increase bleeding during surgery or interfere with anaesthetic agents? Make sure you anaesthetist has a list of all of your medications and supplements, prescribed and over-the-counter.
- Do I need to cease any of my medications or supplements before surgery?
- How will I feel afterwards?
- What are my options for post-surgical pain control?

Some options include intravenous or oral narcotics and oral analgesics, or non-steroidal anti-inflammatory drugs (NSAIDs). A patient-controlled analgesia pump lets you give yourself doses of pain medication into a vein as you need it.

- What measures will you take to prevent nausea or treat it after the procedure?
- Will antibiotics be given routinely?

Ask your anaesthetist to give you a written report of all the medications used during the anaesthetic. This is particularly important if you have an adverse reaction to any of the agents, so you know to avoid them in future. If you handle the anaesthetic well, the report will provide a guide for future anaesthetics, should they be necessary.

If any close relatives have had severe reactions to anaesthesia, it is worth mentioning to the anaesthetist.

Common adverse effects of anaesthesia can include nausea or vomiting, sore throat (related to the breathing tubes in your throat), dizziness, blurred vision, headache, bladder problems, damage to lips and tongue, aches and pains, pain and bruising at injection sites, cognitive (thinking) difficulties such as confusion and memory loss.

Nausea can usually be anticipated and there are medications that can be given to prevent it, or to treat it if it happens. If you have had a severe nausea reaction to anaesthetics in the past, let the anaesthetist know so that they can change the anaesthetic you are to be given, or plan how to prevent the nausea.

Fatigue after anaesthesia is also common and usually passes in a few days or weeks. Fatigue is partly due to the physical and emotional trauma of the surgery, but some of the effect is likely to be due to the anaesthetic agents. Pay attention to your diet to ensure you are getting good nutrition, and a coenzyme Q10 supplement can help relieve fatigue.

It is possible to have an **allergic reaction** to anaesthetic agents and other chemicals and medications used in operations. If you have a history of serious allergic reactions to medications, some anaesthetic departments are able to do allergy testing, injecting under the skin tiny doses of the medications likely to be used, then measuring any reaction. This gives the anaesthetist a guide to which drugs are safe and which ones need to be avoided because of the possibility of an allergic reaction.

We know that general anaesthetics for any type of procedure can cause lingering **cognitive difficulties** in a significant number of people, known as 'post-operative cognitive dysfunction'. This is usually temporary. The risk is greater in older patients and increases with the amount of time under anaesthetic. It is estimated to happen to 30–50 per cent of patients who have had major surgery, making it very common. Healthy nutrition and returning to physical activity as soon as possible are essential.

It is important to keep your brain active with reading, connecting with friends and family, and trying to return to your usual routine as soon as you can during your recovery. Ask your doctor to review your medications to see if any of them can affect your cognitive ability – statins for cholesterol lowering are one example. Sometimes more intensive intervention is necessary.

Case study

John was 75, very active socially and worked as a volunteer with several charities. He needed to have a surgical procedure and was under anaesthetic for four hours. The result of the surgery was very successful, but since the operation he had become anxious, depressed and confused. Months later he was still having severe difficulty managing all but the most basic living skills and relying heavily on his children for help. His family was so concerned that they thought that he may not be able to continue to live independently. John had a comprehensive integrative assessment. He was anxious and depressed, agitated and distracted. He was not eating any vegetables. He was not physically active. He had trouble getting to sleep because of anxiety, and he was waking in the early hours of the morning. He lacked motivation and energy. An integrated treatment plan involved:

- *an anti-depressant medication with anti-anxiety effects*
- *melatonin in the evening*
- *coenzyme Q10 supplement*
- *vitamin D supplement to correct deficiency*
- *fish oil supplement for omega-3 essential fatty acids*
- *an extract of Bacopa (Bacopa monnieri) or brahmi, a herbal medicine used to enhance memory, recall and attention span*
- *diet rich in vegetables and fish with other proteins*
- *daily exercise with morning sunlight exposure.*

Over the following months, John's cognitive function improved, his mood stabilised, sleep cycle returned, and his energy levels recovered. He returned to normal activities and continued with his new healthy lifestyle. Over several months he slowly weaned off the anti-depressant medication.

QUESTIONS TO ASK YOUR SURGEON

If surgery is part of your treatment plan it will be important for you to be informed about what is ahead of you so that you are mentally and physically prepared. Here is a suggested list of questions to ask your surgeon:

- What is the exact name of the procedure?
- What is the aim of the procedure?
- Why is this procedure necessary?
- Are there any other treatment options?

- What is your experience with this procedure?
- How long do you expect the operation to take?
- How long will I be in hospital after surgery?
- What are the possible adverse effects of surgery?
- What can I do to minimise the adverse effects?
- Will I need to have a bladder catheter during and after the operation?
- Are there any long-term nutritional implications of this surgery?
- What can I expect during recovery?
- What are the expected costs?

Check with your health insurance plan about any out-of-pocket expenses if you are having surgery as a private patient.

Chemotherapy

Chemotherapy is the use of chemical substances to treat cancer. It is given as an intravenous drip directly into the bloodstream, or orally in tablet form.

The chemotherapy protocol will be aimed at the eradication of cancer, mopping up after other treatments such as surgery, or palliation (reducing cancer symptoms). Protocols are decided on the basis of the results of clinical trials, and a calculation of which chemotherapy agent or combination of agents is statistically likely to be the best option.

Doctors try to predict whether a treatment is likely to work and what side effects it might cause based on studies of large groups of people with similar cancers, but nobody can tell you for certain how a specific cancer will behave when it is exposed to chemotherapy, or how your body will react.

Chemotherapy drugs are designed to be more toxic to cancer cells than to normal cells in the body. This means that there will be some toxic effects on your body and this is the reason for the adverse effects.

Adjunctive therapies for cancer chemotherapy are designed with a number of purposes in mind and it is important to be clear about your intentions. The adjunctive treatments I am going to discuss are not a replacement for chemotherapy. They are intended to relieve symptoms and side effects, improve the tolerability of chemotherapy, improve your quality of life during chemotherapy treatment and hopefully hasten your recovery, extend your remission, and improve your survival following chemotherapy.

Some adjunctive therapies are safe and recommended to undertake throughout chemotherapy. Some treatments are likely to interact with chemotherapy and should be avoided or timed to be clear of chemotherapy.

Treatments such as meditation, relaxation, yoga, acupuncture, and massage are not going to cause any conflict with chemotherapy at all. If your immune system is compromised or if you have problems such as a low platelet count (which would increase the risk of bleeding or bruising), then you may be advised not to have acupuncture or to have a modified oncology massage technique.

Some supplements and herbal medicines will interact with chemotherapy (favourably or unfavourably), so anything you ingest or inject will need to be checked for interactions.

SIDE EFFECTS OF CHEMOTHERAPY
FATIGUE

Fatigue is a very common adverse effect of chemotherapy. It can also be an effect of the cancer itself.

In the case of chemotherapy delivered in cycles – courses with rest periods in between – the fatigue is usually worse in the days following each cycle of treatment and improves towards the next treatment, when the pattern starts over.

There may be other factors contributing to the fatigue you can experience during chemotherapy, and your general health will need to be monitored throughout treatment. Your doctor will consider other potential causes such as nutritional deficiency, anaemia, medication side effects, insomnia, chronic pain, underlying infection, or depression. Once you have dealt with any treatable underlying factors, here are some strategies for managing fatigue:

- pace your activities – include rest periods interspersed with gentle exercise. Try reading or listening to music as energy-conserving activities
- enlist the help of friends and family or hire help if you can for daily chores
- avoid alcohol, caffeine and tobacco.

See page 263 for more information on managing fatigue.

If you are having difficulty sleeping, see the chapter on sleep for more detailed advice (see page 360).

Supplements

L-carnitine is an amino acid essential for energy production in mitochondria. It has been shown to ameliorate fatigue in 90 per cent of patients receiving chemotherapy with cisplatin.

Melatonin is a naturally occurring hormone that helps to regulate your sleep cycle. Low melatonin levels in the body may be linked to a higher risk of breast and colorectal cancer. Some research suggests that melatonin supplementation can help sleep problems and fatigue related to chemotherapy. A 2012 review found that melatonin given concurrently with chemotherapy for solid tumours substantially improved tumour remission and one-year survival, and alleviated side effects of chemotherapy and radiotherapy, including fatigue. No severe adverse events were reported.

Glutathione is a substance produced naturally by the liver. It is also found in fruits, vegetables and meats. Intravenous glutathione infusions can be provided by specialised clinics to help counter some of the side effects of chemotherapy, including fatigue and nerve damage.

There is also evidence for safety and efficacy of some **herbal medicines** in relieving chemotherapy-related fatigue. These include panax ginseng, astragalus (*Astragalus membranaceus*), withania (*Withania somnifera*), bupleurum (*Bupleurum* spp.) and reishi mushroom (*Ganoderma lucidum*). If you want to use herbal medicines and nutritional supplements to manage your fatigue during chemotherapy, make sure you consult a qualified practitioner with experience in working with people with cancer.

NAUSEA AND VOMITING

Nausea and vomiting are common side effects of chemotherapy. There are non-pharmacological and pharmacological options for treatment.

Potent anti-nausea drugs, which are commonly referred to as 'antiemetics', will usually be necessary to manage chemotherapy-associated nausea and vomiting, and these medications will be prescribed in anticipation so that you are prepared.

Antiemetic medications have improved over recent decades and they are usually very effective. Some are available for intravenous infusion, oral tablet, or as a wafer that dissolves on your tongue. Adjunctive therapies can reduce the amount of antiemetic medication you need, or improve your tolerance of chemotherapy. When your chemotherapy is planned, you will be provided with antiemetic medication such as metoclopramide, ondansetron (Zofran) or others for prevention or relief of nausea.

Other treatments for nausea include acupuncture and specific herbs and supplements:
- **ginger** (*Zingiber officinale*),
- **baical skullcap** (*Scutellaria baicalensis*) or **astragalus,**

- **Vitamin B$_6$** is also often used for pregnancy-induced nausea
- **mind–body techniques** may be useful.

See page 259 for more information on combating nausea.

HAIR LOSS

Chemotherapy can cause you to lose some or all of your hair temporarily because the chemotherapy drugs damage hair follicles as well as cancer cells. Although people are prepared with information about chemotherapy and when it is likely to cause hair loss and reassured that it will grow back, there is a lot of variation in how people respond. In general, women tend to find hair loss more difficult than men.

Ask your oncologist specifically about the possibility of hair loss if you are having chemotherapy. Some people are not too bothered and they buy hats, scarves or wigs to cover their head. But for others it is a source of great distress. And while it isn't in the same league as coping with cancer, I have had some patients tell me that losing their hair was the most upsetting part of the whole treatment process for them.

One woman told me that she was more worried about losing her eyebrows and eyelashes than the hair on her head. If your eyes do not get irritated from wearing them, you can use false eyelashes. You can also buy false eyebrows. You can also lose the hair on your legs, arms and pubic area, but with current fashion trends, that does not tend to cause any concern at all.

There is not a lot we can do to prevent hair loss with some forms of chemotherapy. Some cancer units offer a 'cold cap', which is a strap-on cap cooled in a freezer and worn at each chemotherapy infusion. The cold temperature is thought to reduce hair follicle damage by reducing the amount of exposure of the follicles to chemotherapy drugs. Some people find the cold temperature very uncomfortable.

If your oncologist tells you to expect total hair loss, plan how you will manage this. Think about whether you want people beyond your immediate family to know about your cancer. You may choose to tell your family, friends and work colleagues you are going to have chemotherapy and that you will be losing your hair.

Depending on how 'out' you want to be about your cancer treatment, think about whether you prefer to keep your head uncovered or to conceal the hair loss. I find most people will arrange to have their head shaved once the process of total hair loss begins in order to avoid having clumps of hair falling out in the shower, over their clothes or on their pillow. Once the hair loss starts, it only takes a few days, so you will need to be prepared. It is best to arrange to have a hairdresser shave your head with electric clippers to avoid nicking your own scalp with a razor. This can be an emotionally traumatic moment so make sure you prepare for it by talking to someone you trust, and consider taking along a support person.

Once your head is shaved, that is the end of the hair loss process. Remember to protect your scalp from sunburn with sunscreen and/or a hat whenever you are outdoors.

If your preference is to conceal your hair loss some of the time or all of the time, ask your oncology team for a referral to a specialist wig supplier. You may decide to have your current hairstyle and colour duplicated so that there is no apparent change, or you could opt for a whole new look, or a range of different looks. Even if you don't think you will wear a wig, make enquiries and have a colour and style match done in case you change your mind. Some cancer services have a wig library for people who want to borrow a wig rather than purchasing one. Some people find wigs uncomfortable and instead choose to wear scarves or hats.

When hair grows back, it may be curlier or straighter, thicker or finer, and may be a different colour.

You may be told to expect hair thinning rather than total loss. This again will depend on the type of chemotherapy you are prescribed. Hair thinning is a possible consequence of some of the hormonal treatments for breast cancer, such as tamoxifen, Arimidex, Aromasin and Femara, which are currently prescribed to be taken for over five years. The hair thinning tends to improve after the first year of taking the medication but can persist for the length of time you are on the medication.

If the particular type of chemotherapy is likely to cause hair thinning but not total loss, you can help preserve some of your hair by using a gentle shampoo and conditioner, air dry after washing, or have your hairdryer on a cool setting. Brush or comb your hair gently. Do not apply chemical hair dyes and avoid having your hair straightened.

A lot of people ask me what supplements they can take to encourage healthy hair regrowth. First and foremost it is important to optimise your nutrition through the right mix of foods.

You can encourage healthy hair regrowth by eating a healthy, balanced plant-based diet (see the chapter on nutrition, page 323) with adequate protein. Some examples of foods that encourage healthy hair regrowth include fish for protein and omega-3 healthy fats. You can also try ground flaxseed or flaxseed oil. Other sources of protein include organic eggs and poultry, nuts such as walnuts that contain healthy fats, vitamin E and biotin, and lentils as they contain protein, iron, zinc, and biotin. Also make sure you have a daily source of vitamin C from citrus fruit, blueberries or other fruits.

If you think about taking nutritional supplements to encourage healthy hair growth, seek skilled professional advice because you will need to coordinate all your nutritional needs, including doses and combinations of supplements relevant to your stage of cancer treatment and recovery.

Herbal treatments for hair regrowth are mostly untested for effectiveness and for interactions with other medications so would be best avoided.

See also the chapter on intimacy, sexuality and cancer recovery (page 106).

MUCOSITIS (INFLAMMATION OF MUCOUS MEMBRANES)

Mucositis occurs when cancer chemotherapy breaks down the rapidly dividing cells lining the length of the gastro-intestinal tract from the mouth to the anus, leaving the mucosal tissue vulnerable to ulceration and infection.

Signs of mucositis include: red, swollen gums, sores in the mouth and throat, bleeding from the mouth, difficulty swallowing or talking, burning sensation when eating.

Glutamine is an amino acid that furnishes fuel for the cells of the digestive system. It is usually given as a powder mixed with water, then 'swished and swallowed'. Glutamine increases regeneration of intestinal mucosa which can be damaged by chemotherapy, thereby reducing intestinal damage and decreasing diarrhoea. Protecting and repairing the gut increases intestinal absorption of essential nutrients.

A Mayo Clinic study showed that glutamine reduced the duration and severity of mouth pain related to chemotherapy mucositis. A randomised human study showed glutamine was also able to decrease chemo-induced hepatic veno-occlusive disease and cardiac complications.

REDUCED IMMUNE FUNCTION

Cancer is a sign of a malfunction in your immune system. The cancer itself also challenges your immune system as your body tries to fight to eliminate it.

Chemotherapy damages your immune system by reducing the number of white blood cells produced by your bone marrow. While this is a temporary effect, it can make you vulnerable to infection while your immune system is weakened. If your white cell count is low you will need to take special precautions to avoid infection.

Avoid infectious people

Avoid people who are sick with coughs and colds or a potentially communicable disease. Warn the people around you that they must not approach you closely if they have any sign of a respiratory infection, vomiting or diarrhoea, a fever or any other possible signs of infection. It is best to avoid crowds of people in places like shopping centres, public transport or cinemas while you are going through chemotherapy. Avoid shaking hands and social cheek-kisses while your immunity is compromised.

Immunise yourself and your household members

If it is autumn or winter, arrange to have a flu vaccination. This is an inactivated vaccine and is safe to have if your immunity is compromised, but you will need to avoid live attenuated vaccines. Check with your doctor if any planned vaccines fall into this category. People in your household and friends and family who plan to see you should also make sure their immunisations and boosters are all up to date as much as possible to protect you.

Meticulous food preparation and storage

Food preparation needs to be meticulous. Avoid any foods where there is a likelihood of harmful bacteria being present. To be sure, eat freshly cooked foods and not leftovers, takeaways, pre-wrapped sandwiches from a sandwich bar, soft cheeses, pâté, shellfish or raw or soft eggs. Sort through your pantry and refrigerator regularly and dispose of any foods that are past their use-by date.

Personal hygiene

Have a daily shower or bath and use a fresh towel each day. Wash your hands after going to the toilet, before you prepare or eat food, and after handling pets. If you have pets, wear disposable gloves if you handle their waste.

Report signs of infection urgently

If you feel unwell or develop a fever, you need to report to your doctor as soon as possible. Out of office hours, your cancer care team may have a contact number for you to call, or you should go to your nearest accident and emergency department.

Rehabilitating your immune system

To give your immune system the best chance of recovery, you need to focus intensively on your lifestyle. Optimising your diet; getting enough quality sleep; detoxing from alcohol, tobacco and environmental chemicals; and minimising sources of stress are basic fundamentals.

A healthy gut is essential to a healthy immune system. Chemotherapy may cause damage to the lining of your gut – for example, severe diarrhoea caused by some chemotherapy drugs can break down the gut lining.

Stress management through mind–body interventions can also help to support your immune system during chemotherapy.

Supplements to help boost immunity

A high degree of finesse, care and experience is needed when you are dealing with any products that are 'ingestible or injectable' while you are having chemotherapy. Substances that are biologically active and interactive with your body chemistry will have the potential to interact with chemotherapy agents.

I point this out because it is the reason why some oncologists will tell you not to take anything that is not a prescribed pharmaceutical when you are having chemotherapy. Unfortunately this would mean that you would miss out on some highly effective and safe adjunctive treatments with evidence of reducing side effects and improving tolerability of chemotherapy and supporting your immune system, so making it more likely that you will be able to complete the recommended course.

That being said, adjunctive treatments need to be planned and prescribed carefully by a health professional with expertise and experience in working with patients who are undergoing cancer treatment and recovery.

There is more information on boosting your immunity in the chapter on immunity (see page 355).

Astragalus (huang-qi) is used to enhance the effectiveness of chemotherapy and reduce associated side effects. This herb is also used to enhance immune function. It has a wide safety margin. A Cochrane review of Chinese herbs for chemotherapy side effects in colorectal cancer patients showed that astragalus can reduce nausea, vomiting and leucopenia (low white cell count). Increases in the proportion of T-lymphocyte subsets (CD3, CD4 and CD8) were also reported.

There is a potential role for **withania** as an adjunctive treatment during chemotherapy for the prevention of drug-induced bone marrow suppression.

Selenium has been shown to reduce kidney toxicity, bone

marrow suppression and weight loss associated with cisplatin chemotherapy and it is important to treat selenium deficiency.

A healthy gut is essential to a healthy immune system. Different **probiotics** have different actions and so different probiotics will need to be used depending on what you are trying to achieve.

NERVE TOXICITY/CHEMOTHERAPHY-INDUCED PERIPHERAL NEUROPATHY (CIPN)

Some chemotherapy agents can cause damage to the nerves in your fingers and toes. The chemotherapy classes that are most involved are the taxanes, platinum analogues and vinca alkaloids. Cisplatin, carboplatin and oxaliplatin are particularly notorious for this side effect and it can also occur with the chemotherapy agents vincristine and paclitaxel.

You will receive an information sheet before you start chemotherapy, and this will contain the names of the chemotherapy agents that you are to be given. If you are not sure, ask your oncologist to write down the name and class of chemotherapy agents in your protocol.

Neuropathy, or nerve damage, is estimated to occur in 10–20 per cent of cases treated with these types of chemotherapy.

Symptoms of CIPN include pain (persistent or episodes of shooting pain, like electric shocks), burning sensation, tingling ('pins and needles' feeling), loss or reduction of sensation in fingers and toes, trouble using your fingers to pick up or hold things, dropping things, balance problems, tripping or stumbling while walking, muscle weakness, trouble swallowing, constipation, trouble passing urine, and blood pressure changes.

CIPN is usually diagnosed clinically and then confirmed with nerve conduction studies and other neurological investigations so other causes of nerve damage are ruled out. It is very important to address this particular side effect in advance and try to do whatever you can to prevent it, because once it develops it can be persistent, severe and resistant to treatment. In some cases it can be permanent.

Once this side effect develops it often leads to a reduction in the dose of chemotherapy, or a delay or abandonment of that particular treatment. Many potential treatments for neuropathy have been tried without much success. In particular, pharmaceutical approaches such as antidepressants or analgesic medication are uniformly unhelpful and have side effects of their own.

Treatments for CIPN
Glutathione
Glutathione is a naturally occurring antioxidant within cells. It has many biological functions within cells, playing an important role in detoxifying and eliminating potential toxins. Glutathione levels decrease with age. It also decreases if you smoke or drink alcohol. Low glutathione levels have been reported in a range of neurological conditions such as Parkinson's disease. Glutathione levels are also decreased if you are deficient in vitamin B_{12}, folate and/or vitamin B_6 and if your vitamin C levels are low.

Food sources of glutathione include meat, garlic, fruits and vegetables. Levels in food are reduced by preservatives and processing. Oral glutathione is not well absorbed, so intravenous therapy is usually recommended to achieve the levels you need to counter the effects of chemotherapy.

One double-blind trial studied the nerve-protecting effect of intravenous glutathione during cisplatin treatment for stomach cancer. In this study the glutathione was given intravenously over 15 minutes, just prior to giving cisplatin chemotherapy, then intramuscularly in the following second through to fifth days. After nine weeks, none of the patients out of the 24 receiving glutathione developed neuropathy, but 16 of the 18 patients who received the placebo had developed neuropathy symptoms.

The effectiveness of the chemotherapy was not impaired by the administration of glutathione in this study.

This study was followed by a second randomised, placebo-controlled trial with 52 patients receiving oxaliplatin. Again, the group receiving glutathione developed less neurotoxicity. Both studies reported no difference in tumour response outcomes, but the protective effect of glutathione was significant.

Vitamin E

Vitamin E has potential as a preventive treatment against chemotherapy-induced peripheral neuropathy. Vitamin E has been studied and found to help protect nerves during cisplatin treatment. It was also found to help prevent nerve damage in patients having paclitaxel chemotherapy. The incidence of neuropathy differed significantly between groups, occurring in three out of 16 (18.7 per cent) patients assigned to the vitamin E supplementation group and in 10 out of 16 (62.5 per cent) people who did not receive the vitamin E.

Calcium and magnesium

A study in 2008 looked at patients with colon cancer who were treated with oxaliplatin. Intravenous CaMg (1 g calcium gluconate plus 1 g magnesium sulfate pre- and post-oxaliplatin) was investigated and found to reduce sensory neuropathy. The study was terminated because another trial had suggested that CaMg reduced the effectiveness of cancer treatment. The researchers felt this potential treatment deserved to be looked at further, provided that the issue of whether the cancer-specific treatment was affected or not was clarified. At this stage it is not routinely recommended.

Vitamins B_1, B_6, B_{12}

In the nutrition chapter (see page 323) I look at the importance of quality nutrition. Vitamins B_1 (thiamine), B_6 (pyridoxine) and B_{12} (cobalamin) are particularly important for nerve health. Deficiencies in these B vitamins can increase the risk of peripheral neuropathy (nerve damage) developing with chemotherapy. Deficiencies in these vitamins are also related to low glutathione levels. It is important to correct any deficiencies with food sources as much as possible, but there are many reasons why this might be difficult and supplementation is warranted with professional advice.

Alpha-lipoic acid
Alpha-lipoic acid has been used for many years in Europe as a treatment for peripheral neuropathy. A series of 15 patients with CIPN from oxaliplatin and then another series of 14 patients with CIPN from docetaxel/cisplatin improved with alpha-lipoic acid. The researchers said that alpha-lipoic acid may reduce oxidative stress and have a beneficial effect on blood vessels.

Herbal treatments
In addition to the supplements outlined above, a number of herbal treatments have been studied over the years. A recent review of these studies was published listing 26 relevant studies on five single herbs, one extract, one receptor-agonist, and eight combinations of herbs were identified focusing on the single herbs *Acorus calamus rhizoma*, *Cannabis sativa fructus*, *Chamomilla matricaria*, *Ginkgo biloba*, *Salvia officinalis*, sweet bee venom, *Fritillaria cirrhosae bulbus*, and the Traditional Chinese Medicine herbal combinations Bu Yang Huan Wu, modified Bu Yang Huan Wu plus Liuwei Di Huang, modified Chai Hu Long Gu Mu Li Wan, Geranii herba plus Aconiti lateralis praeparata radix, Niu Che Sen Qi Wan (Goshajinkigan), Gui Zhi Jia Shu Fu Tang (Keishikajutsubuto), Huang Qi Wu Wu Tang (Ogikeishigomotsuto), and Shao Yao Gan Cao Tang (Shakuyakukanzoto).

The reviewers concluded that the knowledge of how the herbs work is still limited, the quality of clinical trials needs further improvement, and studies have not yielded enough evidence to establish a standard practice, but a lot of promising substances have been identified. They added that while CIPN has a number of possible mechanisms, a combination of herbs or other substances might target these mechanisms with the aim of protecting or regenerating nerves damaged by CIPN.

At this stage there is still no standard protocol, but if you are being advised to have chemotherapy likely to cause CIPN, or if you have experienced this side effect, it is certainly worth seeing an experienced professional to discuss an appropriate adjunctive program for you.

Acupuncture

When I was in China in 2012 I had the opportunity to visit a number of clinics and I spoke to Traditional Chinese Medicine doctors who were using acupuncture to prevent and treat peripheral neuropathy. They considered it to be moderately effective in treating nerve damage caused by diabetes. It was also being used in the management of chemotherapy-induced peripheral neuropathy.

According to the Mayo Clinic, acupuncture may reduce symptoms in about three-quarters of people with peripheral neuropathy. A Canadian pilot study showed promising results but it was only a small study.

Acupuncture has yet to undergo large randomised controlled trials but it is worth trying to see if it helps you.

Physical and occupational therapies

Once nerve damage has occurred, physical and occupational therapies can help you retain your gait and balance and assist with your fine motor coordination. It is important for you to maintain your muscle strength so that you avoid falls.

Avoid alcohol

General advice includes avoiding alcohol, which can make peripheral neuropathy worse over time.

INFERTILITY

If you have not had children or you have not completed your family and if chemotherapy is likely to impact on your future fertility, ask your medical team about ways of keeping your options open. An example would be a women having her eggs frozen or sperm being collected for storage for later use.

KIDNEY (RENAL) TOXICITY

Some chemotherapy agents and other treatments such as some antibiotics have the potential to cause kidney damage, which can lead to renal failure. This is most likely to occur in older people, especially those with pre-existing kidney disease, and people taking multiple medications. The anti-cancer drugs most likely to cause kidney damage include cisplatin; carboplatin; nitrosureas, such as carmustine; mitomycin; and methotrexate, especially if high doses are used.

Your kidney function will be assessed before treatment and monitored throughout. If blood tests show that your renal function is being impacted, the dose or the type of chemotherapy will need to be changed.

Signs of renal damage include abnormal blood tests (electrolytes, creatinine, eGFR), passing less urine, swollen hands and feet/ankles, headache, fatigue and weakness, nausea and/or vomiting, increased blood pressure.

To protect your kidneys the medical team may increase intravenous fluids to help flush the drugs through your kidneys.

A medication called amifostine may be given to protect the kidneys when high doses of the chemotherapy agent cisplatin are given.

You will need to maintain oral intake of fluids as well, and avoid eating salty foods including processed foods with added salt. Do not add salt to your cooking or to your prepared food.

Milk thistle (*Silybum marianum* or silymarin)

Milk thistle, which is used to prevent and treat liver toxicity, has been shown to reduce kidney toxicity caused by the chemotherapy agent cisplatin.

Acetyl-L-carnitine

Acetyl-L-carnitine is a naturally occurring compound that combats oxidative stress and inflammation. There are many studies reporting the protective effect of acetyl-L-carnitine against the toxicity of radiotherapy and chemotherapy agents including doxorubicin and cisplatin. One large trial found that patients who received acetyl-L-carnitine (3,000 mg per day) during their taxane-based chemotherapy for breast cancer developed neuropathy more frequently and had more severe neuropathy. So acetyl-L-carnitine should be avoided with taxane chemotherapy.

CARDIOTOXICITY (HEART DAMAGE)

Cardiotoxicity is, literally, the harmful or toxic effect of chemotherapy drugs and molecular targeted therapies on the heart. The effect may be acute, or delayed for months or years.

Drugs most commonly associated with this side effect include the anthracyclines such as doxorubicin (Adriamycin). Alkylating agents such as cyclophosphamide, ifosfamide, cisplatin, carmustine, busulfan, chlormethine and mitomycin have also been associated with cardiotoxicity. Other agents that may induce a cardiac event include paclitaxel, etoposide, teniposide,

the vinca alkaloids, fluorouracil, cytarabine, amsacrine, cladri-
bine, asparaginase, tretinoin and pentostatin. You can see it is
a long list.

You will need to read the information on chemo side effects
that you are provided with by your medical team. It is important
for you to specifically ask your doctor if any of the drugs in your
chemotherapy program has cardiotoxicity as a side effect, and
how to recognise the symptoms.

Symptoms of cardiotoxicity relate to the reduced ability of the
heart muscle to pump effectively. Acute reactions include chest
discomfort and shortness of breath consistent with inflammation
of the heart muscle and surrounding pericardium.

Toxicity can also develop months after the last chemotherapy
dose and typically appears as new onset heart failure with
dysfunction of the left ventricle. Late reactions can sometimes be
seen years after chemotherapy has been completed as new-onset
cardiomyopathy, often in patients who were treated for childhood cancers.

Damage to the heart from chemotherapy can be temporary
or permanent and can range from mild to severe. The situation
becomes even more complicated if you have pre-existing heart
disease.

The dose of the anti-cancer drug administered during each session,
cumulative dose, schedule of delivery, route of administration,
combination of drugs given, and sequence of drug administration
are important factors to be considered to avoid cardiotoxicity.

Your oncologist is likely to arrange heart function tests before
treatment so that you can be monitored for any cardiac problems
during the course of treatment. You may not notice symptoms
at first, so the monitoring during treatment and beyond is very
important. Your chemotherapy treatment will be modified if signs
of cardiotoxicity are noticed.

There may be no symptoms of cardiotoxicity, but it may be identified by changes noticed on an electrocardiograph or cardiac echo. When they do occur, symptoms can include chest pain, shortness of breath or cough, palpitations (awareness of irregular heart rhythm), rapid heart rate or unusually slowed heart rate, trouble lying flat in bed (you may have to sleep on two or more pillows), shortness of breath that may cause you to wake up in the middle of the night, tiredness and reduced exercise tolerance, and puffy or swollen ankles.

Prevention and treatment

Established chemotherapy-induced cardiotoxicity is difficult to treat, so a proactive and preventative approach in the planning stage of cancer treatment is very important.

L-carnitine is an amino acid essential for energy production in mitochondria. This is particularly important in heart muscle cells. Long-term L-carnitine administration 2 g once or twice a day may reduce the cardiotoxic side effects of doxorubicin (Adriamycin). In combination with **alpha-lipoic acid**, L-carnitine can help regenerate the mitochondria, the energy-producing parts inside body cells that are damaged by chemotherapy.

Coenzyme Q10 provides some protection against cardiotoxicity caused by some forms of chemotherapy. Coenzyme Q10 protects the energy-producing mitochondria in heart muscle cells. Studies suggest that coenzyme Q10 given concurrently with chemotherapy treatment does not interfere with the anti-cancer action of anthracyclines (chemotherapy agents such as doxorubicin) and might even enhance their effects, but it is important to get individual professional advice on this.

A range of other dietary components and supplements such as ginkgo biloba, curcumin, resveratrol, vitamin E and grape seed have been investigated and found in experimental models to have some protective effects against cardiotoxicity.

One of the difficulties in providing advice on this is that there is no agreed protocol for protecting the heart from the effects of chemotherapy.

Your heart, like every other major organ in the body, works best if you eat **a healthy diet** low in saturated fats and with plenty of variety of fruit and vegetables. Try to keep your body weight in the healthy range.

Don't smoke. I know this seems like glaringly obvious advice, but one of the most toxic things you can do to your heart is to smoke tobacco. If you are still smoking, quit now.

Avoid alcohol. Alcohol can contribute to heart muscle weakness.

You will need to have your **blood pressure** checked to make sure it is kept in the healthy range – under 135/85 for most people – to minimise strain on your heart.

The condition of your heart will need to be thoroughly assessed and any treatment prescribed by a specialist cardiologist.

HEPATOTOXICITY (LIVER DAMAGE)

Your liver will need to work hard during cancer treatment as it is one of the main organs involved in metabolising the drugs used in chemotherapy as well as medications and supplements used for symptom control, such as paracetamol. In addition, many chemotherapy agents are toxic to liver cells. If there are more toxins passing through the liver than it can cope with, they will accumulate in the liver and this may result in liver damage (hepatotoxicity).

If the liver is damaged, it is unable to perform its usual functions effectively. These functions include the production of bile to aid digestion of fats, excretion of waste products, the processing and storing of vitamins and minerals, fats, glucose and proteins, and the production of clotting factors necessary for blood clotting.

Your medical team will check your liver function prior to treatment as part of the planning and assessment process.

Symptoms of liver damage include abnormal liver function tests, jaundice, fatigue, nausea and vomiting, abdominal pain, and bleeding that does not stop within the usual timeframe of a few minutes.

Protecting your liver

There is no specific medical treatment for liver damage so prevention is essential. The first thing you can do to help your liver cope is to do a **detox** (see page 373 on how to safely detox).

The most important thing you can do to help your liver is to **avoid alcohol** (see the chapter on alcohol, page 295).

Avoid drugs that cause liver damage. Some medications are known to place more strain on the liver than others. These include paracetamol and statins (cholesterol-lowering drugs). If you are taking one of these medications regularly, speak to your doctor about whether it is necessary for you to continue to take them or whether there are other options for you that are less likely to cause liver damage.

In the chapter on **high-dose intravenous vitamin C and other nutrients** (see page 173), I have provided evidence and references for their use throughout chemotherapy.

It is important that you seek detailed advice about the suitability of your situation for intravenous vitamin C.

You will also find information about some treatments in the chapter on herbs and supplements (see page 188) and part five 'Symptoms and side effects of cancer treatment' (see page 245).

'CHEMO BRAIN'

'Chemo brain' is a term used to describe the effect of chemotherapy on your brain's ability to function normally. People with chemo brain describe a sense of mental fogginess, trouble with memory, being forgetful, taking longer than usual to finish things, having trouble multitasking or doing complex tasks, being disorganised and having trouble remembering names and dates. These changes might only last during the course of treatment and for a short time after, or the effect may be prolonged. This side effect seems to be a feature of some, but not all types of chemotherapy.

As you can imagine, chemo brain can have a major effect on your life, not just with day-to-day activities, but also with work performance. It is not always easy to detect more subtle changes in your brain function with standard medical investigations, but you will notice the change.

There can be a direct toxic effect of chemotherapy on brain function, but it is important not to just assume that any problem with thinking or other brain functioning is a result of chemotherapy just because that seems to be the obvious reason.

Many other factors can have an effect on your brain functioning too, and they need to be checked. These include other drugs or medications such as opioid painkillers or hormone treatments, anaemia, nutritional deficiencies such as iron deficiency, infection anywhere (including urinary tract infection), tiredness related to insomnia, cancer-related fatigue and depression.

So far, medical science has not found a way to prevent chemo brain, but there are some ways to manage it:

- see your doctor to work out if there is a treatable underlying cause of your mental fogginess
- get yourself organised with a detailed diary of the things you need to do
- try to focus on one task at a time
- let your close family and friends know what difficulties you are having and let them know what they can do to make things easier for you

- a diet with plenty of antioxidant-rich fruits, omega-3 fats (as found in seafood) and vegetables is important for general health, but particularly important in cancer recovery
- yoga and meditation can help.

Herbs and supplements for chemo brain

Given that medical treatments are very thin on the ground for this distressing side effect, it is worth looking at some low-risk complementary therapies to see if they help you. Most of the information in this next section relates to evidence from age-related cases of cognitive impairment and I am conscious that I am applying this to the chemo brain situation despite the lack of specific research in this area to date. Of course, if you are planning to take herbs for this purpose, particularly in combinations and/or with drugs, then I recommend you see a practitioner who is qualified to prescribe and monitor herbal medicines.

Ginkgo biloba is a popular herb used for improving circulation and enhancing memory and thinking. Ginkgo biloba supplements are considered to be generally safe but they may interact with blood-thinning medications, so if you are taking one of these medications, or if your platelet count is low, let your GP know so that a decision can be made about whether it is safe for you. If you are on warfarin (Coumadin), your blood can be monitored.

There are some preliminary studies showing positive inter-actions with cisplatin and doxorubicin in reducing kidney toxicity, ear toxicity, and cardiotoxicity respectively. But given the lack of information at this stage on interactions between ginkgo and chemotherapy agents, it would be wise to wait until your course of chemotherapy is complete.

Brahmi (*Bacopa monniera*) is a traditional Indian medicinal plant that has multiple effects on the central nervous system. The standardised extract of this plant has been shown to enhance behavioural learning and information processing in healthy volunteers. It has also been shown to be effective in improving age-related memory impairment. While there are studies to show that brahmi improves memory it has not been formally trialled in cases of chemo brain.

Given the lack of information at this stage on interactions between brahmi and chemotherapy agents, it would be wise to wait until your course of chemotherapy is complete.

Fish oil rich in omega-3 fats is used as a cognitive booster, particularly fish oil high in DHA. It also has general anti-cancer benefits.

Other nutrients that may help with chemo brain include acetyl-L-carnitine, coenzyme Q10, phosphatidyl serine and phosphatidylcholine.

Radiotherapy

Radiotherapy is a term that describes a number of types of treatment that use radiation to kill or contain cancer cells. It may be recommended as the only treatment for a cancer, or as part of a combination therapy alongside surgery and/or chemotherapy and/or immunotherapy.

Some people have few or no adverse reactions to radiotherapy, while other people are significantly affected. Whether or not you get side effects will depend on the type and extent of radiation, the part of your body affected and the extent of damage to normal tissues around the cancer.

Recommendations will be made by your cancer specialist team about whether radiotherapy needs to be a part of your treatment protocol, and if so, what doses and numbers of treatments. It is important that you are fully informed about all aspects of your treatment so that you can work out a plan for minimising the possible side effects.

The radiation oncologist will develop your treatment plan based on your scans (CT, MRI, PET and ultrasound) and the results of biopsies or surgical pathology, and the plan will be discussed by your specialist cancer team as part of an overall strategy.

The radiation can be delivered by:

- a machine outside your body
- inserted into the body close to cancer cells (a treatment called brachytherapy), or
- injected into the bloodstream (an example of this is radioactive iodine used to treat thyroid cancer).

There may be only a single treatment, such as the insertion of brachytherapy (radioactive implants) into cancer tissue. Other radiotherapy plans involve many visits over weeks or months. In this case, the radiation oncologist will usually make small permanent tattoo marks in your skin to ensure accuracy for each treatment.

PREPARATION

It is useful to prepare yourself for your first consultation with the radiation oncologist so that you can plan the practical aspects of your treatment. Here are some of the questions you need to ask:

- What is the purpose of the radiotherapy treatment? (Elimination of cancer, adjunctive treatment/management of symptoms.)
- What is the type of radiotherapy?
- What is the schedule of visits?
- How long will each visit last?
- What adverse effects can you expect during treatment?
- What can you do to prevent or treat any potential side effects?
- What follow-up investigations will be done to assess how effective the treatment has been?

- Who do you contact if you have problems related to the radiotherapy?
- If you are taking any medications or supplements, or using any topical creams are they suitable to continue using during radiotherapy?
- If fertility is important to you because you have not had children or completed your family, is this treatment (usually to the pelvic area in a woman or the testes/groin/prostate area in a man) likely to affect future fertility?
- If treatment is likely to affect fertility, what can you do to keep your options open?
- Do the people around you need to take any precautions?
- What are the possible long-term effects?

Diarise your visits and plan to have some rest days after each treatment.

A lot of patients I see are surprised by how tired they feel during radiotherapy treatment so I would also advise you to look at your work and social schedule over the coming months and plan to modify your daily activities to allow for lower energy levels for a while.

FERTILITY

If you have not had children or you have not completed your family and if radiotherapy is likely to impact on your fertility, ask about ways of keeping your options open. An example would be men having sperm frozen and stored prior to radiation treatment for prostate or testicular cancer. For women, the process could be more difficult particularly if time is of the essence, because retrieving eggs involves intensive hormone treatments and fertility procedures sometimes over many months.

DENTAL AND ORAL HEALTH

If you are having radiotherapy around your head, neck or jaw, arrange a visit to a specialist dentist and oral hygienist at least two weeks before treatment starts to try to anticipate and prevent future oral or dental problems.

If you are having radiotherapy to the mouth or jaw area or the abdomen, arrange to see a dietitian in advance so that you can make a plan for maintaining your nutritional status during treatment.

SIDE EFFECTS OF RADIOTHERAPY

In this section I will cover some of the more common side effects of radiotherapy and provide you with some direction about how to prevent or manage them. Whether you have side effects and how significant they are for you will depend on your type of cancer, its position and the dose of radiation. There are effective strategies and adjunctive therapies you can use to help to prevent or diminish adverse effects.

FATIGUE

One of the unexpected side effects of radiotherapy is fatigue that is not immediate, but rather can tend to sneak up on you.

Case study

Angela had just turned 50 when she visited her GP for a check-up. She had no family history of breast cancer and her regular self-examination had not turned up any lumps. Her GP suggested a mammogram. The referral sat in her bag for several months until it fluttered out one day and she thought 'I really should get that done'. She went along for the mammogram, expecting to get the all-clear. She was shocked to be called back for further testing, including a needle biopsy. Even then she thought it had to be all right. When her GP told her that the result showed a breast cancer and she would need to see a surgeon urgently, she was terrified. She had surgery to remove the lump. She was back to work in a week. At her follow-up visit to the surgeon, he referred her to a radiation oncologist for radiotherapy. She thought that she would be able to just continue with her busy life juggling her career and her two teenage children. At first that was true. 'It was the fatigue that crept up on me,' she said. 'For the first week or two I was fine. Then gradually over the weeks, as the treatment went on, I became more and more exhausted. One day I sat in the car outside work and thought, I just cannot go in. I drove home and called work, and they were great about it. They told me to take time off until the treatment was over, and then to come back part time when I felt like I could. I went back to work after a couple of months but I didn't feel like my energy was back to normal for about a year.'

If you experience fatigue while you are having radiotherapy, do not assume the radiotherapy is responsible. It may be, but there might be some other reason that turns out to be the cause, or at least is contributing to the severity of your fatigue.

It is best to explore these possibilities with your GP, who will consider nutritional deficiency, anaemia, medication side effects, insomnia, underlying infection, or depression.

Once you have ruled out correctible causes of fatigue, there are strategies you can put in place that can help, see page 263 for information on combating fatigue.

Intravenous vitamin C can help improve fatigue related to radiotherapy (see page 173).

Supplements which may be helpful for post-radiation fatigue include acetyl-L-carnitine, coenzyme Q10, and panax ginseng. Omega-3 fatty acids from fish oil or flax oil supplements may be used to reduce inflammation caused by radiation.

LYMPHOEDEMA

Lymphoedema occurs when radiotherapy disrupts the lymphatic drainage, usually in one of your limbs. The affected area becomes swollen, heavy, uncomfortable, and less mobile. It can happen early in the course of treatment, or as a delayed consequence of scarring due to radiotherapy

If you develop lymphoedema you will need to see a specialised lymphoedema therapist. The aim of treatment is to control swelling, prevent infection and maintain function as much as possible. Treatment is ideally undertaken by a qualified lymphoedema therapist, but they are in short supply and you might find yourself on the end of a very long waiting list. I have patients who in frustration have resorted to YouTube to learn how to do lymphoedema massage and wrapping. If you can arrange even a few sessions with a therapist to teach you the correct techniques, you may be able to ask a friend or relative to do some of the treatment for you.

A treatment program might need to involve limb exercises, skin care, specialised lymphatic massage, and wearing pressure garments. There are some other treatments you can try, including **low level laser therapy** of the whole limb, at two to five sessions a week for two to three weeks.

Horse chestnut standardised extract is a supplement that contains escin, a plant compound that strengthens the tissues of the lymph vessels, capillaries and veins. It may be useful in supporting treatment for lymphoedema.

Bromelain is routinely used in naturopathic oncology to prevent post-radiation fibrosis and to reduce risk of lymphoedema.

I am often asked whether a diuretic or 'fluid tablet' would help reduce the swelling. Lymphoedema is not the same as the fluid retention you might see from hormonal causes or heart failure or kidney disease. Diuretic medications are not useful for this type of localised oedema swelling caused by mechanical blockage of lymphatic drainage and may have unwanted side effects.

If you have lymphoedema or you are at risk of developing lymphoedema because of surgery or radiotherapy in your armpit or groin, then your will need to be vigilant to avoid injury or infection to the affected limb. Most health professionals are aware, but you may need to remind them to avoid procedures such as blood pressure measurement or taking blood on that arm. If your leg is affected, make sure you wear shoes, even around the house, to avoid trauma to your feet.

RADIATION DERMATITIS

Radiation dermatitis (burns or skin inflammation) is a common side effect of radiotherapy. It may manifest as ulceration, flaking, red or brown discolouration, itching, or blistering of skin in the radiotherapy zone. The dermatitis does heal and fade with time but there are some effective treatments to reduce the severity of the burn and accelerate healing.

There are some practical matters to consider. Wear loose-fitting clothing that is made of soft material and is not scratchy. Avoid using harsh or artificially perfumed products on your skin and replace them with gentle organic ones. When you have a shower or bath, make sure the water is warm but not too hot.

Curcumin (*Curcuma longa*) is an extract from the herb turmeric. It has been shown to reduce dermatitis in patients undergoing radiotherapy for breast cancer. A clinical trial involving 30 women with breast cancer showed that daily oral supplementation with turmeric reduced the severity of radiation dermatitis and other side effects of treatment. Women were randomised to take placebo capsules or four 500 mg capsules of curcumin three times a day. Those taking curcumin had significantly less radiation dermatitis than those in the placebo group. Of those taking curcumin, only 28.6 per cent had moist skin loss at the end of radiation treatment, compared to 87.5 per cent taking the placebo.

Calendula ointment applied twice daily was found to be superior to trolamine (a topical pharmaceutical non-steroidal anti-inflammatory agent) for the prevention of skin toxicity, interruption of treatment, patient satisfaction, pain relief and dermatitis.

Topical aloe vera has also been shown to reduce the intensity of radiation dermatitis.

MOUTH PROBLEMS

Having radiotherapy treatment around your head and neck can affect your mouth. Some of the issues you may encounter can include mouth dryness, ulceration (mucositis), difficulty chewing and swallowing, and dental decay. If radiotherapy is planned in this region, you will need to see a specialist dentist prior to treatment to try to anticipate and prevent future oral or dental problems.

Avoid using over-the-counter mouthwashes during your treatment because the chemicals in the mouthwash can irritate the mucous membranes and worsen ulceration.

Avoid eating spicy foods or foods with a hard texture that could damage the delicate lining of your mouth. You might need to eat softened, puréed or cooked foods for a while. Also avoid food and drink that is too hot or too cold.

If mouth problems are causing difficulty eating some foods, I would recommend you see a dietitian for advice on adjustments to your diet so that you can maintain a good nutritional balance.

If you are having problems with swallowing or speech, then a speech therapist can be enlisted to help you to adjust.

If dry mouth (xerostomia) is a problem, your doctor can recommend an artificial saliva product. Acupuncture has been shown to help relieve the symptoms caused by radiation-induced xerostomia.

NAUSEA AND LOSS OF APPETITE

You can experience nausea and loss of appetite if you are having radiotherapy to your abdominal region. If your cancer specialist anticipates that you might experience nausea, you will be given medication to relieve it.

Small frequent meals will be better than trying to manage larger meals. A dietitian will be able to help you to plan your meals so that you avoid nutritional deficiency.

EMOTIONAL DIFFICULTIES

It is no mystery why going through radiotherapy might be emotionally challenging. Meditation, mindfulness, gentle exercise and relaxation therapy can help you cope. See part two 'Dealing emotionally with cancer' page 63 for a detailed discussion about coping emotionally, including where to get professional help.

HAIR LOSS

It is common to think of hair loss as an inevitable side effect of cancer treatment, but it is not. Radiotherapy only affects the local area that is being treated. If you are having radiotherapy to the scalp region then you may have some hair loss in the region where the radiotherapy is directed, and this may be permanent. See pages 133 for more information.

DO PEOPLE AROUND YOU NEED TO TAKE PRECAUTIONS?

This is a question that often comes up, so it is important for you to know what to advise your family members and other people who are likely to be around you during your radiotherapy treatment.

If you are having external beam radiotherapy, you are *not* radioactive and you do not need to take any special precautions for the people around you.

If you are given a radiopharmaceutical treatment such as radio-active iodine for thyroid cancer, whether orally or intravenously, you *will* need to follow some precautions for the safety of others. You will need to ask your oncologist for advice specific to your situation.

There will be some excretion of radioactivity during your treatment, mainly through your urine, but also through saliva, sweat, and your bowel motions. For the weeks following treat-ment, you will be advised to take some quarantining precautions:

- sleep in a separate bed
- avoid prolonged close contact with infants, children, pregnant women and your pets. Keep a distance of one arm's length between yourself and any others who spend more than two hours near you in any 24-hour period
- wash your hands often with plenty of soap and water, especially after using the toilet
- flush the toilet two or three times after each time you use it
- keep aside your own eating utensils so they are not shared with others, and have them washed separately after each use
- drink plenty of fluids to help flush the radioactive substance from your body
- avoid kissing or any sexual contact for at least two weeks after the treatment.

If you have a permanent internal radioactive implant such as brachytherapy or seed implants for prostate cancer, these use weaker radiation than, say radioactive iodine used to treat thyroid cancer, and patients are usually advised to go home after the implant procedure. The amount of radiation released by the seeds and the duration of treatment depend on the type of seeds used. With these implants you may need to avoid close contact with other people just for the first few days while the radiation is most active.

Ask for specific and detailed advice from your radiation oncologist.

For the first two months after brachytherapy for prostate cancer, advice may include:

- avoiding sexual intercourse for the first two weeks
- after the first two weeks, using a condom during sexual intercourse
- not to have daily close contact with pregnant women or children for more than a few minutes for a few weeks or months.
- not allowing children to sit on your lap for extended periods of time for the first two months.

The amount of radiation emitted will decrease with time and eventually it will be negligible.

HERBS USED WITH RADIOTHERAPY

In Western countries, Chinese herbal treatments are used mainly for the purpose of treating the patient's overall constitution, in order to promote general health and alleviate any discomfort. Western medical practitioners should consult a practitioner trained in herbal medicine to ensure the safety and efficacy of herb–drug combinations and the correct timing of treatment.

Herbs used with radiotherapy include:

- Milk thistle (*Silybum marianum*) – as an antioxidant and liver protectant.

- Green tea (*Camellia sinensis*) – for antioxidant effects.
- Panax ginseng – for symptoms of radiation exposure including fatigue.
- Reishi mushroom (*Ganoderma lucidum*) – for immune effects.
- Holy basil (*Ocimum sanctum*) – for radiation protection.
- Calendula (*Calendula officinalis*) – topical cream, apply externally to radiation-damaged skin, 2–3 times daily.
- High-dose intravenous vitamin C to help reduce the side effects related to radiotherapy (see page 173).

If you are thinking about incorporating herbal medicines into your treatment plan, make sure you seek advice from a qualified health professional who is experienced in working with people having cancer treatment. Doses, combinations and correct timing are extremely important and need to be carefully prescribed.

Immunotherapy

———————————————————————————————————

Cancer immunotherapy is a new class of cancer treatment. It is the new paradigm and is sometimes called biologic therapy. This is a very promising and rapidly evolving area of research and cancer treatment. The aim of the therapy is to harness and support your body's innate immune system to fight cancer.

The treatment involves the use of medications to stimulate your immune system generally with the aim of slowing or stopping cancer growth. Other immune therapies are designed to attack and destroy cancer cells specifically. There are many ways the immune system can be harnessed to fight cancer.

MONOCLONAL ANTIBODIES

Monoclonal antibodies are injected medications that target specific proteins on the surface of cancer cells. An example is trastuzumab (Herceptin) in some types of breast cancer. The antibodies trigger your immune system to attack cancer cells and cause the cancer cell to destroy itself. In other applications, a chemotherapy drug is delivered directly to the cancer cell.

CANCER VACCINES

I want to specifically mention the rapid development of cancer vaccines because it is likely that we will see some dramatic advances in cancer treatment. There are two classes of cancer vaccines: prevention and treatment.

A cancer **prevention vaccine** is given to a person who does not have cancer, in order to prevent the development of a specific type of cancer. The human papillomavirus (HPV) vaccine is one example. It is given to prevent infection with several types of HPV, a virus known to cause cervical cancer and some head and neck cancers.

A cancer **treatment vaccine** helps the body's immune system to recognise and destroy cancer cells. The vaccine may prevent a treated cancer from coming back, it may eliminate any remaining cancer cells after other types of treatment are completed, or stop cancer cell growth. A treatment vaccine is designed to target the cancer cells without affecting healthy cells. The vaccines are developed by taking samples of the cancer and reinjecting them in a modified suspension to stimulate the body's immune system to seek out and destroy the cancer cells. A number of cancer treatment vaccines are in development internationally and currently most are only available through clinical trials.

TARGETED IMMUNE THERAPIES

This new group of therapies unblocks the protective shield that cancers develop to hide from our immune system. The most promising of this group are the checkpoint agents such as ipiliminib, which has shown promising results in some melanoma patients.

QUESTIONS TO ASK

If you are considering immunotherapy for your cancer treatment, there are some questions you will need to ask your medical oncologist:

- Could immunotherapy be part of my cancer treatment plan?
- What is the chance of success in using this treatment for this cancer?
- Will immunotherapy be my only treatment or will it be a part of my treatment plan?
- What type of immunotherapy is proposed? Why?
- What are the aims of this treatment?
- How will I receive immunotherapy treatment and how often?
- What are the possible short-term side effects of immunotherapy?
- What are the possible long-term side effects of immunotherapy?
- How will this treatment affect my daily life?
- Will I be able to work, exercise, and perform my usual activities?
- Are there any clinical trials of immunotherapy available to me?

· PART FOUR ·

Adjunctive therapies

Intravenous Vitamin C and Other Nutrients

I almost didn't include this chapter because it is such a divisive issue among the different practitioners involved in cancer treatment, and because the information is likely to change very rapidly in the next few years as further evidence emerges. But given the widespread popularity of intravenous vitamin C and the growing evidence base for its use as an adjunctive cancer therapy, you need to know about it now, at this stage of your recovery so that you can make decisions about whether you want to include it in your recovery plan.

I became very interested in this area some years ago when several doctors with years of experience in this type of therapy joined my integrative medicine clinic and I saw the level of interest and the numbers of 'word of mouth' referrals from patient to patient. I explored the evidence for efficacy and safety and examined the protocols from clinics in other countries and, mindful of appropriate safeguards, I was eventually sufficiently convinced of its merits to be comfortable in recommending it to patients.

We decided to engage in a research program to formally

monitor the outcomes for our patients and to help fine-tune our protocols. We currently have ethics approval for our first project.

WHY INTRAVENOUS VITAMIN C?

Intravenous nutrient therapy has a number of aims, the most common being:

- to improve wellness
- to boost immunity
- to relieve fatigue related to inflammatory conditions
- to relieve musculoskeletal conditions such as inflammatory arthritis and fibromyalgia
- to treat acute and chronic viral illness
- to assist recovery from surgery or illness
- as an adjunctive therapy for cancer.

When it is used as an adjunctive treatment for cancer, intravenous nutrient therapy is not an alternative to conventional medical cancer treatment. There is some evidence that intravenous vitamin C has some anti-cancer activity of its own, but it is not a 'cure' for cancer. The therapy is thought to work best in the early stages of cancer, in conjunction with chemotherapy and/or radiotherapy.

The aim of intravenous nutrient therapy is to support your body to help you to tolerate chemotherapy and radiotherapy by reducing adverse effects, with the goal of helping you to complete your medically recommended cancer treatment. In some cases there is evidence that it makes chemotherapy and radiotherapy more effective. It is also used to support the body's organs in cases of severe sepsis (overwhelming infection), where the immune system is not able to function. And it is helpful in the recovery phase, to assist your body to recuperate from cancer-specific treatment alongside other adjunctive therapies and lifestyle measures.

You may be considering intravenous nutrient therapy as a 'last resort' if standard cancer treatments have not worked and you have not been given other options for conventional treatment.

THE CONTROVERSY

The use of high dose intravenous vitamin C (IVC) has been the subject of controversy over the years, and remains a subject of some strong disagreement within the medical cancer community. Much of the resistance by oncologists to patients using IVC is the fear of the 'unknown'. By this I mean two things: that which is unknown to some oncologists, and that which is unknown generally because of gaps in knowledge. It is important to make this distinction, and to consider both issues.

High dose vitamin C therapy in cancer patients has been studied since the 1970s, when some original studies by Ewan Cameron and Nobel Prize winner Linus Pauling suggested high doses of intravenous and oral vitamin C substantially prolonged life and improved wellbeing in some patients with advanced cancer. Then in the early 1980s the Mayo Clinic conducted some research and found no anti-cancer effect from high dose vitamin C. This set up the controversy and the use of IVC fell out of favour.

Did this mean that the original research was wrong? Not at all.

In the Mayo Clinic research the researchers used only oral ascorbic acid, not intravenous vitamin C, and the plasma levels of vitamin C were not measured. Most of the dose of vitamin C given orally in the Mayo Clinic study would have been excreted by the gut before it had a chance to reach the bloodstream and therefore the cancer cells. Patients' blood levels of ascorbate in the Cameron–Pauling trial and those in the Mayo Clinic trial would not have been comparable.

Unfortunately, you may not have the luxury of time to wait a decade or so until there is 'enough evidence' in the minds of skeptics to satisfy a change in the more conservative thinking and practice on this.

Many oncologists are concerned about interactions of intravenous vitamin C with chemotherapy agents so in some clinics protocols are arranged to avoid giving it for a few days on either side of 'chemo days'. Other clinics such as the University of Kansas have protocols which give intravenous vitamin C, magnesium and glutathione infusions throughout chemotherapy.

I always recommend honest communication with your GP and oncologist about any adjunctive treatments you decide to use. But you may come up against some resistance or even hostility towards IVC if your oncologist either does not agree with IVC or has not closely examined the evidence supporting the safe use of IVC and other nutrients. You will need to find a doctor working in a clinic that is set up to provide this treatment in a high standard medical environment, ideally as part of a broader healthcare or wellness program.

THE EVIDENCE

There are currently many trials which have looked at the safety and efficacy of high dose IVC. In this section I will refer to just a few, but I would recommend you read more widely around this subject and if you make contact with a clinic that provides high dose IVC, you will be able to ask for more detailed information and studies relating to your specific case.

PLAUSIBILITY

Laboratory research has established an explanation as to why high dose IVC might be an effective adjunctive cancer therapy in certain cancers. We now understand that while vitamin C at low doses is an antioxidant, at high doses it acts as a pro-oxidant, generating hydrogen peroxide (H_2O_2) in cells. The H_2O_2 preferentially kills cancer cells while leaving normal cells unharmed.

CLINICAL EXPERIENCE

Those clinics with extensive experience in providing IVC have amassed many anecdotal reports of effectiveness of high dose IVC in assisting cancer treatment and alleviating adverse effects of cancer treatment. This has led to renewed interest in clinical trials.

LABORATORY STUDIES

On a background of persistent interest in the potential for IVC as an adjunctive and anti-cancer agent, evidence of plausibility and clinical successes, there has been renewed interest in laboratory studies to further knowledge.

Examples of laboratory studies showing that combining vitamin C with chemotherapy improved the effectiveness of chemotherapy include the following:

- ascorbic acid with arsenic trioxide may be more effective in ovarian cancer cells than chemotherapy alone
- ascorbic acid with gemcitabine may be more effective in pancreatic cancer cells than chemotherapy alone
- ascorbic acid with gemcitabine and epigallocatechin-3-gallate (EGCG) may be more effective in malignant mesothelioma cells than chemotherapy alone.

A variety of animal studies have shown promising results.

Researchers at the University of Kansas conducted an animal study of IVC given with chemotherapy for ovarian cancer. They found that the combination of intravenous ascorbate (IVC) with the conventional chemotherapeutic agents carboplatin and paclitaxel synergistically inhibited ovarian cancer and reduced chemotherapy-associated toxicity in patients with ovarian cancer. They concluded: 'On the basis of its potential benefit and minimal toxicity, examination of intravenous ascorbate in combination with standard chemotherapy is justified in larger clinical trials.'

CLINICAL TRIALS

Some clinical studies have been conducted in recent years. I have provided you with a comprehensive list of references so that you can take some time to look at some of the clinical trials for yourself. Here are some examples:

A 2011 study in Germany found that complementary treatment of breast cancer patients with IVC was a well tolerated, improved response to standard cancer specific treatments, and also reduced treatment side effects. IVC administration resulted in a significant reduction of symptoms of the disease and side effects of chemotherapy and radiotherapy, in particular of nausea, loss of appetite, fatigue, depression, sleep disorders, dizziness and bleeding. The researchers found that the overall intensity of symptoms during adjuvant therapy and aftercare was nearly twice as high in the control group compared to the IVC group. Significantly, no side-effects of the IVC administration were documented.

In a 2014 study of 27 patients with advanced ovarian cancer, treatment with chemotherapy alone was compared to chemotherapy along with IVC. Patients who received IVC along with chemotherapy had fewer serious side effects from the chemotherapy.

A series of case reports has indicated that high-dose IVC was associated with long-term tumour regression and unexpectedly long survival in three patients with advanced renal cell carcinoma, bladder carcinoma, or B-cell lymphoma.

A study at the Riordan Clinic in the US showed that IVC reduced cancer-associated inflammation in cancer patients.

High dose IVC has also recently been found to be a safe and promising treatment for inflammation and multi-organ failure in patients with severe sepsis.

In our clinical experience at our Sydney clinic, Sydney Integrative Medicine, the treatment is well tolerated with few side effects, provided that the treatment is appropriately planned and precautions are observed.

As with any decisions about treatment, there is a need to counter these promising and positive outcomes with caution.

According to the National Cancer Institute in the US: 'Vitamin C has been shown to be safe when given to healthy volunteers and cancer patients at doses up to 1.5g/kg, while screening out patients with certain risk factors who should avoid Vitamin C. Studies have also shown that Vitamin C levels in the blood are higher when taken by IV than when taken by mouth, and last for more than 4 hours.'

VITAMIN C

Vitamin C, also called ascorbic acid or ascorbate, is a nutrient that occurs naturally in foods. Humans are not able to make this vitamin in our bodies so we rely on dietary sources such as citrus and other fruits.

People with cancer tend to have depleted levels of vitamin C, however, when you are given megadoses of vitamin C intravenously, the aim is not to correct a deficiency but to use the vitamin C for its therapeutic action, which is only seen at these high doses. Given intravenously, vitamin levels in the blood are much higher than if it is given orally – in fact, 25 to 100 times higher than with maximal oral doses.

PLANNING

In the absence of an international or even a national protocol for the use of intravenous nutrients including high dose vitamin C, different clinics providing this form of treatment have adopted their own protocols to provide individualised doses and combinations depending on the particular circumstances for each person.

I have attempted to draw together some guidelines based on published evidence of the benefits and risks at different stages of cancer treatment, and conversations with colleagues experienced in this form of supportive therapy.

As with any medical intervention, the doctor arranging your high dose IVC will need to know everything about your particular cancer including its type and staging, your treatment plan, results of scans, tumour markers and other blood tests, and any other relevant medical history. You will be asked to have a blood test for biochemistry, full blood count and G6PD deficiency. You will also have a urine test to check that your kidney function is adequate.

G6PD is an enzyme that helps red blood cells function. The blood test is to see if you have an uncommon inherited condition called Glucose-6-phosphate dehydrogenase (G6PD) deficiency, in which the body doesn't have enough of the G6PD enzyme. This condition is more common in African American males and people with a Mediterranean ethnic background including Italians, Greeks, Arabs, and Sephardic Jews. If you have G6PD deficiency, you will not be able to have high dose IVC infusions because it could cause hemolytic anaemia (the destruction of red blood cells).

DELIVERY

The bags of fluid are first warmed to body temperature and the vitamin C is added to the intravenous fluid. Other nutrients such as magnesium may also be added to avoid blood vessel spasm. High dose IVC infusions have to be given slowly to avoid adverse events such as irritation of the vein, nausea, shakes and chills. You will be advised to eat before the IVC infusion to help reduce blood sugar fluctuations.

TIMING

Your chemotherapy and radiotherapy program will be diarised with your medical oncologist and radiation oncologist, and planning for infusions will need to be worked carefully around these dates. Some clinics will give IVC throughout chemo/radiotherapy while others will avoid giving infusions for several days either side of when chemo/radiotherapy are given.

There is some disagreement among experts as to whether it is appropriate to give vitamin C on the same day as, or on days close to, giving chemotherapy and radiotherapy. One of the concerns surrounding the use of antioxidants such as vitamin C is that they have the potential to interfere with the actions of chemotherapy and radiation therapy that rely on the production of reactive oxygen species for their cytotoxic activities.

One clinical study, however, showed that ascorbic acid does not reduce the therapeutic effects of the chemo drugs paclitaxel and carboplatin. Another study found an increase in chemo-associated adverse effects with inadequate intake of vitamin C in children with acute lymphoblastic leukaemia.

The University of Kansas advises giving IVC on the same days as chemotherapy/radiotherapy to augment the effectiveness of those treatments. Their view is this: 'Research has shown that using the vitamin C concurrently with chemotherapy or radiation will not decrease the effectiveness of these treatments. In addition, intravenous vitamin C is not an antioxidant; it is a pro-oxidant and, therefore, seems to augment the effectiveness of chemotherapy or radiation.'

A German study (ii) showed that high dose IVC reduced quality-of-life related side effects of radiotherapy and chemotherapy in women being treated for stages IIa to IIIb breast cancer.

The type of chemotherapy may be important. IVC is not given

in conjunction with methotrexate chemotherapy because of urine pH (acidity) requirements for methotrexate.

The Riordan Clinic in the USA has published their detailed protocol, which is available on the internet. Their view is that: 'A variety of laboratory studies suggest that, at high concentrations, ascorbate does not interfere with chemotherapy or irradiation and may enhance efficacy in some situations.'

Because of the concerns of some oncologists, at this stage our clinic does not give vitamin C infusions on the days of chemotherapy/radiotherapy treatment but several days before and after. We will monitor emerging evidence and adjust our protocols accordingly.

HOW OFTEN AND HOW MANY?

One of the frequently asked questions is: 'How many treatments should I have and how long should I keep up the infusions?' The answer to this question is partly determined by the clinical judgement of the doctor prescribing what is assessed as optimal for you as an individual, and partly comes down to convenience and affordability. The protocols also differ somewhat from one clinic to another.

The protocol at the University of Kansas Infusion Clinic involves two to three infusions per week while there is active disease, including weeks when chemotherapy is administered. For maintenance their protocol is IVC infused once per week. Patients are encouraged to take oral supplemental nutrients on a daily basis and adhere to a whole foods diet free of processed carbohydrates and sugar. After the patient is disease-free, treatment is suggested to continue for one year. Thereafter, slow tapering is recommended with occasional administration of maintenance doses one or two times per month along with close monitoring.

At our clinic we also advise patients to stop having infusions if there is no demonstrable benefit, or when they choose to cease for any reason.

PRECAUTIONS/WHAT TO AVOID

If you are considering IVC as part of your recovery plan, it is not for everyone and there are some precautions, some of which relate to other medical conditions you may have which can impact on the safety of the procedure for you.

- The first precaution is not to believe anyone who tells you that intravenous nutrients can 'cure' your cancer.
- Do not use intravenous nutrients as an alternative to the cancer-specific treatments recommended by your medical oncologist.
- Some medical conditions will exclude some people from IVC (but not other intravenous nutrients). Before you have IVC you will have a standard blood test for Glucose-6-phosphate dehydrogenase (G6PD) deficiency.
- If you have hemochromatosis: this is an inherited condition where the body absorbs and stores more iron than it needs. Vitamin C assists the absorption of iron so high dose vitamin C may not be recommended, although this may not be an absolute contraindication.
- If you have a history of kidney disease, you will need to let your doctor know and you may be advised against high dose IVC because kidney failure has been reported after ascorbic acid treatment in people with existing kidney disease.
- If you have a condition likely to be worsened by fluid overload, such as congestive heart failure, then you may not tolerate an infusion of fluid.
- High dose vitamin C may contribute to the formation of oxalate-type kidney stones because of the metabolic

conversion of vitamin C to oxalic acid. If you have a tendency to develop kidney stones you should discuss this with your doctor as there could be an increased risk of stone formation. It may not be a deal-breaker as you could have your urinary oxalate monitored.

- IVC is not given in conjunction with methotrexate chemotherapy because of urine pH requirements.
- At this stage it is not possible to predict with confidence who will and will not gain clinical benefit from high dose IVC.

POTENTIAL SIDE EFFECTS

Side effects are possible, but they tend to be minor, provided precautions are followed.

Side effects of high dose IVC can include lethargy/fatigue, local vein irritation, muscle cramp (can be prevented by adding magnesium), headache, nausea, transient flu-like syndrome, light-headedness.

OTHER INTRAVENOUS NUTRIENTS

Magnesium

Magnesium is often added to the IVC infusion to reduce the incidence of vein irritation and spasm. It is also used for muscle pain, anxiety, and migraine headaches, as well as to correct mineral imbalances. IV infusions of magnesium need to be given as a slow drip.

Glutathione

Glutathione is a compound comprised of the three amino acids cysteine, glutamic acid, and glycine, which are present in most human tissue. Oral glutathione supplements are not well absorbed, so intravenous therapy is usually recommended to achieve the levels you need to counter the effects of chemotherapy such as fatigue and peripheral neuropathy.

Glutathione is a naturally occurring antioxidant that has many biological functions within cells, playing an important role in detoxifying and eliminating potential toxins by binding to toxins so that they are safely eliminated.

Food sources include meat, garlic, fruits, and vegetables, but glutathione levels in food are reduced by preservatives and processing.

Glutathione levels decrease with age. It also decreases if you smoke or drink alcohol, are deficient in vitamin B_{12}, folate and/or vitamin B_6, and if your vitamin C levels are low.

Glutathione is used as an adjunctive therapy to protect against the adverse effects of some types of chemotherapy. No serious adverse effects have been reported in studies to date. Some people have reported skin rashes.

One particular application of glutathione is in the prevention of peripheral neuropathy from some forms of chemotherapy, such as cisplatin. Peripheral neuropathy is a particularly distressing side effect, causing persistent pain or numbness or tingling in hands and feet, tripping over or dropping things, loss of balance perception and other neurological difficulties.

One double-blind trial studied the nerve protecting effect of intravenous glutathione during cisplatin chemotherapy treatment for stomach cancer. In this study the glutathione was given intravenously over 15 minutes, just prior to giving cisplatin chemotherapy, then intramuscularly in the following days two to five. After nine weeks, none of the patients out of the 24 receiving glutathione developed neuropathy, but 16 of the 18 patients receiving placebo had developed neuropathy symptoms. Effectiveness of the chemotherapy was not impaired by the administration of glutathione in this study.

This study was followed by a second randomised, placebo-controlled trial with 52 patients receiving oxaliplatin for treatment of advanced colorectal cancer. Again, the glutathione group developed less neurotoxicity. In both studies, they reported no difference in tumour response outcomes, but patient numbers were small, however the effect was significant.

Intravenous glutathione may be, and usually is, combined with vitamin C.

B vitamins

B vitamins may reduce the formation of hydrogen peroxide in cancer cells, so it is avoided during chemotherapy/radiotherapy and can be given in the recovery phase once the treatments have concluded.

Iron

Iron deficiency is a common consequence of chronic disease, blood loss from surgery or other causes of bleeding, dietary deficiency, or poor absorption in conditions such as coeliac disease or inflammatory gut disorders. Iron transports oxygen to your body tissues via haemoglobin. It is also involved in many critical enzyme systems such as hormone production and liver detoxification. Without adequate levels, you become pale, tired, irritable, breathless, and lacking in energy.

Iron deficiency is the most common cause of anaemia but you can have symptomatic iron deficiency without the low haemoglobin of anaemia. Low iron stores are demonstrated by a low ferritin level result in your blood test.

If your iron stores are very low, or if you need to increase your iron levels quickly, or you have difficulty absorbing iron from your diet or in oral supplement form, you can have injected iron. Oral iron supplements can cause constipation in many people, which is an added problem you don't need. Do not have intramuscular iron injections, because the pigment in the iron can leave you with a permanent tattoo that looks like a bruise.

Intravenous iron infusions need to be done in clinics that are set up to provide high quality medical supervision. Most hospitals have iron infusion clinics.

A new safer form of iron for intravenous infusion is now available in Australia on the PBS: Ferric carboxymaltose or Ferinject. It should be given mixed with sodium choride in a slow drip infusion. Your doctor will need to monitor your iron levels to check your response.

Herbs and Supplements

———

Taking herbs and supplements is very common among cancer patients and long-term survivors. Herbal medicines form the basis of most traditional medical systems around the world including Traditional Chinese Medicine, Ayurveda, Unani and European. This use of plants as medicines stems from a time predating the modern pharmaceutical industry. Indeed, many of the common pharmaceuticals still in use today arose from herbs within those healing systems. Examples are aspirin (meadowsweet), atropine (*Atropa belladonna*), caffeine (*Camellia sinensis*), digoxin (*Digitalis purpurea*), and the chemotherapy drugs paclitaxel (Pacific yew) and vincristine (Madagascar periwinkle). Many herbal medicines have been scientifically tested for efficacy and safety, while others have not been tested, or have been shown to be ineffective.

If you are considering taking a herbal medicine while you are going through cancer treatment, I would strongly recommend professional advice rather than trying to figure it out yourself and taking the wrong type of preparation or the wrong dose, combination or timing. Consult a medical professional, preferably with training in integrative medicine, before you commence taking any herbal medicines or supplements. A review of 32 studies published between 1999 and 2006 looked at vitamin and mineral supplement use among US adult cancer patients and survivors. In studies combining different cancer sites, 64–81 per cent of survivors reported using vitamin or mineral supplements and 26–77 per cent reported using multivitamins. In contrast, approximately 50 per cent of adults in the US population use dietary supplements and 33 per cent use multivitamin/mineral supplements. Between 14 per cent and 32 per cent of survivors initiated supplement use after their diagnosis, and use differed by the site of their cancer. Breast cancer survivors reported the highest use, whereas prostate cancer survivors reported the least. Interestingly, up to 68 per cent of physicians are unaware of supplement use among their cancer patients.

In other sections of this book I will also specifically refer to herbs and supplements in relations to symtoms and side effects so be sure to check the cross references and index for all the information.

GET PROFESSIONAL ADVICE

There is a growing awareness of interactions between herb and drug, or herb and supplement, or supplement and drug. By far the majority of people who take herbs and supplements as part of their cancer treatment plan do so in conjunction with their medically prescribed cancer-specific treatments, not instead of their prescribed treatments. Their aim in taking the herbs or supplements is usually to relieve the side effects of cancer treatment, to support their immune system or to improve their general wellbeing. In other words, they are used as 'adjunctive' or supportive therapies, not as 'alternatives' to conventional cancer treatment.

Reasons for using herbal medicines include:

- prevention or relief of some of the symptoms of the cancer itself
- alleviating some of the side effects from cancer treatments
- treating an associated condition, such as anxiety or depression
- providing a sense of control or a feeling of active involvement in your cancer treatment.

Some herbs and supplements claim or have been shown to have 'anti-cancer effects'. At this stage in the development of research, these results are usually based on evidence from laboratory or animal research rather than large-scale trials on people with cancer. It is important not to take a leap of logic from reports of some in-vitro anti-cancer activity to a belief that one or other natural therapy will 'cure' your cancer.

Sometimes herbs and supplements are prescribed by health professionals who know what they are doing and are aware of the benefits and risks, and the importance of timing of doses in relation to cancer-specific treatments. Unfortunately, however, some healthcare practitioners lack the necessary training or expertise to coordinate and integrate your complementary therapies safely and effectively.

Ideally you will be able to tell your cancer specialists what other treatments you are using to help you manage the side effects of treatment or assist in your recovery, and hopefully they will support your decision. But this is not always the case. I have seen many examples of patients who have been told by their specialists to 'stop taking everything except your chemotherapy and prescribed drugs' without consideration for the potential benefits of those supplements, including the possibility that you may be better able to tolerate chemotherapy so you are more likely to be able to continue treatment through the full course. It's all about finding the right balance.

CHOOSING HERBAL MEDICINES

The particular type and formulation of herbal medicine selected by the practitioner is vitally important because the quality and effectiveness of herbal medicines can vary significantly. Think about fruit and vegetables you buy at the local markets or super-market: all products of nature, but the flavour and quality varies markedly with the seasons and growing conditions, including the location of farms, the quality of the soil, rainfall, environmental temperatures, storage and other factors. Herbs are also products of nature, so they will vary too depending on these same factors.

You also need to consider the specific species of herb, the part of the plant used, and the harvesting and processing methods. Herbal products might be sourced from leaves, stems, fruit, flowers, seeds, roots, rhizomes (an underground stem) or bark.

Preparations can be in the form of raw herbs, tinctures, liquid extracts, syrups, tablets, capsules or creams. Some herbal medicines come pre-packaged and labelled, while some are sold as raw herbs to be made into tea.

Liquid preparations prescribed and mixed individually should only be prepared by a qualified herbal medicine practitioner.

Good suppliers and manufacturers try to standardise their products as much as possible with chemical analysis and quality control at all stages of production, but some poorer quality products may contain few or none of the active ingredients you think you are buying, and there could also be inconsistency from batch to batch.

You might be struck by the variation in cost of some of the herbal preparations compared with others that seem to be equivalent. That is not to say that because one brand or preparation is vastly more expensive than another that it must essentially be superior, but it is a reason to ask some questions about the source and the quality of the product. Don't assume that a different brand or preparation of herbal medicine will give you equivalent results to a similar one you have tried before.

I have seen patients who started out getting good clinical results with their first course or two of a herbal medicine, only to find the effect 'wore off'. On closer questioning, it wasn't that the effect had worn off but that they had bought a different brand at a discount supplier or over the internet expecting it to be the same because the name of the generic herb on the label was the same. All of those other factors I mentioned, such as the soil the plant was grown in, the processing method, the amount of active ingredients, and the presence of contaminants can affect your result.

There are some important questions you need to ask to be sure you are fully informed about any decisions you make about taking any substances alongside your cancer-specific treatments:

- Who is giving me advice about herbs and supplements and what are their qualifications and experience?
- What is this substance or mixture of substances being recommended?
- What am I trying to achieve by taking this?
- Is the supplement clearly labelled with ingredients and dosages?
- Is the herb/supplement a standardised product from a reputable manufacturer or supplier?
- What is the evidence for effectiveness in my particular type of cancer?
- What is the evidence of safety?
- Are there any potential adverse effects?

- Interactions can be helpful or dangerous. Does this substance have the potential to interact with any of my prescribed medicines?
- Do I have any other medical conditions (such as diabetes or liver or kidney disease) that might be positively or negatively affected by taking this substance?

ADVERSE EFFECTS

Generally speaking, herbal medicines that are processed and used properly are considered very safe, but side effects and interactions can and do happen.

This is particularly important to consider because herbal medicine preparations are widely available in pharmacies, health food stores, in supermarkets and over the internet without professional advice, and it is common to see people self-medicating. You might get it right, but there are pitfalls. The stakes are higher if you have a serious medical condition such as cancer, and especially at times when you might be undergoing cancer-specific treatments, in particular, chemotherapy drugs.

Adverse effects are, literally, any unpleasant, harmful or undesirable effects of a healthcare treatment. There are degrees of severity for adverse effects. An example of a relatively minor adverse effect might be mild nausea that is tolerable and subsides over time or which goes away when you stop the treatment. Generally speaking, a more serious adverse effect might be one that forces you to stop the treatment or seek medical advice, but is reversible when you stop the treatment. The most serious type of adverse effect is one that causes death, permanent damage, birth defects, or requires hospitalisation. Serious adverse effects are rare with herbal medicines.

It is important to read information about adverse effects of a treatment before you take anything new. There are two reasons for this. Firstly, it will help you make an informed decision about whether to start a treatment. Secondly, that information will also make sure that you are alert to the possibility that a treatment could be the cause of a new symptom. This is particularly important for more serious or irreversible adverse effects.

PRECAUTIONS

Be careful about the type of advice you get, and who gives it to you. Be very aware of any practitioner who tries to tell you that a particular herb or supplement will 'cure' your cancer, or that you can abandon your medical advice in favour of some alternative advice.

INTERACTIONS

There are several different outcomes of herb–drug interactions relevant to cancer treatment and recovery:

- a beneficial, protective or additive effect in combination with chemotherapy agents, radiotherapy or immunotherapy
- reduction in potential for drug side effects
- reduction of toxicity of chemotherapy drugs
- increase in potential for drug side effects
- reduction of drug effectiveness
- potentially dangerous increase in drug activity.

Most of the concern about herb–drug interactions in chemotherapy appear to be theoretical or insignificant. Conversely, the evidence for effectiveness of herbal medicines in the management of cancer is currently weak. But it is important to make informed decisions based on the possibility of interactions.

Herbal medicines that are reported to have the potential for significant interaction with drugs include garlic (*Allium sativum*), ginger (*Zingiber officinale*), ginkgo (*Ginkgo biloba*), ginseng (*Panax ginseng*), and St John's wort (*Hypericum perforatum*).

On the other hand, the herb astragalus has no known harmful interactions and is considered safe.

Some drugs, such as warfarin or digoxin, are more likely than others to be affected by herb–drug interactions.

Issues such as combinations, timing of dosage in relation to chemotherapy, taking other medications and dosage ranges are important.

SELF-PRESCRIBING

With easy accessibility to bottles of herbs and supplements in pharmacies, supermarkets, health food stores and via the internet, one of the groups I worry about are the uninformed or under-informed self-prescribers. If you hear from a friend or read in a magazine about a wonderful natural product they suggest you should take because it worked wonders for someone else, always ask a practitioner for advice before you decide to take it. There is a perception that 'natural' products are inherently safe, but it is incorrect. If you self-prescribe without sufficient knowledge or advice, you are taking an unacceptable risk with your health.

Case study

Rick is a 63-year-old man who developed polycythemia, a condition where too many red blood cells are produced in bone marrow. His pharmaceutical treatment was a medication called hydroxyurea, but that wasn't working as it should. His dose was increased, but the red blood cell count did not shift. He came to see me to try to work out what to do. We talked in detail about everything he was doing, and we discovered that he was taking slippery elm to help his bowels. Slippery elm bark powder can, at least theoretically, reduce absorption of some drugs. He hadn't thought it was significant enough to report to his haematologist. We decided he would stop taking it to see what happened. His red cells dropped rapidly and as we monitored his blood count and with advice from his haematologist, his dose of medication had to be halved.

CONTRAINDICATIONS

A contraindication is a specific situation in which a drug, supplement or procedure should not be used because it may be harmful. There are levels of contraindication. A **relative contraindication** is a precaution where the risk needs to be weighed against any potential benefit before a decision is made to proceed. This might be the case when a herb is known to have beneficial effects but might have an impact on the dose of chemotherapy given. An **absolute contraindication** is where the potential risk of a treatment is so great that the particular medicine or procedure should be 'absolutely' avoided. An example would be the prescribing of the herb St John's wort in a patient who is already taking an SSRI antidepressant.

TIMING

Timing is crucial. Some medications or supplements are best taken on an empty stomach, some with food. Some combinations can be taken safely at any time, while others need to be separated by hours or days.

Some substances will affect your sleep quality if they are taken at night. Others will cause drowsiness or sedation if you take them in the morning.

Some food or drinks (including alcohol of course) will impact the safety or effectiveness of medication or supplements.

REGULATIONS FOR QUALITY AND SAFETY

The regulations governing supplements and herbal medicines differ from one part of the world to another. Some countries insist on medical prescription for herbal medicines, some have regulated direct-to-consumer supply, while some countries classify herbal medicines and supplements as foods or dietary supplements. Other countries have virtually no regulation on supply at all.

In the US, since 1994 the Food and Drug Administration has classified herbal medicines as foods. Manufacturers have the responsibility for product safety and they are removed from the market only if there is found to be a safety risk to consumers.

In Canada, herbal medicines are classified as 'natural health products' and products need to be reviewed and obtain a licence before they go to market.

In the United Kingdom, some herbs need a medical prescription, some have to be registered as Traditional Herbal Medicinal Products, while others can be freely used as foods or supplements.

In Australia, there is strict government regulation overseen by the Therapeutic Goods Administration. All herbal products manufactured commercially in Australia must be produced according to the code of Good Manufacturing Practice (GMP), and they are registered with an AUST L or AUST R rating. Most herbal medicines have an AUST L rating, meaning that they are considered low risk and generally safe. You will see one of those terms on the label with a number. Aside from strict manufacturing standards, manufacturers must follow strict regulations about labelling and advertising.

SOME COMMONLY USED HERBAL MEDICINES

The following list of the herbs and supplements that might be relevant to you is not exhaustive but they are some of the more common products or ingredients you could encounter if you are considering an integrated approach to your cancer treatment and recovery and life beyond.

ANDROGRAPHIS

Andrographis is widely used in traditional medicine of India, China and Korea. In Ayurvedic medicine, this herb is traditionally used for anti-cancer, immune-boosting and liver detoxifying and protective effects.

Use in cancer recovery – Andrographis has some anti-cancer and immune-boosting effects. It protects the liver from chemical injury and also helps to detoxify the liver. It may be used to treat viral respiratory infection.

Additionally, preliminary research on the active ingredient, andrographolide, has shown some anti-cancer and immune-boosting effects.

It is also used at lower doses to prevent colds in winter months.

Andrographis is often used in combination with Siberian ginseng as a tonic to assist in recuperation. This combination is called Kan Jang.

The best way to take andrographis is as a tablet, as it is very bitter as a liquid, hence its common name 'king of bitters'.

Interactions – There are some drug interactions, particularly with immunosuppressants, blood thinners and oral diabetes drugs, so check with your GP or herbal medicine practitioner before you take it. If you are taking the blood-thinner warfarin and you plan to start taking andrographis, check your INR to see if you need to adjust your warfarin dose.

If you are taking medication to lower blood pressure, andrographis can have an additive effect, which means your medication dose may have to be reduced.

Cease taking andrographis a week before major surgery because it can cause blood to thin.

There are theoretical but not proven interactions with some chemotherapy drugs.

ARNICA

There is a long history of traditional use of arnica, but there are limited well-conducted clinical trials.

Use in cancer recovery – Used topically on the skin, arnica helps to reduce bruising and swelling, and is used for its anti-inflammatory properties.

You should avoid using it on broken skin.

If the raw herb is taken orally, it can have some serious adverse effects such as allergy, gastrointestinal upset, internal bleeding, fast heart rate, trouble breathing and coma, so I would advise avoiding this form.

ARTEMISIA ANNUA
(Chinese Wormwood, Qing Hao)

In Traditional Chinese Medicine, this herb is used to treat fever. Artemisinin, an active ingredient in *Artemisia annua*, is recommended in the treatment for malaria.

Use in cancer recovery – Two of the components of *Artemisia annua*, artemisinin and artesunate, have been studied as anti-cancer treatments and have been found to have anti-cancer properties, however evidence is not yet sufficient to recommend its use in cancer treatment.

ASTRAGALUS (*Astragalus membranaceus*)

The astragalus root (huang-qi) has been used in Chinese medicine for thousands of years. It is often combined with other herbs to protect and support the immune system, restoring impaired T-cell function in people with cancer. It is quite safe.

Use in cancer recovery – Boosts immunity, enhances the effectiveness and reduces the side effects of chemotherapy. It is also used to reduce fatigue and help recuperation from chemotherapy.

A 2005 Cochrane review of Chinese herbs for chemotherapy side effects in colorectal cancer patients showed that astragalus can reduce nausea and vomiting and reduce the incidence of neutropenia (low white blood cell counts).

Astragalus extracts have been shown to inhibit tumour growth, delay chemical-induced liver cancer in experiments on rats, and have anti-angiogenic property. In vitro, animal, and anecdotal human data show that astragalus reduces immune suppression, a side effect of chemotherapy, and may also enhance the effects of platinum-based chemotherapy.

There is no evidence of harm or serious adverse effects at recommended doses.

Precautions – Astragalus stimulates the immune system, so it may interact with drugs that suppress the immune system, such as tacrolimus or cyclophosphamide. This combination should be avoided.

You need to exercise caution and discuss with your doctor if you have an autoimmune disease such as lupus or rheumatoid arthritis.

In Traditional Chinese Medicine, astragalus is not used to treat the acute phase of an infection.

If you are using astragalus while undergoing chemotherapy for cancer treatment, your cancer specialist will need to know because doses of chemotherapy may need to be adjusted.

Interactions – There is an interaction with the drug lithium, causing an increase in the blood levels of lithium, so that combination is best avoided.

Astragalus appears to lower blood sugar, so if you are on diabetes medication your blood sugar levels will need to be monitored.

BAICAL SKULLCAP
(*Scutellaria baicalensis, Huang Qin*)

Baical skullcap is used in Traditional Chinese Medicine for its anti-inflammatory, anti-allergenic, anti-microbial, diuretic and anti-tumour effects.

Use in cancer recovery – Baical skullcap may be useful as an adjunctive therapy during cancer treatment to reduce nausea and boost your immunity.

Precautions – Baical skullcap can increase the effectiveness of several drugs that have a sedating action including some antidepressants, alcohol and sleeping pills, so you need to check with your doctor before taking it.

BLACK COHOSH
(*Cimicifuga racemosa* **or** *Actea racemosa*)

Use in cancer recovery – Black cohosh may help the symptoms of menopause from adjunctive hormone therapies used in breast cancer treatment. These adjunctive therapies block oestrogen so they will initiate or exacerbate menopause symptoms.

After a diagnosis of breast cancer, most forms of hormone replacement therapy are contraindicated and hot flushes and other menopause symptoms can make hormone suppression after breast cancer intolerable.

There has been a concern in the past about the safety of black cohosh in women who have hormone-sensitive breast cancer. A 2014 review found that current evidence does not support an association between black cohosh and increased risk of breast cancer. This is reassuring and answers the most common question women have when considering this herb after they have had breast cancer.

Black cohosh is well-tolerated when taken simultaneously with tamoxifen and in breast cancer survivors with menopausal hot flushes.

Precautions – If you are currently having chemotherapy treatment for breast cancer, your specialist will need to know if you are taking black cohosh because it might increase the effectiveness of some types of chemotherapy.

Adverse side effects are rare but might include headache and dizziness, and there have been rare isolated reports of liver damage.

It may take weeks or months to show if it is going to work for you. It is frequently used in combination with other herbs such as St John's wort for its mood stabilising affect.

CALENDULA (*Calendula officinalis*)

Calendula cream has antibacterial and anti-inflammatory effects and is great for accelerating wound healing. It also works very well as a burn cream, and as a topical treatment for skin inflammation, bruises, boils and sunburn.

Use in cancer recovery – It has a soothing effect on skin burns from radiotherapy.

Apply calendula topical cream to radiation-damaged skin two to three times daily.

Precautions – Calendula is considered to be very safe. There are occasional reports of allergic reactions. No interactions with other drugs or herbs are known.

CRANBERRY (*Vaccinium macrocarpon*)

Use in cancer recovery – Cranberry may be useful in reducing the incidence of urinary tract infection where a non-pharmaceutical approach is preferred. Cranberry is used for the prevention of recurring urinary tract infections and is available as juice or as tablets. The juice is widely available but if you don't like the taste, or if you don't want the extra calories from the juice, the tablet form is preferable.

Cranberry extract pills have been shown to halve the rate of post-operative urinary tract infections in women having elective gynaecological surgery.

Precautions – Diabetics should use the tablet form rather than the juice because of the sugar content of the juice.

Established urinary tract infections need to be treated medically to avoid kidney complications.

If you are taking warfarin, your doses need to be checked if you start taking high doses of cranberry.

GARLIC (*Allium sativum*)

Garlic is a food and a medicine. It can be used fresh (raw or cooked), or in capsules, tablets, or as an oil.

Garlic has an antibacterial and antiviral effect, and is used to prevent the common cold. It also has an antifungal effect, and can be used to treat tinea infections.

Use in cancer recovery – If you have planned surgery or dental work, stop high dose supplements of garlic a week before. This does not apply to fresh garlic in food. (Garlic does not appear to affect warfarin.)

Side effects – The main problems with garlic is that it can cause bad breath, heartburn and upset stomach, so enteric-coated odourless preparations are usually better tolerated and more socially acceptable.

Precautions – Garlic is safe for most people, but do not take garlic as a medicine without medical advice if you have a clotting or bleeding disorder, or diabetes. Garlic has been found to interfere with the effectiveness of the anti-HIV drugs saquinavir and ritonavir. Allergic reactions are possible.

GINGER (*Zingiber officinalis*)

The most common and well-established use of ginger is in assisting digestion and alleviating symptoms of nausea and vomiting.

Use in cancer recovery – Ginger has been used to help relieve nausea in cancer patients who are having chemotherapy. The evidence for its effectiveness is weak and honestly, it is really asking too much of ginger or a ginger extract to relieve the nausea of chemotherapy on its own. Generally, strong antiemetic (anti-nausea) medication is needed to provide adequate relief. Ginger may help to stimulate your digestive system and improve your appetite but medication will be needed to control vomiting from chemotherapy.

You will also be advised to stop ginger supplements before surgery.

Precautions – Do not take ginger as a herbal medicine without medical advice if you have a bleeding or clotting disorder, or if you are on medication for diabetes or high blood pressure.

GINSENG

Ginseng root has traditional use in Chinese medicine as an energy booster.

Use in cancer recovery – There are different types of ginseng. High doses of pure American ginseng (*Panax quinquefolius*), taken by cancer patients and survivors for just two months, has been shown to significantly improve the severe fatigue often experienced both during and after chemotherapy. Panax ginseng may help fatigue caused by radiation treatment.

GRAPE-SEED EXTRACT (*Vitis vinifera*)

Use in cancer recovery – Antioxidants, such as those found in grape-seed extract, are thought to have a role in reducing the risk of developing cancer. Laboratory in-vitro studies have found that grape-seed extracts may prevent the growth of breast, stomach, colon, prostate and lung cancer cells. But there is no clear evidence yet whether it has this effect in humans, so it is not possible to make practical recommendations in this regard.

Grape-seed extract may also help prevent damage to human liver cells caused by chemotherapy medications.

GREEN TEA (*Camellia sinensis*)

Green tea is a fascinating plant with many reported health benefits. It actually comes from the same plant as black tea and oolong tea, but is processed differently and contains less caffeine. It has a high antioxidant content and has been shown to reduce LDL-cholesterol 'bad cholesterol' and stroke risk.

Green tea may help with weight loss because it reduces appetite and boosts metabolism. It also reduces blood sugar levels, and research suggests it may provide some cancer protective effects.

It can reduce inflammation in inflammatory bowel disease, such as Crohn's disease, and may protect the liver against toxins like excessive alcohol.

Precautions – Tannins in tea can reduce iron absorption, so preferably should not be drunk within two hours of a meal. There is a drug interaction with the blood thinning drug warfarin, so make sure you check your medication level with your doctor if you are taking this as a high dose supplement.

HOLY BASIL (*Ocimum sanctum*)

Holy basil is a popular herb in the traditional medical cultures of India and Southeast Asia. Mostly used as a medicinal tea, it has anti-inflammatory, analgesic, liver-protective, stress-relieving and immune-modulating properties.

Use in cancer recovery – Holy basil is used during radiotherapy to selectively protect normal tissues from being damaged by radiation.

It is safe with low toxicity.

LICORICE (Gan Cao, *Glycyrrhiza glabra,*
Glycyrrhiza uralensis)

Licorice is a common herbal ingredient in Traditional Chinese Medicine combinations. It is used as a tonic, expectorant and a demulcent in Ayurveda. (A demulcent is an agent that forms a soothing film over mucous membranes, relieving minor pain and inflammation. An expectorant thins mucus so it can be more easily coughed up.)

Licorice is often used in combination with other herbs to treat indigestion. It is also used as a flavouring agent.

Precautions – Licorice in known to increase blood pressure. This can be an issue if you have hypertension. If your blood pressure increases, check any herbal medicines you are taking for the presence of licorice. You will be advised to stop taking licorice at least two weeks before scheduled surgery. The deglycyrrinated (DGL) form of licorice does not have this effect on blood pressure.

Whole-herb licorice can also cause water retention and electrolyte imbalances, which can lead to abnormal heart rhythms.

It may interfere with the effectiveness of some chemotherapy agents, such as cisplatin and other medications.

MISTLETOE (*Viscum album L.*)

Use in cancer recovery – Mistletoe extracts are commonly used by cancer patients with the aim of improving survival and quality of life, stimulating the immune system, improving survival and reducing the adverse effects of chemotherapy and radiotherapy. Preparations from the European mistletoe are among the most prescribed drugs in cancer patients in several European countries. There have been more than 50 clinical trials of mistletoe extracts in patients with cancer and most studies report improved quality of life in symptoms such as fatigue, nausea and vomiting, depression, emotional wellbeing, and concentration.

Data on side effects indicated that, depending on the dose, mistletoe extracts were usually well tolerated and had few side effects.

OLIVE LEAF

Olive leaf extract is known for its antioxidant, anti-inflammatory, antiviral, anti-hypertensive and other properties. Leaf extracts have shown some anti-cancer activity in laboratory tests but this has not been tested in humans.

PEPPERMINT (*Mentha piperita*)

Peppermint is used to treat the symptoms of stomach upset and gastrointestinal discomfort. It is popular as a herbal tea and as capsules.

Use in cancer recovery – Peppermint oil given before surgery may be useful in controlling nausea after surgery, usually in conjunction with antiemetic medication. It has been shown to have significant anti-tumour activity in vitro and in some animal studies, but this has not been confirmed in human studies.

Precautions – Do not take peppermint oil if you have gallbladder inflammation or liver disease. This precaution does not apply to peppermint tea.

RED CLOVER

Red clover contains phytoestrogens known as isoflavones. There is a concern that long-term use of HRT in women after menopause may increase the risk of breast cancer and endometrial cancer, so women need to look for other ways of managing their menopause symptoms. The phytoestrogens in red clover can reduce meno-pause symptoms but, unlike black cohosh, we do not have safety data for women who have had breast cancer.

Use in cancer recovery – Red clover may be helpful in managing hot flushes and other menopausal symptoms in some women but current advice does not extend to using it with adjunctive anti-hormone therapies used in the treatment of breast cancer or in women who have had breast cancer, particularly oestrogen-positive cancers.

Precautions – Red clover may interfere with the action of tamoxifen.

REISHI MUSHROOM (*Ganoderma lucidum,* Ling Zhi, Ling Chi, Lin Zi, mushroom of immortality)

Reishi mushroom is used in Traditional Chinese Medicine to treat hypertension, viral infections, inflammation, and liver disorders; to lower high cholesterol; and for immune stimulation in patients with cancer and AIDS.

Use in cancer recovery – A few studies have shown it to have immune-boosting and anti-tumour effects.

Meta-analysis results showed that patients who had been given reishi mushroom alongside chemotherapy and radiotherapy were more likely to respond positively compared to the treatments alone.

RESVERATROL

Resveratrol is a compound found in the skin of red grapes and is usually taken as a supplement for its antioxidant and anti-inflammatory properties. This compound is thought to limit the spread of cancer cells.

Use in cancer recovery – From animal studies it is thought that resveratrol may protect against chemotherapy-induced cardiotoxicity, but there have been very few studies of the effect of resveratrol in humans, and particularly on humans with cancer.

ST JOHN'S WORT (*Hypericum perforatum*)

St John's wort is a yellow-flowered plant. Its use as a medicine dates back to Ancient Greece, where it was used for the treatment of nervous conditions, and it has been known in Europe as a treatment for anxiety and depression since the sixteenth century. Extensive scientific testing has concluded that it is at least as effective as pharmaceutical antidepressants for the treatment of depression, with fewer side effects. It is also useful for the irritability of premenstrual syndrome and menopause.

The main active constituents are hyperforin and hypericin.

Use in cancer recovery – St John's wort can be used to treat the anxiety and depression that may be experienced following cancer treatment. Because of potential interactions with other medications, treatment should not be started until chemotherapy is concluded.

Precautions – There are multiple potential drug interactions, particularly the SSRI class of antidepressants and some chemotherapy agents. Preparations with lower hyperforin content (such as ZE117) are less likely to cause drug interactions.

ST MARY'S THISTLE (*Silybum marianum*)

St Mary's thistle, also known as milk thistle, is a popular herb used to protect the liver against toxins such as alcohol and medications like paracetamol, and helps to repair liver damage. The active constituent in milk thistle is silymarin.

Use in cancer recovery – Laboratory studies demonstrate that silymarin functions as an antioxidant, stabilises cell membranes (preventing toxic chemicals from entering the cell), stimulates detoxification pathways, stimulates regeneration of liver tissue, inhibits the growth of certain cancer cell lines, exerts direct cytotoxic activity towards certain cancer cell lines, and may increase the effectiveness of some chemotherapy agents. It is also known to neutralise a number of free radicals.

It is commonly used in detox protocols.

No human clinical trials on milk thistle or silymarin as a cancer treatment or as an adjunctive therapy in individuals with cancer have been published, but it is generally regarded as safe.

SAW PALMETTO (*Serenoa repens*)

Saw palmetto is the most popular herbal therapy to reduce benign enlargement of the prostate. Many studies report that saw palmetto may be as effective as the pharmaceutical hormonal agent finasteride (Proscar) and may cause fewer side effects when used to treat bladder problems.

Use in cancer recovery – Many older men will be familiar with the symptoms of an enlarged prostate gland, most significantly trouble in passing urine. Saw palmetto is a popular herbal remedy, often used in combination with other herbs, to relieve the symptoms of benign prostatic hypertrophy (BPH). It does not prevent prostate cancer. One of its advantages is that it can reduce benign prostate swelling without altering the PSA level, the marker for prostate cancer. So if prostate cancer were to develop or worsen, the PSA level would reflect that. You can expect it to take a month or two to show a benefit.

Saw palmetto may benefit men with chronic bacterial prostatitis if it is taken in combination with stinging nettle (*Urtica dioica*), curcumin (from turmeric), and quercetin (a flavonol found in fruits, vegetables, grains and leaves).

Precautions – Urinary symptoms need to be investigated to check for infection, prostate enlargement or prostate cancer.

Interaction with finasteride – Saw palmetto may work similarly to finasteride, so you should not use this herb in combination with finasteride or other medications used to treat BPH unless directed by your doctor.

SIBERIAN GINSENG (*Eleutherococcus senticosus*)

Siberian ginseng is different from American ginseng or Korean ginseng. It is known as an adaptogen, helping the body to adapt to times of emotional and physical stress. It is prescribed in times of exhaustion or during convalescence.

Use in cancer recovery – Siberian ginseng has an immune stimulating effect and is used to combat fatigue and to increase energy and alertness.

Precautions – Siberian ginseng has some possible side effects, such as increased blood pressure, trouble sleeping, headache and irregular heartbeat. It may interact with a number of medications including blood thinners, sedatives, diabetes medicines, digoxin, steroids and lithium, so you need to check with your pharmacist or doctor before taking it.

SLIPPERY ELM (*Ulmus rubra*)

Slippery elm bark powder is another very useful herbal medicine. We recommend it for relieving the symptoms of a range of gut problems including gastritis, dyspepsia, gastro-oesophageal reflux, peptic ulcer, irritable bowel syndrome and Crohn's disease.

Use in cancer recovery – Slippery elm is used orally to soothe irritation or ulceration of the stomach and intestines.

Precautions – No adverse reactions or drug interactions have been reported following use of slippery elm, but it may interfere with the absorption of some medications, so is best taken at a different time of the day from medicines that need careful monitoring of dosages, such as digoxin, lithium, warfarin and epilepsy medications.

TURMERIC (*Curcuma longa*)

Turmeric is a member of the ginger family grown in India, Asia and Africa and it is used as a powder or in capsules, teas or liquid extracts. The active ingredient is curcumin. Turmeric is approved in Europe for use in digestive problems. It has been shown to improve remission rates in ulcerative colitis.

Use in cancer recovery – Turmeric has anti-inflammatory, anti-cancer and antioxidant properties. Laboratory studies have shown that curcumin interferes with several important molecular pathways involved in cancer development, growth and spread. Curcumin can kill cancer cells in laboratory dishes and also slows the growth of the surviving cells. But human studies on the effect of curcumin in cancer prevention and treatment are still in their early stages.

Curcumin is not well absorbed by the gut, so high doses are needed to have a systemic effect, although it does absorb into the colon lining and into cancerous tissues in the colon.

Precaution – Turmeric should be ceased two weeks before surgery. It can interact with blood-thinning medications and can lower blood pressure. High doses can cause stomach upset. You should avoid turmeric if you have had bile duct blockage, gallstones, or stomach ulcers.

VALERIAN (*Valeriana officinalis*)

Use in cancer recovery – Valerian is a very popular herbal medicine dating back to Hippocrates and Galen. It is a useful alternative to benzodiazepine medications used to relieve insomnia and reduce anxiety, and is often used in combination with other herbs such as passionflower. Some studies have shown it is as effective as benzodiazepine drugs for people with trouble falling asleep. The herb works differently from the benzodiazepines, in that it becomes more effective over a couple of weeks of regular use. It does not cause drowsiness the next day and it is not considered to be addictive.

WITHANIA (*Withania somnifera,* Ashwagandha, Indian ginseng)

Withania, or ashwagandha, is a popular Ayurvedic herb. It is one of the herbs known as adaptogens, used to improve wellbeing during times of physical and emotional exhaustion and during convalescence. Withania is often used in formulations prescribed for stress, strain, fatigue, pain, skin diseases, diabetes and gastro-intestinal disease.

Use in cancer recovery – There is a potential role for withania as an adjunctive treatment during chemotherapy for the prevention of drug-induced bone marrow suppression.

It has been shown to improve chemotherapy-induced fatigue and improve quality of life in women being treated for breast cancer.

OTHER SUPPLEMENTS

The safe and most effective use of supplements requires experience and a knowledge of the evidence for benefits and pitfalls. Some patients I see have been told by their oncologist not to take any supplements, and this can mean an unnecessarily difficult struggle with treatment side effects. Other patients arrive with a suitcase full of supplements and no logical plan for what supplements they might need and what to avoid. This section of the book is not intended as a replacement for professional advice but it is meant to assist you to understand what help may be available for you and some rationale for the responsible and careful use of supplements to assist your recovery. I have consciously avoided including dosage information because prescribing of supplements, particularly in combinations, is individualised and mindful of your nutritional status, medications and other therapies. Remember that many supplement preparations are in combinations with other substances so it will be important for you to be aware of the ingredients and doses in any and every preparation and avoid overdosing or self-prescribing.

THE BIG ANTIOXIDANT DEBATE: FRIEND OR FOE DURING CANCER TREATMENT?

There is an ongoing debate about the use of antioxidant supplements during chemotherapy and radiotherapy and this may cause you confusion if you are getting conflicting advice.

If you find the debate confusing, you are not alone. A 2015 survey of North American Cancer centres found that only 5 per cent had policies on antioxidant use while 69 per cent provided guidelines. Specific antioxidant supplements were generally not recommended by cancer institutions, and this is certainly the Australian experience. Official policies and guidelines on antioxidant supplements during treatment were not particularly evidence-based, and were generally more restrictive than the research evidence might suggest, adding to the complexity of their optimal and safe use.

Antioxidants include Vitamin A, carotenoids, alpha-lipoic acid, vitamin C, Vitamin E, selenium and glutathione. Some oncologists will tell you to avoid all antioxidants until cancer-specific treatment is completed. Others believe that antioxidant support is important to improve the tolerability of cancer treatment. Clinical trials have not tested every antioxidant with every chemotherapy agent and every cancer type. However, evidence to date supports the view that most antioxidants do not interfere with cancer treatment and may have beneficial effects.

Meanwhile, the FDA has approved the use of a potent pharmaceutical antioxidant, amifostine, to protect sensitive tissues during radiotherapy and chemotherapy.

There are some exceptions based on current knowledge:

- avoid high dose vitamin C with methotrexate and dacarbazine
- avoid Vitamin A, vitamin C, selenium, and N-acetylcysteine, with doxorubicin
- avoid betacarotene with 5FU
- avoid N-acetylcysteine with cisplatin
- avoid citrus bioflavinoid supplements with tamoxifen.

I have tried to distil useful and practical information for you based on the current state of evidence, bearing in mind that there are strong conflicting opinions within the medical community on the use of antioxidant supplements during treatment with chemotherapy and radiotherapy. There is much less resistance to the use of antioxidant supplements in recovery and recuperation after treatment.

There is strong consensus on the importance of dietary sources of antioxidants at all stages of cancer treatment.

ALPHA-LIPOIC ACID

Alpha-lipoic acid is an antioxidant present in every cell of the body and helps turn glucose into energy. It appears to help in the recycling of other antioxidants. The main food sources are potato, spinach, liver, red meat, broccoli, potatoes, yams, carrots, beets.

Use in cancer recovery – Researchers have begun to look at whether alpha-lipoic acid can help prevent nerve damage and heart muscle damage from the use of some chemotherapy drugs.

If you are undergoing cancer-specific treatment, make sure you get professional advice on timing of supplementation with alpha-lipoic acid. It may also protect against the tissue damage caused by radiation.

Precautions – High doses of alpha-lipoic acid supplements may lower blood sugar levels. You need to be aware of this if you are taking medications for diabetes.

B VITAMINS

B group vitamins are essential to many functions of the body. Supplements are usually taken in combinations and are recommended for pregnant women, the elderly and people with nutritional deficiency and nutrient absorption problems.

Different genetic types deal with B vitamins differently, so your genetic type might determine the effect of these vitamins on your personal cancer risk.

Use in cancer recovery – Low folate is linked to higher risk of several cancers.

Low vitamin B_6 intake has been found to be associated with a risk of colorectal cancer. Vitamin B_6 deficiency is more common in elderly people and in heavy alcohol drinkers.

Vitamin B_{12} deficiency is a risk in people who have had stomach surgery (gastrectomy), or removal of the end of the small bowel (terminal ileum). Ask your medical oncologist if the chemotherapy recommended for you has the potential to cause nerve damage (peripheral neuropathy) Vitamins B_1, B_6 and B_{12} in particular are essential for nerve health and may reduce your risk of this complication.

BETACAROTENE

Betacarotene, also known as provitamin A, may help decrease the risk of developing cancer. It is thought to have a cancer-preventive effect by enhancing the white blood cells in your immune system. White blood cells work to block cell-damaging free radicals. Food sources include dark green leafy and yellow-orange fruits and vegetables, such as carrots, squash, spinach, sweet potatoes.

Use in cancer recovery – Eating foods rich in betacarotene is recommended to decrease the risk of recurrence of stomach, lung, prostate, breast, and head and neck cancer. But more research is needed before a definite recommendation on betacarotene consumption can be made, particularly by supplementation.

Precautions – Large doses can cause your skin to turn a yellow-orange colour, a condition called carotenosis. High intake of betacarotene in supplement form was shown in one Finnish study to increase the risk of lung cancer in male smokers, so current information is that supplementation should be avoided if you smoke until this risk is clarified with further research.

CALCIUM

Adequate calcium from diet and supplements is important to prevent osteoporosis. Food sources include dairy products, leafy green vegetables and fish with bones.

Use in cancer recovery – Several studies have suggested that foods high in calcium might help reduce the risk for colorectal cancer and precancerous polyps. Some studies have found that women with higher calcium intake in their diet (not from supplements) seem to have a lower risk of breast cancer.

A randomised clinical trial reported in 2007 found lower risk for all cancers combined in women given calcium supplements than in women taking the placebo. Cancer risk was even lower among women taking both calcium and vitamin D.

During cancer treatment, bones can be particularly vulnerable. Hormonal therapies used in the treatment of breast or prostate cancer commonly cause osteoporosis.

The chemotherapy drugs methotrexate and doxorubicin may directly damage bones. Radiation therapy can cause osteopenia (bone thinning) within the area being treated. If chemotherapy medications reduce your appetite or cause nausea and vomiting, this can result in osteopenia.

Adequate calcium intake is essential for bone health in cancer treatment and recovery. Physical activity and general nutrition are also important for bone health and these can be compromised during cancer treatment and the recovery phase. If adequate dietary calcium intake is difficult or impossible, supplementation including vitamin D and magnesium will be necessary.

Precautions – Medications that lower stomach acid (proton pump inhibitors) reduce calcium carbonate absorption. Calcium citrate is better absorbed in this situation.

Calcium can affect the absorption of some other minerals, so it is important for you to get advice about combining supplements and timing of doses.

Calcium levels can become elevated in people with some types of advanced cancers (such as myeloma), but not in earlier cancers. Diarrhoea and dehydration can also increase calcium levels.

COENZYME Q10

As supplements go, coenzyme Q10 (CoQ10 or ubiquinone) is a quiet achiever. A powerful antioxidant, CoQ10 is generated naturally in the body and a small amount comes from the diet in foods such as meat, poultry and seafood, whole grains, soybeans and nuts.

CoQ10 plays an essential role in manufacturing energy in every cell in the body. It is a powerful antioxidant responsible for helping to convert food into energy, and for protecting cells from damage. It supports the body's immune system and provides protection against some infections and some forms of cancer. It is also proving to be something of a 'wonder-supplement' in various types of heart disease.

The symptoms that suggest you may be deficient in CoQ10 can be quite subtle. They include physical fatigue, muscle weakness, tiredness after a short amount of exercise, trouble concentrating, foggy thinking, irritability and difficulty dealing with stress. You may also notice an increased susceptibility to infections like colds and flu, and gum disease.

Who is most at risk of CoQ10 deficiency?

- CoQ10 levels decrease as you get older.
- Some people are born with an inability to make CoQ10.
- There may not be enough CoQ10 in your diet. This is especially the case with vegetarians.
- There may be too much demand for CoQ10 by your body, such as a serious medical condition or intensive exercise.
- Some medications, such as cholesterol-lowering drugs called statins, but also the oral contraceptive pill, beta-blockers and tricyclic antidepressants, interfere with the production of CoQ10 in your body.
- Some studies have shown that CoQ10 levels are lower in people who are obese.

CoQ10 was first discovered in 1957 and there are indications that this could be one of the most useful supplements we have for a range of health problems. It has been shown to help prevent heart failure, lower cholesterol and slow the progress of some neurological diseases.

If you are likely to have a CoQ10 deficiency, it can be supplemented with capsules or tablets. The usual dose is 100–200 mg per day, but higher doses are recommended in some conditions.

Use in cancer recovery – According to the National Cancer Institute in the US, interest in CoQ10 as a possible adjunctive treatment for cancer began in 1961, when it was found that some cancer patients had a lower than normal amount of it in their blood. Low blood levels of CoQ10 have been found in patients with myeloma, lymphoma, and cancers of the breast, lung, prostate, pancreas, colon, kidney and head and neck. CoQ10 is used as an adjunctive therapy alongside conventional cancer treatments, but timing with respect to chemotherapy may be important. CoQ10 protects the heart from damage caused by some chemotherapy drugs.

CoQ10 provides some protection against hepatotoxicity (liver damage) during cancer treatment and against cardiotoxicity (heart damage) caused by some forms of chemotherapy.

Precautions – CoQ10 should always be taken with a meal containing a small amount of fat, such as oily fish, fish oil supplements or cheese, to help absorption.

While CoQ10 is generally considered to be very safe with few side effects, its safety has not been established in pregnancy or breastfeeding. It is not appropriate for children under the age of 18 except on medical advice. Nor is it advisable to take high doses of vitamin E with CoQ10.

If you are taking the blood thinner warfarin, you will need to have your levels monitored for several weeks after you start taking CoQ10 supplements.

FISH OIL

Fish oil is an important source of omega-3 fatty acids. According to the Cancer Council NSW, there is some evidence suggesting a protective effect of fish consumption with a reduced risk of breast, rectal and prostate cancer. The recommendation is to eat fish, preferably oily fish, at least two times per week and include some plant foods and oils rich in omega-3 fatty acids in your diet. Eating fish also contributes healthy proteins to your diet.

You may not be able to eat enough fish to gain the protective effect of omega-3 fatty acids, so a fish oil supplement may be necessary.

GLUTAMINE

Glutamine is an amino acid. It is a major component of tissue of the skeletal muscles and it is a major source of energy for cells lining the gut. It is also a nutrient in muscle protein metabolism in response to infection, inflammation and muscle trauma. Food sources of glutamine are dairy products, fish and green leafy vegetables.

Use in cancer recovery – Cancer produces a state of glutamine deficiency, which is further magnified by the toxic effects of chemotherapy agents. This leads to increased tolerance of the tumour to chemotherapy as well as reduced tolerance of normal tissues to the side effects of chemotherapy. Other states of physiologic stress such as severe sepsis and surgery are characterised by a relative deficiency of glutamine.

Chemotherapy doses are limited by toxicity to normal tissues. Intravenous glutamine protects liver cells from oxidant injury. It may also protect the heart and nervous system from the toxic effects of chemotherapy.

Glutamine used as a mouthwash can help reduce the effects of mucositis (mouth ulcers) caused by chemotherapy.

Research also suggests that oral glutamine supplementation enhances the ability of anti-tumour drugs to selectively target cancer cells by protecting normal tissues from and possibly sensitising tumour cells to radiation-induced and chemotherapy treatment-related injury.

There are no known drug interactions and glutamine is considered safe to use during chemotherapy and radiotherapy.

GLUTATHIONE

Glutathione is an important antioxidant composed of three amino acids (cysteine, glutamic acid and glycine) found in almost all cells in the body. It helps to destroy toxins in the body and prevent cell damage. The main food sources are garlic, fruits, vegetables and meat.

Use in cancer recovery – Glutathione intravenous infusions may help prevent the toxic side effects of chemotherapy and have been used to repair nerve damage caused by some forms of chemotherapy. These are arranged through a clinic with specialised expertise in nutrient infusion.

See page 184 for more information on glutathione.

INDOLE-3-CARBINOL

Cruciferous indoles/indole-3-carbinol (I3C) is found in cruciferous vegetables and is also available as a supplement. Food sources are cabbage, broccoli, Brussels sprouts, Chinese cabbage, horseradish, arugula and kale.

Use in cancer recovery – There is some laboratory evidence that I3C has anti-cancer activity. Human clinical trials showed that it is effective in the treatment of precancerous cervical dysplasia shown on abnormal Pap smears and vulvar intraepithelial neoplasia, the precursor to vulval cancer.

L-CARNITINE

L-carnitine is an amino acid essential for energy production in mitochondria, the energy generators in every cell.

Use in cancer recovery – Long-term L-carnitine administration may reduce the cardiotoxic (heart muscle toxicity) side effect of the chemotherapy drug adriamycin. L-carnitine has been shown to improve cancer-related fatigue and quality of life in people undergoing cancer treatment.

LYCOPENE

Lycopene is a carotenoid antioxidant compound that gives red fruits and vegetables their colour. Food sources include tomato (especially cooked tomato products), strawberries, watermelon, apricots, guava and papaya.

Some studies have found that people who have diets rich in tomatoes appear to have a lower risk of cancers of the lung, prostate, stomach, bladder, cervix and skin. Studies have also demonstrated that populations with high intake of dietary lycopene have lower risks of prostate cancer.

In vitro (laboratory studies), lycopene inhibits androgen receptor expression in prostate cancer cells and reduces prostate cancer cell proliferation. It is not clear what effect consuming lycopene-containing foods will have on someone who has already developed a cancer, but lycopene is most likely to be effective as a component in a balanced healthy diet containing an adequate range of fruits and vegetables.

MAGNESIUM

Magnesium is an essential mineral, and deficiency is common. It may be deficient because of an inadequate diet, the use of some medications, drinking alcohol, diabetes, an unhealthy gut or digestive system and older age. Symptoms of magnesium deficiency include anxiety, restless leg syndrome (RLS), insomnia, irritability, abnormal heart rhythms, muscle twitching or spasm, muscle weakness and insomnia. Food sources include green leafy vegetables, avocado, sunflower seeds and pumpkin seeds.

Use in cancer recovery – The possibility of magnesium deficiency needs to be on the diagnostic radar and suspected or conformed deficiency should be treated with dietary changes and supplementation. A study published in the *European Journal of Clinical Nutrition* showed that a higher intake of dietary magnesium was associated with a lower risk of colorectal tumours. Magnesium may be added to intravenous vitamin C infusions to prevent vascular spasm.

MELATONIN

Melatonin is a hormone with antioxidant properties, and is produced by the pineal gland at the base of the brain. It is probably best known for its role in helping to regulate sleep cycles. Melatonin supplements may help to regulate sleep cycles where sleep routine is disrupted. For this reason it is used to overcome jet lag.

Use in cancer recovery – People who work night shifts have been found to have an increased risk for some cancers, and it has been suggested that this is associated with lower melatonin levels. Women with breast cancer tend to have lower levels of melatonin than those without the disease.

Melatonin has been used alone and combined with chemotherapy, radiation therapy, hormone therapy (such as tamoxifen for breast cancer), and immunotherapy (such as interleukin-2) in a number of studies involving different types of cancer. It can be used safely as an adjuvant breast cancer treatment with the anti-oestrogen and aromatase-inhibiting hormone therapies. Some studies have suggested that melatonin may extend survival and improve quality of life for people with certain types of untreatable cancers such as advanced lung cancer and melanoma.

Melatonin may decrease surgery-associated anxiety and pain. It has virtually no contraindications.

The usual dose range is 2–6 mg at sundown for immune support and sleep. Higher doses are often used under professional supervision after a cancer diagnosis.

PREBIOTICS

Prebiotics are non-digestible fibres that serve as the food to keep your 'good' bacteria healthy. You can either consume prebiotic-rich foods (such as asparagus, garlic, leek, onion, banana and artichoke) or take a prebiotic supplement. See page 417 for more information on prebiotics.

PROBIOTICS

Probiotics are beneficial live microorganisms inhabiting the gut that seem to change how the immune system reacts to invading microorganisms. They compete with harmful bacteria and enhance the activity of the immune system. They also help calm the immune system if it is overactive, and they may help restore or maintain a healthy balance of bacteria in the gut, which can be upset by antibiotics.

There are many different types of probiotic and they are referred to according to their species. Each one can have a quite different activity in the human gut. Some examples of commonly used types are *Lactobacillus acidophilus*, *Bifidobacterium lactis*, *Lactobacillus plantarum 299v*, *Lactobacillus rhamnosus* and *Saccharomyces boulardii*.

Use in cancer recovery – Probiotics are very useful in helping to maintain healthy gut function. Many medical treatments, including chemotherapy and antibiotics can drastically alter the balance of gut microbes. Probiotics help to detoxify the body and assist in the elimination of carcinogens.

They may increase the body's ability to respond to immunotherapy or chemotherapy. Probiotics assist in absorption of nutrients and the synthesis of some vitamins. They also have a role in reducing systemic inflammation and in maintaining the immune system.

SELENIUM

Selenium (Se) is an essential micronutrient that reduces the toxicity of heavy metals such as mercury, lead, arsenic, silver and cadmium by forming inert complexes.

Selenium deficiency has been associated with an increased risk for cancer and heart disease, thyroid disease, depression and anxiety. Inadequate selenium levels can impair your immune system and increase your vulnerability to infection.

Food sources include Brazil nuts, wholegrains and cereals, meat, fish and poultry. The selenium content in foods varies depending on the amount of selenium in agricultural soils. Many parts of the world are considered selenium deficient.

Use in cancer recovery – It is important for you to avoid selenium deficiency. Although the epidemiological data are somewhat controversial, it does appear that selenium deficiency is a cancer risk factor. It also appears that selenium may be an anti-metastastatic element (preventing the spread of cancer) in addition to being a cancer preventative agent.

Selenium has been shown to reduce kidney toxicity, bone marrow suppression and weight loss associated with cisplatin chemotherapy. There is not enough evidence to say whether selenium might reduce the side effects of surgery, radiation therapy, or other forms of chemotherapy.

Selenium supplements are considered safe in moderation but can be toxic in high doses. A total selenium intake from supplements should not exceed a maximum of 150 µg per day. Long-term, excessive doses (over 1000 µg per day) can cause fatigue, depression, arthritis, hair loss, body odour and gastrointestinal symptoms.

VITAMIN C

Vitamin C is an important antioxidant. Unlike other mammals, humans are not able to synthesise their own vitamin C and we rely solely on food sources. A varied and high fruit and vegetable intake, including foods containing vitamin C, is protective against cancer. But vitamin C content in foods is destroyed by cooking, exposure to light, heat, oxygen and storage.

At very high doses, which are achieved through intravenous infusion (IVC), vitamin C has a profound stimulating effect on your immune system and is preferentially toxic to cancer cells. It has been shown to improve wellbeing in people with cancer. It may also protect healthy cells from damage arising from cancer treatment.

Whether to give IVC through chemotherapy is currently controversial. Some clinics believe it is safe and effective while others have a more cautious approach, preferring to avoid chemotherapy days.

High dose vitamin C should be avoided with some forms of chemotherapy, specifically methotrexate, DTIC (dacarbazine) and doxorubicin because of concerns about potential adverse interactions.

What is not controversial is the need to maintain adequate levels of dietary vitamn C intake.

For more information, see the chapter Intravenous Vitamin C and Other Nutrients, page 173.

VITAMIN E (*alpha-tocopherol*)

Vitamin E is a fat-soluble nutrient with antioxidant activity. It is used by your body to regulate gene expression and immune function. There are eight natural forms of vitamin E, the most active form for the human body is alpha-tocopherol. Food sources include vegetable oils, sunflower seeds, nuts, green leafy vegetables, egg yolks, whole grains and cereals.

Use in cancer recovery – Vitamin E has been extensively studied. Overall evidence from research has shown that vitamin E supplements do not lower the risk of heart disease or cancer.

Vitamin E supplementation is effective therapy for vitamin E deficiency which is rare. Deficiency can occur with bile flow blockage and severe protein-kilojoule malnutrition (starvation), and in people with reduced fat absorption through the gut due to surgery, Crohn's disease or cystic fibrosis. Vitamin E deficiency is probably not an issue for most people, but may be a problem for some people with cancer. Symptoms include muscle weakness, vision problems, immune system changes, and neurological signs such as numbness, trouble walking, tremors and problems with balance. Vitamin E supplementation may help prevent some adverse effects of chemotherapy, such as nerve damage.

Vitamin E has been suggested as an element of combination therapy to prevent complications such as nerve pain due to cisplatin chemotherapy. See page 140 the section on neuropathy.

A synthetic form of a vitamin E is available as a supplement.

Precautions – Large doses of vitamin E from supplements are not recommended if you are taking blood thinners and some other medications, as the vitamin can interfere with the action of some medications. Very high doses of vitamin E can also interfere with the way other fat-soluble vitamins work.

Some oncologists believe that vitamin E can help reduce side effects of chemotherapy and radiotherapy while others disagree (see my note on the antioxidant debate on page 214).

ZINC

Zinc is one of the fundamental minerals used by the immune system. It improves immune function and also functions as an antioxidant and anti-inflammatory agent. It is necessary for wound healing, and taste and smell sensation.

Zinc deficiency is very prevalent, particularly in vegetarians and the elderly. Vegetarians commonly eat a lot of legumes and whole grains. These foods contain phytates that inhibit the absorption of zinc in the body. Deficiency may cause problems with growth, diarrhoea, skin dryness, hair loss, loss of taste and smell, fertility and poor immune function.

Because zinc deficiency causes loss of taste sensation, a zinc taste test is one method that is used to detect deficiency. A solution of zinc sulfate in purified water is swished around in the mouth. If there is a strong initial taste, you have adequate zinc and you do not require supplementation. If you have delayed or no taste sensation from the solution, then you may have a zinc deficiency.

Food sources include seafood, poultry, meat, nuts, eggs, legumes, cheese and grains. Supplements come in different forms: zinc gluconate, zinc sulfate, zinc acetate, zinc picolinate.

Use in cancer recovery – Because cancer treatment affects your immune function, you need to make sure you have optimal zinc levels to support your immune system to fight infection and other illnesses.

Zinc deficiency should be treated with nutritional correction and supplementation. Evidence suggests that it may be of particular importance in the body's defence against the initiation and progression of cancer.

Zinc is also an important nutrient for the prostate gland. Cancerous prostate glands seem to have less zinc than normal prostate glands and some studies show that adequate dietary zinc is associated with a lower incidence of prostate cancer. Zinc supplementation may be of benefit in preventing mucositis (mouth ulcers) in oral cancer patients receiving radiation. Zinc sulfate has also been shown to help people who had radiation therapy for head and neck cancer to recover their taste sensation.

Precautions – Excessive zinc supplementation can lead to nausea and vomiting, headache and fatigue. Zinc supplementation can interfere with your body's absorption of magnesium, copper and iron from foods and supplements.

Other Therapies

MEDICAL CANNABIS

Back in 1996 I was working as the medical reporter for the *Today Show* on the Nine Network in Australia. We headed to San Francisco to investigate Proposition 215, the move in California to legalise marijuana (cannabis) for medical use. California was the first state in the US to establish a medical marijuana program, effectively allowing legal access to cannabis for people with cancer, AIDS, multiple sclerosis and some other medical conditions provided that they had a doctor's recommendation.

The law has been through a number of iterations since 1996, but California continues to have a medical access program for patients who are likely to benefit from cannabis.

Canada, Switzerland, the Netherlands and Israel have legalised programs for medical cannabis. In the Netherlands there is an official tolerance policy for possession of small amounts of cannabis for personal use. Conversely, cannabis is treated as a serious illicit drug in other countries such as Indonesia, with a conviction for importing large quantities attracting the death penalty. I make this point because if you are considering using cannabis to help manage your cancer symptoms or treatment side effects, you will need to take into consideration the legal situation in your country or state. There may be severe penalties, including jail in some jurisdictions, for seeking or supplying cannabis even for medical purposes.

In Australia, the debate about legalisation of cannabis for medical use is being revisited as I write. Several senior politicians are supporting it and popular opinion is in favour of legalisation. Several states have announced their intention to support trials of medical use of cannabis in the near future. The medical profession is divided, with many doctors rightly concerned about the potential for harm, balanced against the potential for benefit. This is particularly the case for smoking cannabis. Pharmaceutical preparations of cannabinoids have been used successfully to treat pain from neuropathic, post-operative and rheumatoid arthritis causes, multiple sclerosis and cancer, and also for nausea and appetite loss in HIV and cancer.

Then there is the valid argument comparing the potential harm from cannabis preparations to the potential harm from existing legal treatments such as strong opioid medications.

HOW CANNABIS IS USED

The most common ways cannabis is used is by inhalation or oral ingestion.

Smoking is a common method but the smoke can cause damage to your lungs and airways and cause inflammation in your nose, throat and sinuses. In countries with medical cannabis programs, inhalation is recommended via a specific type of medical vaporiser. The Dutch government's cannabis bureau has published guidelines on use of vaporised cannabis.

Cannabis can be made into a tea, or used as an ingredient in cookies or brownies and eaten. In this form the effect is less intense and takes longer to initiate, but is longer lasting. As a tea it takes 30 to 90 minutes to start to have an effect. The effect reaches a peak after two or three hours and it wears off after four to eight hours. Absorption is increased if you eat high-fat food with the tea.

A growing number of clinical trials are studying medicines made from a whole-plant extract of cannabis that contains specific amounts of cannabinoids. This medicine is sprayed under the tongue in controlled doses.

EVIDENCE FOR EFFICACY

Some people with cancer use cannabis to relieve nausea and cancer pain, to stimulate appetite and prevent weight loss, other people use it to reduce anxiety and aid sleep. There is evidence for cannabis being effective in treating a number of difficult cancer-related conditions such as nausea, loss of appetite, weight loss and debilitation. It has been shown to be effective in relieving nausea and vomiting related to chemotherapy. It is also effective in treating some forms of chronic pain, including nerve pain.

Cannabis will not cure the underlying problem, but may help in managing the symptoms and reducing the reliance on medication.

In places where medicinal cannabis programs operate, generally doctors will only recommend it where standard medical treatments are not giving adequate relief or where medications are causing unacceptable side effects.

Cannabis contains a number of active substances, including tetrahydrocannabinol (THC) and cannabidiol (CBD). THC is mostly responsible for the therapeutic effects of cannabis, where other constituents such as CBD may influence the effectiveness of the drug.

According to the patient information provided by the Dutch medicinal cannabis bureau, inhaling cannabis with a high CBD content is more effective for patients with inflammatory conditions, for relief of chronic nerve pain and muscle spasm in conditions like multiple sclerosis. Cannabis with high levels of THC is preferred for treating weight loss, nausea and vomiting.

If you look at the reasons for smoking cannabis either recreationally or for medicinal purpose, the euphoric effect is high on the list. Maximum euphoria typically occurs within 15 minutes after smoking and generally takes longer if it is eaten.

SIDE EFFECTS

Like any active drug or herbal medicine, cannabis use does have some risks. Side effects of cannabis include depression, hallucinations, paranoia, triggering of psychosis (particularly in young people), dizziness, heart palpitations, fits of laughter (this may be a desirable side effect), hunger, altered perception, confusion, slower reaction times, and addiction (this is less likely with the lower doses used for medical purposes compared with the higher doses generally used recreationally).

It is important to note that different crops and strains of cannabis/marijuana have different effects. Medicinal marijuana must not contain any pesticides, heavy metals, fungi, bacteria or other contaminants.

Increased risk of lung cancer

Smoking cannabis brings with it some of the same risks of lung disease as tobacco. A New Zealand study involving people under the age of 55 found that long-term cannabis smoking increased the risk of lung cancer. Another study found that men who smoked the same amount of tobacco had double the risk of lung cancer if they also used marijuana.

Marijuana and other cancers

Evidence of a link with cancer is inconsistent and conflicting. Marijuana possibly increases the risk of testicular cancer, prostate cancer, cervical cancer, and a type of brain tumour. But a large review by Health Canada concluded that while there are carcinogens in cannabis and a theoretical basis for a link between marijuana and cancer, that link is, at this stage, inconclusive.

Marijuana and immunity

There is no convincing clinical evidence that usual doses of cannabis damage the immune system.

Withdrawal effects

If you use cannabis at high doses regularly for weeks or months, physical dependence is a real possibility and if you stop using it, you can experience a withdrawal syndrome. Withdrawal effects include several days of irritability, restlessness, sleeping problems, nausea and hot flushes.

GENERAL ADVICE

If you are thinking about using cannabis for medical reasons, consider the possible legal issues in your country or state as possession for cannabis, even for medical purposes, could result in prosecution and possibly a jail sentence. Be clear about why you are considering wanting to use cannabis. Could your symptoms have a legal, safe and effective remedy?

The aim is to use small doses to the point of symptom relief. Higher doses will achieve a 'high', but are more likely to cause unwanted side effects.

If you have any medical condition affecting your lungs or breathing capacity, smoking tobacco or cannabis can make it worse. If you have a medical recommendation to inhale cannabis, a vaporiser is the safer and more reliable method.

Be mindful of the theoretical increased risk of some cancers associated with cannabis use. As you are recovering from one cancer, you need to do all you can to reduce your risk factors for others.

Different types of cannabis plants have different effects and side effects. If you live in a country which does not have a medical marijuana program that tests and regulates the quality of the product, you may not know what you are buying.

If you decide to use cannabis, do not combine it with alcohol as the alcohol may exacerbate the side effects of cannabis.

If you are using cannabis your reaction times may be slower for hours, so driving or operating machinery could be dangerous.

Do not use cannabis in any form if you are pregnant or planning a pregnancy as it can damage a foetus and may increase the risk of some future childhood cancers. THC also crosses into breast milk, so cannabis use is contraindicated while you are breastfeeding.

If you have a family history of schizophrenia or other psychotic illness, cannabis is best avoided.

If you have a history of heart disease you need to be cautious because the adverse effects of cannabis on heart disease are not known.

ONCOLOGY MASSAGE

Massage can play an important role during your treatment and recovery from cancer. The largest published report on therapeutic massage was conducted at the Memorial Sloan Kettering Cancer Center in New York City. Patients were asked to report their symptoms before and after massage therapy using a 0–10 rating scale for pain, fatigue, stress/anxiety, nausea, depression and 'other'. Over a three-year period, 1290 patients were treated. Symptom scores were reduced by approximately 50 per cent. Outpatients improved about 10 per cent more than inpatients and benefits persisted throughout the duration of 48-hour follow-up. These data provided the first significant evidence that massage therapy provides a substantive and measurable improvement in cancer patients' symptoms.

The type of massage and the training of the massage therapist assume a far greater importance in the context of a cancer diagnosis. Oncology massage is a specialised modification of massage techniques to take into account the effects of the cancer itself and the various types and stages of cancer treatment.

Trained oncology massage therapists will consider the way a cancer affects the body and the side effects of cancer treatments, such as medications, surgery, chemotherapy and radiation, and modify their massage techniques in order to adapt for these factors. They will need to consider the amount of pressure to apply, what areas to avoid, how to adapt your position on the bed for comfort, how to adapt their style around recently formed scar tissue, and understand the possible effects of chemotherapy or medication on the potential for, say, bruising.

PURPOSE

If you have used massage in the past to ease muscular spasm, that may still be an aim of treatment. Massage can also be used as a part of a detox process, to help increase the range of motion of your spine or joints, relaxation, to help with anxiety management or depression, and to improve fatigue.

WHAT YOU NEED TO KNOW

Before looking for a massage therapist, ask your medical oncologist or GP if there is any contraindication to you having massage.

You need to ask about the qualifications of the massage therapist and where they studied. Different countries will have different qualifications. For massage therapists working with cancer patients, a higher level of training and experience is very important.

To find a qualified therapist, you could ask for a recommendation from your doctors, your local cancer support organisation or contact one of the professional massage associations. Ask specifically for a qualified oncology massage therapist.

It is important for you to be clear about what you want to achieve from the massage and to communicate that to the therapist. The therapist can then adjust their technique and treatment plan to accommodate your objective. Once you have progressed in your survivorship, meaning that you are past the acute treatment and recovery phase or you are in remission with normal blood counts, then you can resume regular types of massage therapy.

WHAT YOUR MASSAGE THERAPIST WILL NEED TO KNOW

The massage therapist will need information about you to work out the most appropriate treatment for you, but also to make sure the treatment is safe for you.

Make sure you have the following information:

- the site and type of cancer
- the type and timing of previous treatments such as surgery, radiotherapy or chemotherapy
- the type and timing of your current treatments
- whether you have a blood coagulation disorder, making you more vulnerable to bruising and internal haemorrhage

- if you are taking prescribed medications likely to increase the risk of bruising or bleeding: Coumadin, aspirin, clopidogrel, or heparin or the newer agents rivaroxaban and dabigatran etexilate
- if you have a low platelet count, as this also increases the risk of bruising or bleeding
- if you have metastases in bone or a recent fracture site
- whether you have any open wounds or areas of radiation dermatitis
- whether you have any physical mobility restrictions that will require special positioning for comfort.

In many of these situations, the oncology massage therapist will plan to avoid massage in some areas, or lighten the touch over regions of risk.

There is no evidence to suggest that massage therapy can spread cancer, although avoiding direct pressure over a tumour site is a sensible precaution. See page 235 for more information.

PET THERAPY

Our family includes two absolutely divine and devoted toy poodles, Paris and Lulu.

I know from speaking to patients who have pets that they are not only important members of the family but, like our poodles, they provide much-needed emotional support at times of sickness, loneliness, or sadness. To put it simply, they just make you feel better.

This primal connection has been used in different ways in health care in a mode of treatment variously known as pet therapy or animal activities therapy (AAT).

The use of pets in clinical situations has been studied in various aspects of cancer care. Animal-assisted therapy, including visits from certified therapy dogs, has been found to address some of the unmet needs in cancer patients. Research studies have shown positive benefits in reducing pain, psychological distress, and fatigue.

Pet therapy may be offered by your cancer care team at various stages and you could discuss with them whether it would be likely to benefit you.

If you have a pet, or you are thinking about pet ownership, there are some important considerations to keep in mind such as your ability to continue to care for the pet during your treatment.

If your immune system is likely to be compromised in any way, it is particularly important to make sure your animal has a veterinary check-up to ensure it is not carrying any potentially infectious diseases and its immunisations are up to date. Make sure claws are clipped short to avoid your skin being inadvertently scratched.

YOGA

I often recommend yoga to patients undergoing cancer treatment, not only as a form of physical exercise but also as a mind–body practice. Yoga originated in India about 5000 years ago, and was first described in Sanskrit. It was originally developed as a philosophy of living requiring significant personal effort and self-discipline, with the ultimate aim of reaching spiritual enlightenment. The underpinning philosophy is to replace old unconscious habits and thought patterns with new, more helpful patterns.

Yoga practice has become increasingly popular in the Western world as a form of exercise and relaxation since the late twentieth century. In practical terms, yoga combines breathing techniques, specific postures and movements, and meditation. There is a spectrum of yoga practice, from simply doing the postures and breathing through to adopting the yoga philosophy as a comprehensive lifestyle incorporating diet, physical movements, meditation and ethical living.

There are dozens of different types of yoga. Hatha yoga is the most commonly practised form in Western countries and it focuses mainly on postures (*asana*) and breathing exercises (*pranayama*). This style of yoga is fairly slow-paced and gentle, and involves basic yoga poses. Some of the other major styles of yoga you might encounter include:

- **Vinyasa** – Refers to breath-synchronised movement. It is more energetic than Hatha.
- **Ashtanga** – Fast paced and intense, a series of poses is performed flowing from one to the next in the same order each time.
- **Bikram** – A series of 26 postures practised in a very hot room to produce profuse sweating.
- **Iyengar** – Poses are held for a longer time, and may use equipment such as blocks or straps to adjust body alignment.
- **Viniyoga** – A one-on-one process of teaching where a personalised program is developed based on your age, state of health and physical condition.
- **Kundalini** – A form of yoga focusing on meditation and the effect of breathing on posture.

BENEFITS OF YOGA FOR CANCER
While yoga has been popular as a health philosophy for thousands of years on the Indian subcontinent, and as a wellness activity for

decades in the Western world, it is only recently that we have seen a concerted effort to apply scientific research methods to identify and prove the specific health benefits. Some of these efforts have been focused on the effect of yoga practice on symptom management, quality of life, and other measures for people during and after cancer treatment.

Yoga and radiotherapy for breast cancer

Radiotherapy is a common cancer-specific treatment used in women with breast cancer. A 2014 study at the University of Texas MD Anderson Cancer Center looked at the effect of yoga on women undergoing radiotherapy for breast cancer. One group was assigned to a yoga program, while a comparison group did stretching three times a week for the six weeks of radiotherapy. Yoga improved quality of life and day-to-day physical functioning, and reduced fatigue and depression. Yoga also reduced the level of the 'stress response hormone' cortisol. These benefits were still evident six months later in the yoga group.

Yoga and sleep

Between 30 to 90 per cent of cancer survivors have impaired sleep quality following treatment. A 2013 study in the US looked at the effect of yoga on sleep quality of cancer survivors who participated in a four-week yoga program consisting of *pranayama* (breathing exercises), sixteen gentle Hatha and restorative yoga *asanas* (postures), and meditation. People who participated in the yoga program reported that they had improved sleep quality and daytime functioning, and reduced use of sleep medication.

Yoga, fatigue and inflammation

According to research studies, practising yoga for as little as three months can reduce fatigue and lower inflammation in breast cancer survivors. At the six-month point of the study – three months after the formal yoga practice had ended – results showed that on average, fatigue was 57 per cent lower in women who had practised yoga compared to the non-yoga group, and their inflammation was reduced by up to 20 per cent.

The other health benefits of yoga:

- improves blood pressure and circulation
- improves general fitness
- helps stress management
- increases sense of wellbeing
- improves digestion
- may help improve asthma control
- increases joint flexibility, reducing stiffness
- reduces anxiety
- helps prevent osteoporosis (weight-bearing postures)
- helps prevent falls (improves balance).

PRECAUTIONS

If you are over 40, have not exercised for a long time, or your cancer or its treatment has limited your range of movement, consult your GP or seek out a yoga teacher who is accustomed to working with people with medical problems before you start a yoga program. Choose a yoga class and form of yoga to suit your age, state of health, and previous yoga experience, and inform your yoga teacher if you have any medical problems or injuries so he or she can adjust poses for you if necessary, or tell you which particular *asanas* to avoid.

Let your yoga teacher know if you are pregnant. Do not do bikram (hot) yoga if you are pregnant, or likely to be in the early stages of pregnancy.

You should always avoid postures or stretches that cause you pain.

Do not go to a yoga class within three or four hours of a meal.

Yoga is – or at least should be – non-competitive. You do not have to achieve the same level of performance as other, more experienced, yoga participants.

AROMATHERAPY MASSAGE

Aromatherapy massage is the addition of essential oils to massage oil. A major research review found that massage and aromatherapy massage confer short-term benefits on psychological wellbeing, and there was also some evidence of an effect on anxiety. Evidence is mixed as to whether aromatherapy enhances the effects of massage. The point is that there is no harm, so if you enjoy the aromas as part of the massage experience then go for it.

MUSIC THERAPY

Music therapy is a specialised healthcare discipline with university-trained therapists. Music therapy activities might involve passive listening, or active involvement in writing songs, discussing lyrics, or making music.

Music therapy has undergone some scientific scrutiny. A number of clinical trials have shown the benefit of music therapy for short-term pain, including cancer pain. Some studies have suggested that music therapy might help you decrease the need for pain medication.

Music therapy is available as a group experience, including in hospitals or community palliative care services. It is also available on an individual basis where the music therapist will select music based on your taste and preferences and the effect you want. For example, the music or activity might be designed to have a calming or an energising effect.

· PART FIVE ·

Symptoms and side effects of cancer treatment

Symptom Management

Where you are advised to have any cancer-specific treatment, you will need to have a comprehensive discussion about the possible side effects of the treatment and how to manage them as you go through the various stages of treatment.

Symptoms you are experiencing now, or symptoms you might expect to experience can be related to the activity of the cancer itself, or to its treatment – surgery, radiotherapy, chemotherapy, immunotherapy, or hormone therapy. The symptoms or health problems you experience as a result of treatment are called side effects, or adverse effects.

While the main goal of treatment is to eradicate or control your cancer, you need a parallel strategy to minimise or eliminate any uncomfortable or distressing symptoms that can occur as a consequence of the treatment.

We will step through the side effects and look at an integrative approach to managing each one. You may have one symptom or side effect, but it's more than likely you will experience a combination of several side effects. If you are able to take some preventive action, and if you get any side effects under control during the treatment process, you are more likely to be able to complete the full cancer-specific treatment plan. If a cancer treatment is too distressing, the treatment protocol may need to be altered or discontinued, so you can see how important it is to anticipate and manage adverse side effects.

Your cancer team will monitor your progress during treatment and you will be warned about signs or symptoms of a serious problem needing urgent medical assessment. Do not try to ride out these symptoms or manage them yourself without first seeking medical advice.

Symptoms and side effects needing urgent medical assessment include:

- elevated temperature of 38° C (100.4° F) or above
- shivering
- chest pain
- trouble breathing
- flu-like symptoms, such as muscle aches and pain
- bleeding gums
- nosebleeds or bleeding from other parts of the body
- mouth ulcers that stop you eating or drinking
- vomiting that continues despite taking anti-sickness medication
- loose bowel motions, or four or more bowel movements a day
- abdominal pain.

PAIN

I am going to deal with the issue of pain management first because pain is one of the most common, most feared and most distressing symptoms experienced by someone with cancer. Pain may be a direct result of the cancer itself, or related to the treatment of cancer, such as post-surgical pain.

When we look at how to best control cancer pain, we need to bear in mind all of the various physical, psychological, emotional, social, cultural, and spiritual factors that might be involved in your experience of pain. So that you can understand how to achieve the most effective pain relief, it is important to look at the cause of the pain as well as its mechanism, because different pain types respond differently to specific medications and other interventions, and can therefore guide decisions about the treatment you receive.

CAUSE OF PAIN

Pain can be:

- cancer-related – examples include metastatic disease in bone (or bone secondaries) and infiltration of nerves or organs by the cancer
- treatment-related – for example, painful mouth ulcers occurring as a side effect of chemotherapy
- non-cancer related – for example, from a pre-existing condition.

PAIN DIARY

Keep an accurate diary of your symptoms. This will help your doctor and other healthcare professionals to work out the cause of your pain. Make a note of the:

- **Location** – Where is the pain located in your body? Can you point to it, or is it difficult to localise? Does it travel from one part of your body to another?
- **Timing** – Does it happen during the day? Does it come on at night?
- **Onset** – What sets it off or makes it worse? For example, is it worse after meals? Do certain movements or postures make the pain worse?

- **Duration** – How long do the episodes of pain last? Is it intermittent, occasional, constant, always present with exacerbations?
- **Quality** – Would you describe the pain as dull, stabbing, aching, crushing, cramping?
- **Intensity** – How would you rate the intensity of the pain on a scale of 1–10 (10 being the worst pain)?
- **Relieving factors** – What relieves or finishes the pain? Does a particular movement or position help the pain to go away? Does the pain just go away after a time no matter what you do?
- **Associated features** – Are there any associated features such as nausea, vomiting, tingling, or numbness?
- **Treatments** – What treatments have you tried that worked? What treatments have you tried that did not work? Is your pain breaking through your current treatments?

INVESTIGATIONS

For your doctor, the most important part of working out what is causing your pain and what to do about it is to listen to your descriptions and look at the details in your diary. Sometimes the answer will be very obvious, but often you will need to have targeted investigations to work out the cause of the pain or the extent of the problem, or to confirm the clinical impression about what is going on. Ideally, there will be a correctable underlying problem.

Investigations usually involve some form of radiological imaging, such as X-ray, ultrasound, CT or MRI scanning. Your doctor might also want to arrange blood or urine tests or other pathology. The choice of investigations will be determined by what your doctor is looking for.

Starting effective pain relief or changing your current pain management plan should not be delayed while you are waiting for the results of these investigations.

INTEGRATIVE PAIN MANAGEMENT

Because of the range of factors that impact on pain, your pain management team will need to comprise practitioners with expertise in medical, surgical, psychological, pharmacological, anaesthetics, allied health, and integrative assessment and treatment. The choice of treatment or combination of therapies you decide on will depend on the underlying cause of your pain, how severe it is, the availability of skilled practitioners, what your treatment preference is, and what you are able to afford.

There may be a treatable cause of the pain which solves the problem so the first step is diagnosis. The goals of your treatment plan are first and foremost to relieve your pain, but also to help you to keep on with as many of your daily activities as possible and also to cope with the emotional or psychological consequences of pain.

Useful treatment modalities for you might include regional anaesthesia techniques involving nerve blocks, pharmaceutical pain relievers, acupuncture, herbal or nutritional remedies, and a variety of mind–body techniques.

The cancer treatment facility looking after your cancer-specific treatment will have some of these practitioners but may not be able to provide all the potentially useful treatments. For example, the hospital-based team may have an anaesthetist and other doctors who are skilled at pharmacological techniques, but they may not be able to provide acupuncture or meditation techniques. Your GP may be able to direct you to skilled practitioners in these disciplines.

So let's familiarise you with some of the available pain management techniques. Some will be very familiar to you already, while others may provide you with some new ideas.

NON-PHARMACOLOGICAL

I will go through the non-pharmacological therapies for pain management first. I recommend that you check with your medical team to make sure the treatments you choose are suitable for your condition, and whether there are any safety precautions you should be aware of. In addition to the non-pharmacological therapies listed here, aromatherapy (see page 243) and music therapy (see page 243) may also be useful in pain management.

Heat packs

You can buy hot packs or heating pads. You may find that a hot pack gives you some relief of musculoskeletal pain. Make sure you wrap the heat source in a towel to avoid direct contact with your skin, which may cause accidental burns. Take particular care if you have reduced sensation.

Do not use heat treatments on areas where you have recently had radiotherapy.

Cold packs

Cold packs can help to reduce swelling related to inflammation. Flexible, reusable cold packs conform to your body shape. Wrap the cold pack in a small towel to avoid direct contact with your skin. Remove the cold pack after fifteen minutes.

Avoid the use of cold packs if you have peripheral vascular disease (poor circulation in your extremities), or on tissue that has been damaged by radiotherapy.

Exercise

If you are suffering pain, the last thing you may feel like doing is exercise. By exercise, I mean movement. Movement helps to strengthen your muscles, improve your balance and coordination, improve circulation, and get stiff joints working. If you have significant physical health challenges, it is wise to see an exercise physiologist or rehabilitation physiotherapist who can tailor an activity or rehabilitation program that is mindful of your limitations but suitable for your condition. If there is a possibility of bone fracture, in particular if you have bone metastases, you will need careful and specific advice about resistance training and you will need to limit weight training.

You will also need medical advice on a suitable exercise program if you have anaemia, a low white cell count, a low platelet count, a fever or active infection, or if you have balance problems. If you do have any of these conditions, you will need the guidance of an experienced exercise physiologist to plan a safe exercise program for you. See more information in the chapter on exercise, page 307.

Yoga

A gentle yoga program may be a suitable activity at most stages of your treatment and recovery. You will need to let your yoga teacher know about your current health condition, and your program will need to be adjusted to account for any restrictions on your physical ability. See page 239 for more information about yoga.

Tai Chi

I often recommend tai chi or qi gong to patients who need to find a form of safe and gentle exercise to build their strength and fitness, or for people who need help to manage stress and anxiety. They are also fantastic forms of exercise for people who are a bit exercise-averse. You can get a really effective workout without feeling like you have been working too hard.

Both of these carefully choreographed mind–body practices originated in China as a martial art and are also known as 'moving meditation'. You can usually recognise a tai chi group. They will be outdoors in the early morning, with all the participants silently and slowly moving their arms and legs in coordinated, precise flowing movements.

The part of tai chi you cannot see is the meditative effect of the practice on the mind. It appears to be particularly good for improving psychological wellbeing, reducing stress, anxiety, depression and mood disturbance, and increasing self-esteem.

The physical benefits include improved bone density, heart and lung function, physical functioning, improved balance and reduced risk of falls, and improved immunity. With improved function and less pain, the need for pharmaceutical medication is also reduced, thereby reducing the risk of falls and adverse drug events, particularly in vulnerable elderly people.

I strongly advise you find an experienced teacher and have private lessons, or join a group. You can contact the Tai Chi Association for a recommendation. There are some excellent instructional DVDs too.

Transcutaneous Electrical Nerve Stimulation (TENS)

TENS machines can be useful for people with localised pain, usually as part of a comprehensive cancer pain management strategy. They are small battery-operated devices that send a low-voltage electrical current through the skin. This is thought to relieve pain in several ways: it makes the body release its own natural pain relievers called endorphins, and stimulates non-pain nerves that carry messages to the brain. This stimulation effectively scrambles or overwhelms the pain messages trying to get to the brain and reduces the perception of pain.

TENS is a low-risk intervention for pain. Your cancer treatment team will be able to advise on whether it is likely to be helpful for you. They can also give you instructions on the proper use of the machine. You may be able to borrow one for a short time to see if it works for you.

Acupuncture

Acupuncture is a part of Traditional Chinese Medicine that has been used for thousands of years. It has become increasingly popular in the West since the 1970s, and is now considered by most healthcare professionals to be a mainstream treatment.

Acupuncture involves the insertion of very fine needles into specific combinations of points on your body. The theory is that acupuncture changes the flow of energy (Qi) in your body to encourage the body to heal itself. It can also change your perception of pain. Sometimes a herb called moxa is heated over acupuncture points, a technique called 'moxibustion'.

Many of my patients use acupuncture for a variety of health problems, including symptomatic treatment of cancer pain. Some acupuncturists are qualified in Traditional Chinese Medicine, while some healthcare professionals such as doctors or physiotherapists have studied acupuncture techniques as a post-graduate qualification and integrate it into their treatment approaches.

At this stage, the formal research into the effectiveness of acupuncture in cancer care is lagging behind its popularity. But research studies are suggesting that acupuncture has a positive effect in managing cancer-related pain.

Select a well-qualified practitioner who is experienced in working with people with cancer and try a few sessions of acupuncture to see if it is effective for you.

Massage

Massage appears to be of benefit in reducing pain and the anxiety associated with it. If you have had cancer you need to make sure that your massage therapist has specific qualifications and experience in massage for people with cancer. (See also oncology massage, on page 235.)

Mind–body techniques
Other strategies for helping to manage pain include hypno-therapy, meditation, relaxation and guided imagery. These techniques need to be taught by a qualified professional, usually a registered psychologist.

Natural treatments
There are many herbs and natural supplements that can be bene-ficial for pain management. These include supplements such as fish oil, curcumin (an extract of turmeric root), and magnesium. Studies on these natural therapies are promising although more research is needed. When choosing a supplement it is important to seek professional advice from a qualified practitioner to ensure it is safe and that you are not wasting your money.

Some supplements may interact with your cancer or mainstream drug treatments (for example, curcumin and cyclo-phosphamide). Also, supplements vary in quality from brand to brand and need to be taken at appropriate doses to be effective and safe. See the chapter on herbs and supplements page 188.

PHARMACOLOGICAL PAIN MANAGEMENT
It is important to get your pain management right. Pain medica-tions do have side effects such as constipation and drowsiness, so non-pharmacological methods are very important in helping to minimise the amount of drug treatment you need to control your pain.

The use of medication will need to be individualised and constantly reviewed depending on your need for pain relief. I would advise you to discuss your pain management with your cancer-specific specialists at every visit. It is essential to adequately control pain and not try to 'grin and bear it'.

The choice of medication at any given time will depend on the level of severity of pain, the likely cause of your pain, the medications you have already tried and whether or not they have worked for you, and any previous or potential side effects.

It is important that you have adequate supplies of the medications you need for acute situations, chronic pain and breakthrough pain. You will need detailed written instructions on what medication to use and when.

Simple analgesics

Paracetamol is available without prescription and can provide useful pain relief alone for mild pain or used in combination with other drugs for more severe pain. Newer preparations enable three eight-hourly doses a day to provide 24 hours of cover. It is important not to exceed maximum recommended doses.

Non-steroidal anti-inflammatory drugs (NSAIDs) can be useful. I mention this class of drugs because they are commonly prescribed when the possibility of an inflammatory or musculo-skeletal component to the pain exists. Examples of NSAIDs include ibuprofen, naproxen, diclofenac and celecoxib.

Serious side effects can be a problem with NSAIDs and this is the main impediment to them being prescribed as first line analgesics. Side effects of particular concern are stomach and gut irritation and bleeding, increased blood pressure, reduced kidney function, and fluid retention.

Opioids

Opioids are the mainstay of cancer pain management. Opioids include tramadol, morphine, codeine, oxycodone and pethidine. Your cancer care team will speak to you in detail about these medications but it is important to be aware of some basic information about them:

- 'Start low, go slow.' Use the lowest effective dose and increase slowly, depending on your response, and only under careful supervision.
- Opioids should be used around the clock rather than 'as needed'. This has become much easier with the availability of slow-release preparations of morphine, oxycodone, fentanyl and similar drugs.
- Use 'breakthrough' medications to deal with exacerbations or breakthroughs of pain. These medications will be in rapid-acting form rather than slow-acting or slow-release form.
- Prevent constipation. Most people will experience constipation with opioids. You will probably need to take regular laxatives at the same time as the opioids.
- Be aware of the common side effects of taking opioids, such as constipation, nausea and drowsiness, and talk to your doctor about them.
- When you start or increase the dose of an opioid, your ability to drive safely can be affected. Once the dose is stable, you will be advised when it is safe to drive, provided you are not drowsy.
- Alcohol will increase the sedative effect of an opioid.
- Opioids have a high potential for dependence and addiction so your use and withdrawal of medication will need to be closely monitored by your pain management team.

Adjuvant drugs
Sometimes simple analgesics and opioid drugs are not enough on their own. This is particularly the case with nerve pain.

The traditional classes of drugs that can be added are the anti-convulsants and tricyclic antidepressants. Anticonvulsants are the drugs primarily used for treatment of epilepsy, such as carbamaze-pine, sodium valproate, and gabapentin. All these drugs have side effects and the potential for drug interactions, and some require monitoring of levels or other blood tests.

NAUSEA AND VOMITING

Nausea and vomiting are common side effects of chemotherapy. As is the case with pain management, there are non-pharmaco-logical and pharmacological options available.

Potent anti-nausea drugs (antiemetics) such as metoclopra-mide or ondansetron (Zofran) will often be necessary to manage chemotherapy-associated nausea and vomiting, and these medications will be prescribed in anticipation so that you are prepared. Antiemetics have improved enormously over recent decades and some are available in intravenous, tablet or wafer form.

Adjunctive therapies can reduce the amount of medication you need, or improve your tolerance of chemotherapy. They include:

- **Acupuncture** and acupuncture point stimulation can be very effective and safe in relieving nausea associated with chemotherapy. Like all treatments, acupuncture works better for some people than for others. It is worth trying.
- **Ginger** (*Zingiber officinale*) has an anti-nausea effect. It has a long history of use in Traditional Chinese Medicine, Ayurveda, and Arabic herbal traditions. It has been used to help digestion and treat stomach upset, diarrhoea and nausea for more than 2000 years. It can be taken as dried root or as a tea infusion (4–6 slices steeped for 30 minutes in boiling water). It is unlikely to be effective on its own for

chemo-related nausea and vomiting. Tell your doctor if you are taking ginger before having surgery.

- **Baical skullcap** (*Scutellaria baicalensis*) is a herb with an antiemetic effect, which suggests a role in managing nausea and vomiting. It can be taken in conjunction with ondansetron, as there are no reported interactions between these two substances.

- **Astragalus** – A Cochrane review of Chinese herbs for chemotherapy side effects in colorectal cancer patients showed that astragalus can reduce nausea, vomiting and leucopenia (lowered white blood cell count). It can be taken in conjunction with ondansetron, as there are no reported interactions between these two substances.

- **Vitamin B$_6$** is often used for pregnancy-induced nausea and may also have benefit in combating nausea from chemotherapy. One study showed benefit when vitamin B$_6$ injections were given with acupuncture in ovarian cancer patients.

- **Mind–body techniques** such as hypnosis and mindfulness meditation may help you to cope with nausea. These need to be taught to you by a qualified professional.

- **Nutrition** – When you have periods of nausea you will need to try to maintain your nutrition.

- **Cold food** or food at room temperature may be more appealing than hot food, as the smell of cooked food may trigger nausea. Try to choose foods that do not have a strong aroma.

- **Small quantities of food** at frequent intervals during the day may be easier to manage than larger quantities, and eat slowly, chewing thoroughly.

- Nausea can be reduced by eating small amounts of **salty or**

sour foods, such as lemon or sour pickles. Avoid fatty or sweet foods.

- **Cool drinks** – Regular sips of clear, cool drinks can help to reduce nausea. Drink between meals rather than with food.

ANXIETY AND DEPRESSION

Treatment for cancer is often physically and emotionally taxing. Beyond the sense of fear and sadness you might expect, clinically diagnosed anxiety and depression are frequently associated with a diagnosis of cancer and its treatment.

Research shows that 20–35 per cent of people with cancer experience ongoing depression, and 15–23 per cent experience anxiety. So you and your support team need to anticipate its possibility and be aware of the early signs.

Anxiety, depression and substance-use disorder often occur in combination. For example, substances like alcohol or cannabis might be used as a form of self-medication in an attempt to relieve symptoms, or a person with disabling anxiety may develop depression.

SYMPTOMS OF DEPRESSION

You need to be able to recognise the symptoms of depression:

- a deep feeling of sadness or a marked loss of interest or pleasure in activities
- changes in appetite that result in weight loss or gain
- insomnia or oversleeping
- loss of energy or increased fatigue
- restlessness or irritability
- feelings of worthlessness or inappropriate guilt
- difficulty thinking, concentrating or making decisions
- thoughts of death or suicide or attempts at suicide.

For more information about anxiety, depression and emotionally coping with cancer see part two, 'Dealing with cancer emotionally'.

WHERE TO GET HELP

Your GP is a good place to start. If you are diagnosed with anxiety or depression, you will qualify for a mental healthcare plan. Under these plans, Medicare in Australia provides some subsidy for counselling with a qualified psychologist.

Counselling will help you to identify and understand early life traumas or recent life circumstances, including your cancer, that might be contributing to your feelings. A psychologist will also help you to think differently about situations in a way that helps you manage and avoid anxiety. This is called cognitive behaviour therapy, or CBT. You may also learn self-treating techniques such as breathing exercises and relaxation.

Activities like tai chi and yoga can also be helpful.

Mindfulness is a thinking technique that helps you to alleviate anxiety and depression and more fully engage with life here and now. This needs to be taught by an expert.

Massage therapy can be useful for relaxation and easing of muscle tension. Medical or psychological assessment will determine if antidepressant medication is necessary.

OTHER SUPPORT

To help build your defence against depression and anxiety, if you have time try to set up your support network at the time of your cancer diagnosis and definitely before treatment commences. In addition to a support network, it is important to have at least some preliminary counselling to help you understand exactly what the treatment process involves and to help prepare you for the practical ways of managing any side effects, including the emotional repercussions of treatment.

FATIGUE

Fatigue associated with chemotherapy and radiotherapy is common and often underestimated. Cancer-related fatigue is different to the usual 'oh I've had such a busy day today!' brand of tiredness. Simple day-to-day activities like making a phone call or doing the grocery shopping can become formidable tasks. You may feel physically weak or exhausted, even after a long sleep. Your limbs might feel heavy and hard to move. You might feel irritable or frustrated and have trouble concentrating.

In the case of chemotherapy delivered in cycles, the fatigue is usually at its worst in the days following each cycle of treatment, and improves towards the next treatment, when the pattern starts over. With radiotherapy, fatigue usually gets worse over the course of treatment and it can then take several months to get your usual energy levels back.

Surgery, hormone therapy, and immunotherapy can also create fatigue as a side effect. Sometimes the cancer itself is the reason for the fatigue.

The causes of fatigue are biological and psychological. It is likely that inflammatory substances called cytokines (in particular TNFa and IL-6) in your body are related to fatigue. There may be several causes of fatigue and treating one may not entirely solve the problem. In many cases a specific treatable cause is not found, so you have to keep trying to figure out the best way to manage this debilitating symptom.

Some of the underlying causes of fatigue that can be corrected include nutritional deficiency, anaemia, medication side effects, insomnia, underlying infection and depression. So the first thing you need to do is let your GP know that fatigue is a problem and he or she will arrange investigations to see if there is an underlying cause. Investigations might include a full blood analysis, iron studies, vitamin B_{12} level, thyroid function tests, scans and other tests that will be decided upon based on your medical history and what the GP suspects might be the problem.

Some medications and adjuvant therapies such as hormone-suppressing treatments can cause fatigue. If this is the case, discuss it with your GP or oncologist and see if there is a different medication or treatment that might give the same benefits without the fatigue side effect, or if there are complementary treatments that can counter the side effect.

MANAGING CANCER-RELATED FATIGUE

Anticipate that fatigue is likely to be a factor during treatment and modify your planned activities in advance. This will mean taking some time off work, reducing your exercise intensity, and making sure you get plenty of sleep. Check your diary for any unnecessary or burdensome activities or responsibilities and cancel them or delegate to others for the time being. In addition:

- Identify and treat any underlying causes of fatigue where that is possible.
- Pace your activities and intersperse rest periods with gentle exercise. Try reading or listening to music as energy-conserving activities too.
- Enlist the help of friends and family for daily chores where possible.
- Avoid alcohol, caffeine and tobacco.
- Check your nutrition and ensure you include plenty of fluids and fresh organic fruit and vegetables, as well as nutrient-rich foods and complex carbohydrates. A dietitian will be able to assess your nutritional input to see if there is anything that you can do to optimise your nutritional status.

- If you are having difficulty sleeping, see the chapter on sleep (page 360) for more detailed advice.
- Cognitive behavior therapy with a qualified psychologist will help you to address underlying anxiety and fear.

HERBS AND SUPPLEMENTS FOR FATIGUE

American ginseng (*Panax quinquefolius*)

American ginseng taken twice daily has been shown to improve fatigue in people undergoing cancer treatment. In a recent study, researchers demonstrated a strong clinical benefit equivalent to at least a 30 per cent improvement compared with people taking a placebo.

Chinese medicinal mushroom or reishi mushroom (*Ganoderma lucidum*)

In a recent pilot study the spores of the popular Ganoderma mushroom showed promise in relieving fatigue in cancer survivors, particularly in breast cancer survivors suffering from the side effects of oestrogen-blocking therapies such as tamoxifen. A study in China found that a preparation of Ganoderma spores reduced the levels of inflammatory cytokines TNFa and IL-6 and improved fatigue in women with breast cancer who were taking tamoxifen.

Curcumin (*turmeric*)

Curcumin has known anti-inflammatory properties and preliminary studies are showing that it has potential in relieving cancer-related fatigue.

Astragalus

Astragalus is a herb used frequently as an adjuvant in cancer care. A special preparation of astragalus has been shown to have a positive benefit in combating cancer-related fatigue. This study was looking at an intravenous infusion, but astragalus is most commonly taken orally.

L-carnitine
L-carnitine (taken orally, 6 g per day for four weeks) has been shown to improve cancer-related fatigue and quality of life in people undergoing cancer treatment.

ACUPUNCTURE
Acupuncture does seem to help some people with cancer-related fatigue. Some studies have certainly found a benefit, but at this stage the evidence of its effectiveness is not strong overall. My advice if you want to try acupuncture would be to have some sessions with an experienced acupuncturist to see if it helps you.

PHARMACOLOGICAL
Pharmacological approaches to cancer-related fatigue (such as Ritalin or corticosteroids) have so far been limited by ineffectiveness or adverse side effects. Similarly, antidepressant medications have not been shown to be effective for cancer-related fatigue.

CHEMO BRAIN
'Chemo brain' is a term used to describe the effect of chemotherapy on your brain's ability to function normally. These changes might only last during the course of treatment and for a short time after, or the effect may be prolonged. This side effect seems to be a feature of some types of chemotherapy. See page 150 for a fuller discussion.

CONSTIPATION

Constipation is a term used to describe infrequent bowel movements with a hard consistency or difficulty passing stools, and is a common symptom associated with cancer and cancer treatment. Most cases can be simply managed with diet and lifestyle changes, but for the more resistant cases constipation needs to be treated with medication.

Constipation associated with cancer can be caused by low food intake, low fluid intake, medication side effect (especially opioid painkillers), lack of exercise, depression, and reluctance to open your bowels because it is painful or inconvenient.

APPROACHES TO MANAGING CONSTIPATION

Your GP will consider all possible causes for your constipation, but it is important to address the most common causes first, as the solution can be simple and practical:

- Fibre intake. Look at the amount of grains, cereals and fibre in your diet. You can add psyllium or oats, and make sure there is plenty of variety of fruits and vegetables.
- Eat frequent small amounts during the day, chewing thoroughly.
- Drink at least six cups of fluids during the day including water, herbal teas, tea, coffee, fruit juices, soup or other liquids.
- Attempt to increase your physical activity if you can.
- If you have been prescribed opioid (codeine or morphine) medications, you can expect constipation is likely to be a problem and make changes to your diet and start taking a laxative as a preventive.

MEASURES TO PREVENT
AND MANAGE CONSTIPATION

Remember that laxatives are only a symptom-relieving measure and will not actually address any underlying cause of your constipation, although as a temporary or even long-term measure they can provide welcome relief.

Bulk-forming laxatives include psyllium mixed with water or sprinkled into cereal, or Metamucil (processed and flavoured psyllium), flaxseed (*Linum usitatissimum*) powder or seeds, fenugreek (*Trigonella foenum-graecum*) or barley.

Stimulant laxatives such as senna (*Cassia acutifolia, C. angustifolia, C. senna*) and *Cascara segrada*. Senna is a component of some laxatives and should not be taken long-term.

Rhubarb root (*Rheum officinale* or *R. palmatum*) can also be used as a stimulating laxative.

Osmotic laxatives such as lactulose or magnesium citrate or **stool softeners** (Coloxyl or Coloxyl with Senna) might be useful.

Probiotic supplementation with lactobacillus and bifidobacterium can assist gut function.

You may find that constipation continues to be a problem. Your GP may arrange further investigations.

There are specialised laboratories that can run a detailed analysis of your stool sample to see whether you have the right balance of microflora or good bacteria in your gut. This test can help to tailor the correct probiotic, probiotic mix, or dietary changes to return your gut to normal function.

LYMPHOEDEMA

The lymphatic system forms an essential part of the circulation of fluids in the body and is part of the immune system. It involves a network of tiny channels throughout the body that carry a clear fluid called lymph. Lymphatic fluid collects viruses, bacteria and other waste material then drains back to the lymph nodes, which respond by filtering out these harmful substances.

Lymphoedema can develop when the delicate lymphatic vessels are damaged by a procedure such as surgery or radiotherapy, disrupting the normal lymphatic drainage. The lymphatic circulation can also be blocked when a tumour grows and blocks the lymphatic channels.

When lymphoedema develops, the affected area becomes swollen, heavy, uncomfortable and less mobile. Lymphoedema usually involves a limb, although it can affect more central body areas, and can occur during or soon after treatment, or sometimes its onset can be delayed.

A common example is lymphoedema in the arm following treatment for breast cancer, where one or more of the lymph nodes in the armpit are removed to assess whether the cancer has spread there. If the remaining lymphatic vessels are unable to compensate, or if the removal of lymphatic tissue is extensive, the arm on that side is likely to swell up.

PREVENTION

It is not always possible to prevent lymphoedema, but there are some things you can do to reduce the risk of infection developing:

- Scrupulous attention to skincare, including twice daily moisturising.
- Carry a topical antiseptic and apply it to any small cuts or grazes in your skin.
- Careful nail hygiene, including careful manicuring and never ever biting your nails or the skin around your cuticles.
- Wear gloves for activities where your hands are likely to suffer minor injuries (gardening and cooking).

- Avoid sunburn.
- Wear comfortable shoes with no pressure areas.
- Wear shoes when you are outdoors to avoid injury.
- Select socks (preferably cotton) carefully so they do not have tight bands or pressure areas.
- Avoid restrictive clothing such as tight stockings, socks, underwear.
- Remind health professionals to avoid procedures such as blood pressure measurement, injections or taking blood on the side that has previously been subject to lymphatic damage, whether you have lymphoedema or not.
- Report any signs of infection in the affected limb (redness, pain, swelling, elevated temperature) immediately to your GP.

TREATMENT

The aim of lymphoedema treatment is to control swelling, prevent infection, decrease pain and other complications, and maintain the function of your limbs. You will need to see a specially qualified lymphoedema therapist who will advise you on a comprehensive treatment program that might involve specialised massage, elastic bandaging, exercises and skin care.

Specialised lymphoedema massage

Manual lymphatic drainage is combined with specialised multi-layered bandaging to reduce swelling. The massage technique uses directed, very light-touch pressure rhythmically to the skin to stimulate the opening of lymphatic channels. At the conclusion of the massage session, the bandaging is applied. When the limb volume is reduced as far as possible, a pressure garment (stocking or sleeve) will be custom-fitted and worn every day.

Pressure garments

Lymphoedema sleeves or stockings need to be accurately fitted to your individual size. They are designed so that there is a gradient pressure difference, with highest pressure near the fingers or toes, reducing up the limb to encourage movement of lymphatic fluid towards the body.

Exercise for lymphoedema

Exercise is important for general wellbeing, emotional health and improved survival after a cancer diagnosis. (See the chapter on exercise, page 307.) Looking at lymphoedema specifically, gentle muscle contraction will help lymphatic drainage and aerobic exercise encourages lymph vessels to flow more efficiently.

You might feel reluctant to start exercising if you have lymphoedema, but studies on women after breast cancer treatment have shown that you can safely do aerobic (including upper body) exercises, even if you have lymphoedema.

Weight training is also safe. It reduces symptoms of lymphoedema and increases muscle strength. Remember not to be too ambitious at the start, and build up gradually. I would advise you to see an exercise physiologist or physiotherapist for a supervised safe exercise program, at least initially.

Healthy weight

There is some evidence that lymphoedema will improve if you lose weight when you have been overweight, either through reduced energy intake or a low-fat diet. Weight loss also improves the responsiveness to lymphoedema treatment.

Low-level laser therapy

Low-level laser therapy of the whole limb, two to five sessions a week for two to three weeks is worth trying. A study found that low-level laser to the armpit of women who had lymphoedema after breast cancer treatment was effective in reducing the volume of the affected limb, reducing fluid excess in the tissues, and improving tissue softening in about one-third of cases.

HERBAL THERAPIES

Horse chestnut standardised extract contains escin, a plant compound that is well tolerated and has traditional use in strengthening the tissues of the lymph vessels, capillaries, and veins. It may be useful as an adjunctive treatment for lymphoedema and does not have any known side effects.

Citrus bioflavonoids have also shown benefit. One study has shown efficacy of bioflavonoids and a bioflavonoid-rich herb, butcher's broom, for lymphoedema post breast cancer surgery.

PHARMACEUTICAL THERAPIES

There are no pharmaceutical medications that have been shown to reduce lymphoedema. Do not take diuretic medications because they don't work for this type of swelling.

You will need to be alert to early signs of infection and start appropriate antibiotics promptly. For more serious infections, intravenous antibiotics might be necessary.

NUTRITIONAL DEFICIENCY

The side effects of chemotherapy include loss of appetite, nausea, and an altered sense of taste and smell. These symptoms can impact on your nutritional status, because it can be hard to eat a wide enough range of healthy foods if you just don't feel like eating.

During chemotherapy you will need to follow medical advice about controlling nausea and vomiting. When you do have nausea and vomiting, you need to pay particular attention to nutrition.

You can adjust your diet to emphasise the foods you are able to eat that will give you energy and important micronutrients. A pre-emptive visit to a dietitian with experience in dealing with people going through cancer treatment is a good idea.

See page 323, the chapter on nutrition for more information.

MOUTH ULCERS

Mouth ulcers from cancer treatment are painful and can make it difficult to talk, breathe, eat and swallow. While it may not be possible to completely prevent mouth ulcers, there are some measures you can take prior to treatment to reduce the number and severity. For example, if you smoke, even just occasionally, now is the time to stop.

Arrange a dental check and thorough dental hygiene treatment before chemotherapy, or radiotherapy aimed at the head and neck. Good oral hygiene will be essential throughout treatment. Some other steps you can take include:

- Rinse your mouth with filtered water (with a small amount of added salt or bicarbonate of soda) every two hours while you are awake.
- Low-dose oral glutamine supplementation during and after chemotherapy significantly reduces both the duration and severity of chemotherapy-associated stomatitis (mouth inflammation). Swish the solution around your mouth and swallow.
- Use a soft-bristle toothbrush to clean your teeth after every meal. If your platelet count is adequate, floss with unwaxed floss daily.
- Use an oral lubricant.
- Avoid mouthwashes containing alcohol as they irritate the mouth lining.
- It is best to avoid drinking alcohol (including medication

containing alcohol) while you are undergoing any treatments that are likely to cause mouth inflammation or ulcers.

- Apply lip balm regularly.
- Maintain a good nutrition level focused on high-protein and high-calorie foods that are soft and/or semi-liquid, and soft or cooked fruit and vegetables.
- Avoid foods that are sharp or brittle, spicy, or hot.
- Avoid acidic food, such as tomatoes, citrus fruits, soft drinks, etc
- Carafate (sucralfate) can be applied directly to ulcers to assist in healing.

Mouth ulcers can also be the result of infection with the fungus candida. If this is the case, ask your doctor or cancer nurse to confirm that candida is present and if so, you will need to treat it with antifungal lozenges, drops or oral tablets. Examples of antifungals include nystatin or oral tablets called diflucan for more extensive infections.

Acupuncture has been shown to help relieve the symptoms caused by radiation-induced dry mouth (xerostomia). Low-energy laser therapy is used in some specialised facilities to heal ulcers.

SKIN INFLAMMATION FROM RADIOTHERAPY

Radiation dermatitis is a skin inflammation caused by burns from radiotherapy. The dermatitis does heal and fade with time but there are some effective treatments.

Curcumin (*Curcuma longa*) from the herb turmeric, may be able to reduce the burden of dermatitis in patients undergoing radiotherapy for breast cancer. A clinical trial involving 30 women with breast cancer showed that daily oral supplementation with turmeric reduced the severity of radiation dermatitis and other side effects of treatment. The patients taking curcumin had significantly less radiation dermatitis than those in the placebo group. Of those taking curcumin, only 28.6 per cent had moist skin loss at the end of radiation treatment, compared to 87.5 per cent taking placebo.

Calendula ointment applied twice daily was found to be superior to trolamine (a topical pharmaceutical non-steroidal anti-inflammatory agent) for the prevention of skin toxicity, interruption of treatment, patient satisfaction, pain relief and dermatitis.

Also topical **aloe vera** has shown a benefit in relieving radiation-induced dermatitis.

REDUCED IMMUNE FUNCTION

Your immune system inevitably takes a beating during cancer treatment. Not only are your body's defences working overtime to try to battle the cancer, but cancer-specific treatments also depress your immune function.

Lifestyle measures are important. (See the chapter on immunity, page 355.)

STRESS MANAGEMENT AND IMMUNITY

Stress management through a variety of mind–body interventions can help to support your immune system during cancer treatment. (See the chapter on mental health, page 65.)

HERBS FOR IMMUNE SUPPORT

Some herbs are useful in boosting your immunity alongside your cancer-specific treatment.

ASTRAGALUS (HUANG-QI)

Astragalus (huang-qi) is considered very safe and is commonly used by cancer patients to enhance the effectiveness of chemotherapy and reduce its associated side effects. It is also used to boost immune function.

Baical skullcap and withania might be useful to combat reduced immune function also.

A Cochrane review of Chinese herbs for chemotherapy side effects in colorectal cancer patients showed that astragalus can reduce nausea, vomiting, and prevent a low white cell count.

HEPATOTOXICITY

Milk thistle (*Silybum marianum* or **silymarin**) has a liver protective effect in chemotherapy, speeding up the regeneration of new liver cells.

Placebo-controlled clinical studies have shown that silymarin is effective in lowering raised liver enzymes in alcoholic liver disease and it has also been shown to be useful for liver cirrhosis. Milk thistle has been shown to reduce liver toxicity associated with chemotherapy in children with acute lymphoblastic leukaemia and cisplatin-induced kidney toxicity.

Coenzyme Q10 provides some protection against hepatotoxicity during cancer treatment.

KIDNEY (RENAL) TOXICITY

Some chemotherapy agents and other treatments such as antibiotics have the potential to cause kidney damage, which can lead to renal failure. This is most likely to occur in older people, especially those with pre-existing kidney disease, and people taking multiple medications. The anti-cancer drugs most likely to cause kidney damage include cisplatin, carboplatin, and nitrosureas (such as carmustine lomustine [CCNU] and semustine), mitomycin and methotrexate – especially if high doses are used.

Your kidney function will be assessed before treatment and monitored throughout. If blood tests show that your renal function is being impacted, the dose or the type of chemotherapy will be changed.

Signs of renal damage include abnormal blood tests (electrolytes, creatinine, eGFR), passing less urine, swollen hands and feet/ankles, headache, fatigue and weakness, nausea and/or vomiting, and increased blood pressure.

PROTECTING YOUR KIDNEYS

The medical team may increase intravenous fluids to help flush chemotherapy through your kidneys. You will need to maintain oral intake of fluids too.

Avoid salty foods including processed foods with added salt, and do not add salt to your cooking or to your prepared food.

An antioxidant medication called amifostine may be given to protect the kidneys when high doses of the chemotherapy agent cisplatin are given.

HERBS AND SUPPLEMENTS

Milk thistle (*Silybum marianum* or silymarin) is used to prevent and treat liver toxicity and has also been shown to reduce kidney toxicity caused by the chemotherapy agent cisplatin.

L-carnitine is a naturally occurring compound that combats oxidative stress and inflammation. There are many studies reporting the protective effect of L-carnitine against the toxicity of radiotherapy and chemotherapy agents, including doxorubicin and cisplatin. One animal study compared the protective capacity of L-carnitine with amifostine and found that L-carnitine worked better.

HAIR LOSS

Chemotherapy can cause some hair loss. See page 133 for information on hair loss.

INTRAVENOUS VITAMIN C

Vitamin C is a powerful antioxidant, but when used in high doses that can only be achieved intravenously it acts as 'pro-oxidant' and has been shown to have toxic effects against cancer cells.

High dose vitamin C should be avoided with chemotherapy agents methotrexate, DTIC and doxorubicin.

See page 173 for further information on intravenous vitamin C.

POSSIBLE ORAL COMPLICATIONS OF CANCER TREATMENT

Oral complications occur in virtually all patients receiving radiation for head and neck malignancies, in approximately 80 per cent of haematopoietic (blood-forming) stem cell transplant recipients, and in nearly 40 per cent of patients receiving chemotherapy.

Some problems are temporary and only occur during the actual treatment process. Other problems created as a side effect of treatment are permanent. These will need to be prevented where possible and managed long term.

The possible problems you could experience with your mouth as a result of cancer treatment include soreness and ulceration, bleeding gums, infection, alterations in taste, dental decay, poor nutrition and dry mouth (xerostomia).

Chemotherapy can cause you to develop a dry mouth due to thickened saliva, or the reduced or absent flow of saliva. Dryness of the mouth increases your risk of infection and compromises your ability to speak, chew or swallow. Persistent dry mouth also increases your risk of dental decay.

Medications other than chemotherapy can also affect the function of your salivary glands. The most common culprits are some types of antidepressants, antihistamines, decongestants, blood pressure medications, and drugs for urinary incontinence and Parkinson's disease. Smoking can worsen dry mouth symptoms.

High-dose radiotherapy in the head and neck region can damage salivary glands and cause lifelong problems with dry mouth and dental decay. If you have permanent damage to your salivary glands resulting in dry mouth, you will be advised to do daily fluoride application, ensure healthy nutrition, and maintain careful oral hygiene for the rest of your life.

TRISMUS

Trismus is a tight contraction of your jaw muscles, which makes it difficult or impossible to open your mouth or chew food or clean your teeth. Trismus hampers speech because your jaw is clenched shut, and it also makes it very difficult to have any dental procedures.

Trismus tends to develop slowly over time and can occur as a result of scarring or swelling from surgery or inflammation, and scarring in the region of the jaw from radiotherapy. The tumours related to this type of radiation include the nasopharynx, base of the tongue, salivary gland, and cancers of the maxilla (cheekbones) or mandible (jawbone).

Managing trismus

If you are noticing signs of trismus during treatment, alert your medical team sooner rather than later. Early treatment, before scar tissue hardens, will give you the best chance of maintaining your ability to move your jaw. There are physical therapies and trismus devices available that will carefully and gradually stretch your mouth open. The cost of devices and treatments varies widely.

TASTE ALTERATIONS

You might experience changes in your perception of the taste of foods, ranging from unpleasant to tasteless. This side effect is not inevitable and depends on the type of chemotherapy, the stage of treatment, and the type of tumour that is being treated.

Caffeinated foods and drinks, red meat, and citrus fruits or juices are the foods most likely to be reported as 'aversive' during chemotherapy.

NEUROTOXICITY (NERVE DAMAGE)

Neurotoxicity can cause persistent deep aching and burning pain that can feel like a toothache, but no dental or mucosal source can be found. This can be a side effect of some classes of chemotherapy drugs, such as the vinca alkaloids vinblastine, vincristine, vindesine and vinorelbine.

POOR NUTRITION

If you have difficulty with chewing and swallowing because of any of the mouth problems caused by cancer and its treatment, it is likely to affect your ability to eat a range of foods. Whether it is from loss or change of your sense of taste, or pain and discomfort of your mouth tissues, or trouble chewing because of restriction of jaw movement, being unable to eat comfortably will affect your ability to maintain the healthy nutrition you need to get through treatment and recover your wellness so it needs to be anticipated and steps taken to prevent oral problems where possible.

STEPS YOU CAN TAKE
VISIT YOUR DENTIST

Make a preventive dental health visit to your dentist, taking with you the plan and dates for your treatment including the type of chemotherapy and the site and dose of radiotherapy. If possible, make the appointment at least a month before the start of chemotherapy. This is an opportunity for your dentist to identify and treat any tooth decay or gum disease.

BUY A NEW EXTRA-SOFT TOOTHBRUSH

If the bristles on your toothbrush are too harsh, they can cause trauma to delicate oral tissues and make inflammation and ulceration worse.

GLUTAMINE 'SWISH AND SWALLOW'

Glutamine is an amino acid that is an essential part of your diet, found mostly in dairy products, eggs, soybeans, fish, miso, yoghurt and green leafy vegetables.

Experimental studies have shown that oral supplementation with glutamine can significantly decrease the severity of chemotherapy-induced stomatitis (mouth inflammation). Glutamine powder can be mixed as a suspension and then swished around the mouth and swallowed.

RIBOFLAVIN (VITAMIN B$_2$)

One of the symptoms of riboflavin (vitamin B$_2$) deficiency is mouth ulcers (oral mucositis). Chemotherapy is known to interfere with the action of riboflavin, so it follows that riboflavin supplementation may help prevent the mouth ulcers caused by some forms of chemotherapy.

MOUTHWASH

Avoid commercial mouthwashes while you are having chemotherapy, particularly the ones containing alcohol. Rinse your mouth with a baking soda and salt solution, followed by a plain water rinse several times a day. (Use ¼ teaspoon each of baking soda and salt in 500 ml of warm water.) Leave out the salt if you have mouth ulcers.

FLOSS

Floss between your teeth gently every day, especially after eating. If your gums are sore, avoid those areas but keep flossing the other teeth. If your gums are bleeding, ask your doctor or cancer nurse to check your platelet level as a low platelet count can cause gum bleeding.

FLUORIDE GEL

Ask your dentist about a fluoride gel to use each day. This can be applied with a toothbrush as a ribbon of gel, or placed in a mouthguard tray and left in place over your teeth for 10 minutes. Do not eat or drink for 30 minutes after applying the fluoride.

JAW EXERCISES

Exercise the jaw muscles three times a day to prevent and treat jaw stiffness from radiation. Open and close the mouth as far as possible without causing pain; repeat 20 times.

DIET

The right foods are needed for healing to take place. A preparatory visit to a dietitian is worthwhile to make an eating plan. Ensure you are eating plenty of fruit and vegetables and that you have high-quality sources of protein such as eggs, organic chicken or meat, fish and tofu. Fruit and vegetables might have to be mashed, softened or cooked while you have active mouth sores.

Prepare moist softened foods rather than hard crunchy foods while you are at risk of mouth sores. Eat foods and drink fluids that are at room temperature rather than too hot or too cold, which might be uncomfortable for your mouth.

Use a straw to drink. This will reduce contact with painful areas in your mouth.

WATCH OUT FOR CANDIDA

The fungal infection candidiasis or thrush is common during chemotherapy treatment. It shows up as white patches on the tongue, cheeks or palate. Candida can be treated with antifungal medication in the form of drops in your mouth, or oral medication if there is a suspicion that the fungal infection extends beyond your mouth. Candida infection may be prevented by swishing a suspension of probiotic, such as lactobacillus/bifidobacterium, three times a day.

MEDICATION

An intravenous pharmaceutical medication called palifermin (Kepivance) stimulates the growth of cells on the surface of your mouth. This is approved for the treatment of mouth ulcers caused by treatment for blood cancers. Kepivance is a man-made form of a naturally occurring substance called Keratinocyte Growth Factor, sometimes shortened to KGF, which stimulates the growth of the uppermost layer of cells that line your mouth, digestive tract and skin.

Topical anaesthetic gel can help to reduce severe pain from ulceration but does not heal the ulcer.

WHAT TO AVOID

In a simple checklist:

- alcohol
- mouthwashes containing alcohol as the alcohol will irritate your mouth lining and exacerbate dryness

- candy, chewing gum, and carbonated sweet drinks
- spicy, crunchy, sharp, salty, or acidic foods
- toothpicks, to avoid damaging your gum
- smoking. Stop smoking. Right now. Avoid all tobacco products. Forever.

· PART SIX ·

Lifestyle adjustments to support recovery

· PART SIX ·

Why your Environment and Lifestyle Matter

In 2013 I presented a paper at the Global Health Futures Conference in Bangalore, India. Just prior to the conference, a small number of us met with His Royal Highness The Prince of Wales, a long-term passionate advocate for an integrative approach to health and healing, to discuss our ideas about tackling the future burden of chronic disease facing developed and developing countries. The topics we covered included environmental sustainability, building healthy communities, and encouraging lifestyle measures such as healthy nutrition.

He delivered a message to the conference in which he said, rather more poetically than I could have put it: 'John Donne reminds us that no man is an island. Our healing, our resilience and our health are very much connected to our social and physical environment. Too often, however, our society and its stresses are themselves a major cause of illness . . . there is as much truth in the idea that we are what we are surrounded by as we are what we eat.'

This is a concept we call 'epigenetics'. The genes you are born with are not fixed for life. From years of research we now know that there is a vast array of switches that could turn gene activity on or off depending not only on your own environment and activities but also on the environment and activities of your ancestors. The diet or lifestyle habits of your grandparents could be affecting you now, and your environment and lifestyle can also control the behaviour of your own genes and also those of the genes of the generations that follow you.

What we call 'cancer' is not a single disease with a common set of causes. Rather, the truth is that the cause of cancer is a complex intermingling of your genetics, factors in your environment, and the way you live your life. I explain this to you because it is important to your motivation to understand that, at a genetic level, improvements in your lifestyle are worth the effort, because lifestyle changes can alter the activity of the genes that cause cancer to occur or recur.

Professor Dean Ornish from University of Southern California San Francisco led a groundbreaking study which found that intensive lifestyle changes could affect the progression of prostate cancer. One group in the study:

- ate a vegan diet based primarily on fruit, vegetables, beans, and soy protein
- exercised 30 minutes daily
- practised yoga or meditation for an hour daily and
- boosted their social support networks.

In this group, prostate specific antigen (PSA) levels, a measure of the activity of prostate cancer, began to go down. In the comparison group, the PSA levels increased, that is the activity of their prostate cancer got worse.

While we can't turn the clock back to a time before your cancer first started, we do have a growing understanding of how your lifestyle and your environment might cause cancer, and how changing your lifestyle might arrest or even reverse cancer growth in the future.

The advice in this part of the book is intended to influence you to do all you can to encourage your epigenome to turn all the right switches on or off to assist your cancer recovery.

RESOURCE

Check out the National Human Genome Research Institute: www.genome.gov/27532724#al-1

Cancer and Your Environment

Many of my patients who are diagnosed with cancer are very interested in learning about ways of altering their environment so they can reduce the risk of cancer recurrence or future cancer risk for themselves and their families. There are various ways in which your environment can increase the risk of cancer and also some well-recognised major household and environmental cancer hazards.

SECONDHAND SMOKE

There are so many established and well-known health consequences of exposure to secondhand smoke for adults and children including impact on the heart and blood vessels and irritation and damage to airways that I probably don't need to elaborate too much. We know that secondhand smoke contains hundreds of chemicals known to be carcinogenic.

Regular and long-standing exposure to passive smoking increases the risk of some forms of lung and throat cancer in non-smokers. For those with heavy exposure, the risk is nearly doubled. There is also a link between secondhand smoke and nasal sinus cancer and breast cancer in younger women.

Avoiding regular contact with passive smoking is strongly recommended because there is no safe level of exposure.

AIR POLLUTION

The International Agency for Research on Cancer has classified outdoor pollution as a Group 1 carcinogen. Heavy air pollution contributes to cancer risk, predominantly lung cancer, but it is also linked to an increased risk for bladder cancer. The most recent data indicate that in 2010, there were 223,000 deaths from lung cancer worldwide which resulted from air pollution.

Diesel is more problematic than other pollutants. Diesel is a type of fuel distilled from crude oil and contains at least 19 potential carcinogens. The World Health Organization has declared that diesel engine exhaust is a 'known carcinogen', in the same category as arsenic and asbestos.

It is a particular concern if you are in an occupation where you are exposed to car, truck or machinery exhaust. For example, a study of 12,000 miners showed that non-smoking miners who were heavily exposed to diesel fumes for years had seven times the normal lung cancer risk of non-smokers.

If you have a diesel car, consider changing it to a hybrid or petrol version and avoid inhaling its exhaust. If you are in an occupation with heavy diesel fume exposure, look at how you might be able to modify your exposure or consider a change of occupation.

ASBESTOS FIBRE

Asbestos was a common building and insulation material used in the past. When asbestos materials are released into the air, tiny fibres can be inhaled and lead to a type of lung cancer (mesothelioma) and throat cancer. Some studies have also suggested an association between asbestos exposure and gastrointestinal and colorectal cancers, as well as an elevated risk for cancers of the kidney, oesophagus, and gallbladder, although the evidence is inconclusive.

If your work or a renovation project has the potential to bring you into contact with asbestos, make sure you seek expert advice on handling of asbestos materials, use all the necessary protective equipment, that everyone on the site uses it, and that you follow all recommended safety practices and procedures.

PESTICIDES, INSECTICIDES AND WEEDKILLERS

Exposure to a range of household, garden and agricultural chemicals is associated with a higher risk of a variety of cancers, including lymphoma, leukaemia, and prostate, skin and lung cancers. Farmers are at particular risk.

For the farmers' sake as well as for consumers like you and me, I would really like to see more and more farms transitioning to organic farming techniques.

Fruit and vegetables sometimes contain very small amounts of pesticide residue, so it is a good idea to rinse fruit and vegetables in filtered water before eating them. There is no evidence that these small amounts of pesticide residue once the food is washed, will increase the risk of cancer if you eat it. Remember that fruit and vegetables are an important part of a balanced diet, providing vitamins, minerals and fibre – and eating plenty of both is likely to lower your cancer risk.

Correct use and storage of chemicals in your home and garden is crucially important. Only use them if it's absolutely necessary. If possible, to minimise the need to use chemicals, use natural methods such as chemical-free pesticides and pest control measures, companion planting and mulching to control weeds. I'd suggest you use as little of any chemicals in your

home and garden as possible, read and follow all safety precautions, wear protective clothing, wash clothes after using
chemicals and keep chemicals locked away from children as
good general rules.

HOUSEHOLD CLEANERS, SOLVENTS AND CHEMICALS

There is not nearly enough research into the potentially harmful
effects of many household products, but we do know that products
containing benzene and methylene chloride, which is present in
some paint strippers and paints, can cause an increased risk of
cancer.

The best advice is to be cautious but not alarmed. Use products
containing these chemicals sparingly and use environmentally
friendly products wherever possible. Take appropriate precautions and ventilate the area adequately where the chemicals are
being used, avoid contact with your skin, wash your skin after
use and store items safely.

X-RAYS

X-rays and other medical imaging are essential to diagnosis and
monitoring of disease. Having a simple procedure like a chest
X-ray has been assumed to be safe. However X-rays are classified
as a known human carcinogen in the US Report on Carcinogens
and the International Agency for Cancer Research. For most
people the benefit of medical diagnostic radiation far outweighs
the risk, but the story may not be the same for those with a strong
genetic predisposition to cancer. For example, women with breast
cancer genes (BRCA1/2) have double the risk of getting breast
cancer if they have had a chest X-ray, and if they had the chest
X-ray before the age of 20 then the risk was increased fourfold.
This may be because it takes relatively less radiation exposure to

cause DNA damage in genetically predisposed individuals. This should be taken into account before having radiological tests and avoiding unnecessary medical radiation. Try to minimise the use of radiation by discussing with your doctors whether other imaging techniques such as ultrasound or MRI can be used instead.

If you are having dental X-rays, insist on a thyroid shield.

Always let the radiologist know before you have an abdominal X-ray or medical imaging if there is any possibility you could be pregnant.

ULTRAVIOLET RADIATION

Sun exposure is probably the most dangerous form of radiation. Sunburn increases the risk of malignant melanoma, and high-level sun exposure increases the risk of less dangerous skin cancers. Regular and moderate sun exposure without sunburn, however, reduces the risk of a variety of other cancers, probably because of its beneficial effects on increasing vitamin D, regulating melatonin, increasing immunity, improving mood and encouraging a healthier outdoor lifestyle.

RESOURCES

General practice: the integrative approach, Phelps K. and Hassed C., Elsevier 2011.

For more information on X-rays and cancer risk: Cancer Council Western Australia has a helpful fact sheet. www.cancerwa. asn.au/resources/cancermyths/medical-imaging-myth/

Alcohol

When you have been diagnosed with cancer, one of the decisions you will face if you drink alcohol is how much you will continue to drink, or whether you will decide to stop altogether. These are some of the questions that might come up for you once you have been diagnosed with cancer:

- What is the association between alcohol and your risk of recovery from this cancer, a cancer recurrence, or a future cancer?
- Is alcohol safe during your cancer treatment?
- Are there times when you should avoid alcohol completely?
- Do your 'safe' alcohol limits change after your cancer treatment has finished?

In normal circumstances, alcohol is considered by most people to be a legal and socially acceptable drug in 'moderation', or within 'safe' limits. But the ground shifts when you are physically and psychologically dealing with the effects of cancer and its treatment, and there are more issues to consider. We just don't know what 'safe' levels are when it comes to alcohol post-recovery.

So if alcohol is legally available and nearly everyone you know drinks it, then it can't be that bad for you, can it? Let's take a look at the evidence on alcohol and cancer.

WHY THE CONCERN ABOUT ALCOHOL AND CANCER?

Health experts have been looking at the association between alcohol and an increase in the risk of various types of cancer. The International Agency for Cancer Research classifies alcohol as a Group 1 carcinogen. This places alcohol in a category of other carcinogens, including asbestos, gamma radiation, tobacco, human papillomavirus and arsenic.

The more alcohol you consume over your lifetime, the greater the risk of developing alcohol-related cancers. According to the World Cancer Research Fund a convincing link has now been established between chronic alcohol consumption and cancers of the mouth, throat, larynx, oesophagus, liver, colon, rectum, and, in women, breast; and an association is suspected for cancers of the pancreas and lung. Additionally, the evidence does not show any minimum 'safe threshold' of intake and cancer risk, and the type of drink is irrelevant because risk is related to the ethanol content rather than whether it is in the form of beer, wine or spirits, or a cocktail with an umbrella.

The Million Women Study showed that in women, low to moderate alcohol consumption increased the risk for cancers of the mouth and throat, oesophagus, larynx, rectum, liver, breast, and total numbers of cancer cases. While the study also showed that the risk of thyroid cancer, non-Hodgkin's lymphoma, and kidney cancer decreased with increased alcohol consumption, total cancer risk increased by 6 per cent for every standard drink per day.

Once you know you have had a cancer, one of the biggest

questions you face is about whether you can improve your chances of survival and quality of life by changing your previous habits, including your drinking pattern.

ISN'T A SMALL AMOUNT OF ALCOHOL SUPPOSED TO BE GOOD FOR YOU?

There has been a lot of publicity over the years which has tried to make the case that a small amount of alcohol, or drinking within recommended 'safe' levels has health benefits, particularly in prevention of heart disease. The experts have looked at all the research on this and reached the conclusion that 'existing evidence does not justify the promotion of alcohol use to prevent coronary heart disease, and that the previously reported role of alcohol in reducing heart disease risk in light-to-moderate drinkers appears to have been overestimated.' Any benefits are mainly related to middle-aged or older people, and only occur with consumption levels of about half a standard drink a day.

Clearly, when you have a cancer diagnosis the stakes are high, and the cancer will need to be your highest priority. Getting your life back means doing whatever you can reasonably do to stay well and avoid other types of illness where you can. So it makes sense that if you have already been diagnosed with an alcohol-associated cancer, or indeed any cancer, you will need to consider very carefully if, or how much, you drink in the future.

In this chapter we will explore this link further to help you make a decision about your future use of alcohol. Start by having a look at the answers in your health audit about how much you drink (see page 28). Many of my patients are shocked when they tally up the number of alcoholic drinks they have each week. Once you have assessed your alcohol intake and decided you need to make changes, work out if you want to do a full detox or take a cut-down approach.

WORKING OUT STANDARD DRINKS

How much is a standard drink?	
Can/Stubbie low-strength beer	= 0.8 standard drink
Can/Stubbie mid-strength beer	= 1 standard drink
Can/Stubbie full-strength beer	= 1.4 standard drinks
100 ml wine (13.5% alcohol)	= 1 standard drink
30 ml nip spirits	= 1 standard drink
Can spirits (approx 5% alcohol)	= 1.2 to 1.7 standard drinks
Can spirits (approx 7% alcohol)	= 1.6 to 2.4 standard drinks

HOW DOES ALCOHOL CAUSE CANCER?

Alcohol-related cancer is due to DNA damage caused by the action of a chemical called acetaldehyde, which is produced when the ethanol in alcohol is metabolised.

Alcohol can also work with other carcinogens to cause cancer. For example, tobacco smoking and alcohol together are risk factors for 75 per cent of head and neck cancers. Alcohol also increases weight gain and acts as a risk factor for obesity, which in turn increases risk for cancers in the oesophagus, pancreas, bowel, breast and endometrium.

Folate is a B vitamin found in high concentrations in green leafy vegetables and has an important role in repairing DNA damage. Alcohol can interfere with the transport and metabolism of folate, which in turn affects cell function. Alcohol can affect intestinal absorption, transport of folate into tissues, folate storage, and release by the liver. If transport of folate into tissues is affected, then its role in repairing DNA damage is affected, inducing the formation of cancers.

DURING CANCER TREATMENT

If you have a history of using alcohol as an escape or a way of coping with stress, there will be the temptation to follow that pattern again in an effort to relieve the stress of dealing with the cancer. Whether you are a regular drinker or an occasional social drinker, now is the time to look at other ways of relieving your stress.

Aside from the potential for DNA damage caused by alcohol, most of the medications used in cancer treatment and symptom management will make extra demands on your liver because your liver is the organ responsible for processing all the toxins in your body, including chemotherapy and other drugs. If you combine those medications with alcohol, then your liver's ability to metabolise toxins will be impaired.

During treatment, your liver function will be monitored. You may see an increase in your levels of liver enzymes, called 'transaminases'. If your liver transaminases – liver enzymes released by damaged liver cells – are shown to be elevated on a blood test result, it is a signal that your liver is not coping with the load of toxins, whether from medications, alcohol, chemotherapy or other chemicals. Your liver will be working overtime, even if the blood test results are in the normal range. Liver function tests can also be elevated if there are cancer metastases involving the liver.

Alcohol interacts with many of the drugs used during cancer treatment and some of these interactions can be potentially dangerous, particularly the stronger pain killers or sedatives. Additionally, alcohol can irritate and worsen mouth ulcers caused by chemotherapy.

AFTER TREATMENT IS COMPLETED

After treatment is completed, you might ask if there is a safe level of alcohol consumption. To be fair, different doctors will have differing views on this. By now you will have figured out that my advice to you is to avoid drinking completely and indefinitely, to give yourself the best possible chance of cancer-free survival.

The standard 'safe' levels of drinking are intended for a general population with no particular health risks in mind. There has not been a 'safe' level of alcohol consumption established for people who have had a significant cancer diagnosis.

If avoiding alcohol is not realistic for you or you simply do not want to do that in the long term, then that is a decision you need to make based on your careful assessment of risk. Certainly during active treatment with chemotherapy, and radiotherapy, if you are taking pain medications, and in the recovery phase after surgery it will help your recovery to be as free of avoidable toxins – including alcohol – as possible. Once treatment is completed, it is more important than ever to keep under the current maximum recommended daily limit of two standard drinks.

That is a maximum of two standard drinks or one-quarter of a bottle of wine in a 24-hour period, no more than five days a week. If you think that doesn't sound like very much . . . a bottle of wine contains an average of around eight standard drinks, so if you share one bottle of wine between two people, which is a common practice, then that is double the maximum recommended limit. You need to be particularly careful of cocktails, which contain two to three standard drinks.

Case Study

Alicia was just 30 when she was diagnosed with breast cancer. She and her partner Max had been serious party people, but she got the fright of her life when she found out about the cancer. She decided to change a lot of her habits, get regular exercise, eat organic food and quit drinking alcohol and taking party drugs. Her partner went along with the plan, for moral support. A year went by and Alicia had completed her radiotherapy and chemo-therapy and her one-year check-up went well. Alicia and Max decided to celebrate. And celebrate. And celebrate. Alicia came for her next check-up looking pale and thin. Her liver function tests had all crept up into the hundreds where the normal range was down under thirty. Elevated transaminase levels indicate a degree of liver cell damage. Fortunately her tumour markers were stable. Her liver scan showed no metastases. On questioning, Alicia said that she had been drinking a bottle of wine and half a dozen beers a night on Fridays, Saturdays and Sundays. Her diet had 'relaxed'. We talked about the impact this was having on her general health, but also the long-term impact on her cancer-free survival. She decided to rein in the binge drinking but said she would just feel too left out of her group of friends if she didn't have a few drinks on a weekend. She agreed to stop drinking until her liver function tests returned to normal, but then she wanted to go back to drinking but would keep it in the low range.

There are two risky patterns of drinking alcohol: episodes of binge drinking and long-term excessive drinking.

BINGE DRINKING

Cancer has been found to be more common in binge drinkers. Large doses of alcohol also increase the risk of the DNA damage that can cause cancerous changes in cells.

TECHNIQUES FOR CUTTING DOWN

- Decide to stop drinking on most weekdays.
- Eat before you drink alcohol.
- If you are thirsty, drink water first, rather than using alcohol as a thirst-quencher.
- Sip, don't gulp.

- Invest in a spirit measure for when you are drinking at home as it can be easy to underestimate the amount of alcohol in a nip. Each nip equals one standard drink.
- Try substituting at least each second drink with a non-alcoholic drink or water. This reduces the amount of alcohol you consume and also keeps up your hydration.
- You may need to change your social patterns for a period of time to adjust your drinking habits.
- Avoid drinking in 'shouts' or 'rounds' because that locks you into the quantity the group drinks, rather than your own limit.
- If there are only two of you, order wine by the glass or half-bottle rather than sharing a full bottle.
- Don't let waiters or hosts top up your glass before it is empty. If they do, you cannot count how much you are drinking.

LONG-TERM ALCOHOL-RELATED PROBLEMS

The longer you drink to excess, the more likely it will be for you to develop an alcohol-related health problem. Since your diagnosis with cancer, considering the amount of alcohol you drink has become more important than ever.

I have already discussed the consumption of alcohol and how it relates to an increased risk of cancer. There are the non-specific effects of chronic low-grade toxicity and withdrawal, but we also see an increased risk of high blood pressure, heart disease and stroke, cirrhosis of the liver, pancreatitis, alcohol dependence and malnutrition.

ALCOHOL AND NUTRITION

Alcohol has a direct effect on your gut and digestive system, so in addition to the nutritional burden of your cancer and cancer treatment, drinking alcohol creates more potential nutritional deficiencies. And the more you drink, the greater the nutritional deficiencies are likely to be. If your cancer or cancer treatment has caused any digestive problems, you will need professional advice about how to correct this with diet and supplements.

A dietitian can work out the nutrient quality of your diet and help you to correct your eating patterns, and your GP can arrange blood tests for some nutrient levels such as iron, vitamin B_{12} and folate. Some tests for nutrients are difficult to access and are unreliable.

Deficiencies will need to be corrected with supplements, and you will need professional advice on combinations and doses. This is extremely important during cancer treatment, and if you continue to take medications for symptoms management once treatment is completed. As a general guide only, the most common alcohol-related nutritional deficiencies you will need to consider are protein, folate, B vitamins, vitamin C, calcium, magnesium and zinc.

ARE YOU A HIGH RISK DRINKER?

You might be a high-risk drinker if you:

- suffer withdrawal symptoms when you stop drinking
- crave alcohol and become irritable if you can't get a drink
- cannot stop drinking once you have started
- can't remember events or conversations
- have had problems with the law related to your drinking
- have had difficulty maintaining a relationship
- have had trouble keeping a job
- drink alone or secretively
- have liver damage, nerve damage, or significant nutritional deficiencies related to alcohol.

You may be ready to hear the message about alcohol and do something about it. Once you have been diagnosed with cancer you don't have the luxury of time to think about it for a while before you are ready to make the changes that will benefit your long-term health. It is likely that within weeks of diagnosis you will be undergoing surgery, chemotherapy, radiotherapy, or other cancer-specific treatment and so stopping alcohol will be an important part of your cancer prehabilitation.

SLAMMING ON THE BRAKES

Because your liver is one of the key organs responsible for detoxifying your body, you will need it to be in the best possible working order for the job it needs to do. So I would advise you to avoid alcohol throughout the phase of cancer-specific treatments. This becomes even more important if your liver function tests have been abnormal, or if you are taking on-going medication for cancer that needs to be metabolised by your liver. If you are a regular moderate to heavy drinker and you stop drinking abruptly, ask your doctor about an injection of high dose B vitamins (thiamine is particularly important) to help you manage withdrawal.

WITHDRAWAL EFFECTS

If you have been drinking more than is healthy for you, you may be able to just stop without suffering any noticeable withdrawal effects. If you pay close attention to the days immediately after you have been drinking, particularly, say, if you have been drinking heavily on weekends, you may notice a variety of withdrawal effects over the following days when you are not drinking, including fatigue, anxiety, depression, clouded thinking, trouble concentrating, irritability and jitteriness. More severe effects might include sweating, headaches, trouble sleeping, nausea, rapid heart rate and tremor.

The most severe form of withdrawal is called delirium tremens (DTs), with agitation, confusion, hallucinations, and the possibility of seizures. If there is a risk of DTs because of heavy drinking, withdrawal will need to be managed under supervision in a medical setting, usually a hospital.

There are medications, such as disulfiram and acamprosate, that can be prescribed by doctors to help manage alcohol cravings and withdrawal symptoms. But again, close supervision is important so that one potentially addictive substance is not replaced with another.

Once the cancer-specific treatment is completed, you can make a decision about what level of alcohol you want to resume. Ideally, you won't take it up again because, as I pointed out earlier, alcohol has a role in causing the DNA damage that causes cancers to form. So, playing it safe, you might decide to keep it to zero.

If you do decide to drink alcohol again, we don't know if there is a safe threshold once you have had cancer, but certainly no more than one or two standard drinks in a 24-hour period no more than five days a week.

If you are a heavy regular drinker you will need some help to stop, and I would recommend seeking individual professional advice. It would be wise to discuss a plan of action with your GP. This is particularly the case if you have significant medical problems as well as the cancer, if you are on pharmaceutical medication, or you intend to take a combination of supplements. It will also be necessary if you have tried to reduce or quit drinking in the past and found it difficult. Your GP can give you an injection of B vitamins, with thiamine being particularly important to help reduce the effects of stopping heavy alcohol consumption.

As a general guide only, the following supplements may be recommended. This will need to be modified depending on whether you are undergoing cancer-specific treatment. If your GP is trained in nutritional or complementary therapies, then they will also be able to advise you about supplements which might include: a multivitamin containing B vitamins, magnesium and zinc, vitamin C, L-glutamine, or probiotics and the herb silymarin (St Mary's thistle).

TREATMENT FOR HIGH-RISK DRINKERS

If you are a high-risk drinker, you might need specialised alcohol rehabilitation. The effect of withdrawal on the body can be intolerably uncomfortable, and psychological and behavioural therapy can help reduce the risk of relapsing into old habits. The process will need to be fast-tracked if you need to go straight into cancer-specific treatment.

Regular exercise helps to relieve anxiety and depression, which might be part of your reason for drinking, or a consequence of your drinking. Counselling and support groups can help you to figure out why you drink excessively and to stay the course.

The Cancer Council Australia recommends that to reduce your risk of cancer, limit your consumption of alcohol, or better still, avoid alcohol altogether. If you do choose to drink alcohol, the recommendation is to drink only within the National Health and Medical Research Council guidelines for alcohol consumption.

RESOURCE

For general information on alcohol and health, go to the National Health and Medical Research Council website: www.nhmrc.gov.au/health-topics/alcohol-guidelines/alcohol-faq

Exercise

It is now accepted wisdom that physical activity is a positive thing for your general health, including the prevention of cancer. It is also an essential part of your recovery from cancer even through treatment. We are starting to understand much more about how to go beyond the initial specific treatment of the cancer and approach recovery with the aim of feeling as good or even better than you did before your diagnosis by adopting a well-planned commitment to exercise. That approach may also increase survival.

Exercise not only helps with preventing and managing cancer, but also with many symptoms common among cancer patients. It helps to reduce fatigue, improve quality of life, reduce emotional distress, improve immunity, and improve aerobic capacity and muscle strength. Exercise can also help with other symptoms common in cancer, such as chronic pain. The reduction in pain is largely due to the fact that exercise induces endorphins but it also has positive effects on mood, muscle relaxation, and has an anti-inflammatory effect.

A review of the role of physical activity in cancer prevention, treatment, recovery, and survivorship concluded that exercise can decrease the severity of side effects of cancer treatment and aid in rehabilitation. It is important not to leave your plans for an exercise program until after your treatment is over, even if it takes a monumental physical and mental effort to get moving. Although you may be limited by fatigue or other physical restrictions, I advise making a plan that keeps you involved in some form of regular physical activity throughout the treatment process and beyond as an integral part of cancer treatment. Please do not regard this plan as an optional extra.

After a cancer diagnosis, regular exercise will improve the outcome of surgery, reduce some of the symptoms common in cancer patients, and help you to manage the side effects of chemotherapy and radiotherapy. Exercise also helps to maintain your physical functioning and reduce the likelihood of muscle wasting and bone loss that come with prolonged inactivity and some medical treatments.

Clearly, you will need to check with your GP or oncologist to make sure your plan for exercise is medically safe for you.

HOW EXERCISE HELPS CANCER RECOVERY

A major review of research into the effect of exercise on cancer recovery looked at strength training, resistance training, walking, cycling, yoga, qi gong and tai chi. The research found that exercise may have beneficial effects on health-related quality of life including cancer-specific concerns (for example, breast cancer), body image and self-esteem, emotional wellbeing, sexuality, sleep disturbance, social functioning, anxiety, fatigue and pain.

INCREASED ENERGY

Fatigue is a common side effect of cancer-specific treatment and this will affect the amount and type of exercise you feel like doing, and the amount of exercise that will be appropriate for you to do at different stages along the way. If you do the right type and amount of exercise, expending some energy actually gives you energy. Think of it like this. Fitness is about efficiency. Exercise increases muscle strength and improves your heart and lung function. The improved delivery of oxygen and other essential nutrients to every cell in your body in turn helps those body cells to perform their essential functions more efficiently, improving energy production. Let's look at a few examples.

Johns Hopkins Hospital in Baltimore, US conducted a study of a self-paced home walking program for women having radiotherapy for breast cancer. Fatigue was the most frequent and intense symptom they reported. The women who exercised throughout their treatment scored significantly higher for physical functioning and had reduced symptom intensity, particularly fatigue, anxiety, and difficulty sleeping.

Another study in Portland, Oregon, looked at whether exercise had an effect on fatigue over the first three cycles of chemotherapy in women receiving treatment for breast cancer. They found that women who exercised daily during treatment had significantly reduced levels of fatigue, and as the duration of exercise increased, the intensity of fatigue declined.

A recent meta-analysis found that exercise is effective in managing cancer-related fatigue and also helped to relieve depression and improve sleep quality in cancer patients.

BETTER SLEEP

Getting enough sleep can be a challenge for you during and after cancer treatment (see the chapter on sleep, page 360). Exercising regularly improves your sleep quality at night and wakefulness in the day. The type and timing of exercise is important. For example, it is better to exercise earlier in the day or to have a period of several hours of quiet activity between exercising and when you go to bed. Vigorous exercise too close to bedtime activates your sympathetic nervous system and increases your alertness, making it more difficult to get to sleep.

A Canadian study looked at the effect of the amounts and different types of exercise on sleep quality in women with breast cancer who were undergoing chemotherapy. Supervised exercise during chemotherapy consisted of either a standard dose of 25–30 minutes of aerobic exercise, a higher dose of 50–60 minutes of aerobic exercise, or a combined dose of 50–60 minutes of aerobic and resistance exercise three times a week.

The group with the higher dose of aerobic exercise found it easier to get to sleep, felt they had slept better and had better overall sleep quality than the group with the standard dose. Compared to a standard volume of aerobic exercise, higher volumes of both aerobic and combined exercise improved some aspects of sleep quality during breast cancer chemotherapy.

Cancer and its treatment can cause tiredness and fatigue, regardless of the amount of sleep you get. Try setting an alarm at a reasonable time in the morning that will allow you enough sleep, but also allow for some morning activity. Rather than trying to get more sleep in an attempt to raise your energy level, often what you need is planned activity in your day incorporating aerobic and resistance components, allowing for rest periods and a regular evening bed time.

EXERCISE LIFTS YOUR MOOD

A cancer diagnosis presents all sorts of physical and emotional challenges, and a flat or depressed mood is understandably common. It can be difficult to muster the motivation to be physically active when you are feeling unwell.

If you lack the confidence or the motivation to get started

on an exercise program, try organising to meet up with a friend for a walk or a swim. Some cancer units offer group exercise classes that might involve gentle movement or modified yoga or tai chi. A program supervised by an exercise physiologist or physiotherapist will guide you at a pace, frequency, and intensity suitable for your physical ability.

Aerobic exercise, with its huff and puff, appears to be the most effective in improving mental health. High-intensity exercise seems to be more effective for this than low-intensity exercise but the level of intensity you can manage will be dictated by your current state of wellbeing.

You get an immediate mood lift during an exercise session, but you will only experience sustained mood elevation with a sustained exercise habit. There are a number of explanations for this, including the release of endorphins, the calming effect of an increase in body temperature, improved blood circulation in your brain, and the impact on the hypothalamic-pituitary-adrenal axis modifying your physiological reaction to stress. The lift might also have something to do with distraction from your worries. Exercise lifts your mood by:

- improving your general health, physical fitness, and sense of wellbeing
- improving quality of sleep
- making you feel better about yourself through a sense of mastery over aspects of physical function
- distracting you from problems, thereby temporarily providing relief from worries
- helping to release negative or destructive emotions such as anger, hostility and frustration
- enabling greater social engagement, especially in shared activities or team/club sports

- increasing brain neurotransmitters, such as serotonin
- reducing the need for medications used to manage symptoms of pain, depression and anxiety.

EXERCISE IMPROVES YOUR BODY STRENGTH, FUNCTION AND FITNESS

Exercise improves your wellbeing, whatever state of health you are in. Regular exercise increases muscle strength and endurance, and maintains bone density. Exercise also boosts your immune system, improves digestion and reduces constipation.

EXERCISE HELPS YOUR SEX LIFE

There is not a lot of research on the link between cancer, physical exercise, and sexual functioning. Prostate cancer is a possible exception, where the question of sexual functioning is one of the prominent outcome measures after treatment. It makes sense that if you have less fatigue and you are physically stronger then sexual function will be better. However other issues such as possible nerve damage during surgery will also determine sexual functioning after prostate cancer treatment.

EXERCISE AND CANCER PREVENTION

Evidence for the role of exercise in the prevention and management of cancer is significant and growing. The World Cancer Research Fund reviewed the vast body of research on exercise and its association with cancer and declared that physical inactivity is clearly a risk factor for cancer.

Regular moderate exercise reduces the risk of several cancers, including cancers of the bowel, prostate, and breast, and has been shown to prolong survival for those who already have cancer as well as improve quality of life. Over 30 studies have shown a protective relationship between physical activity and colon cancer mortality. This protective effect also extends to precancerous bowel polyps. The reduction of bowel cancer risk with regular exercise is around 50 per cent.

Large-scale Norwegian studies show a 37 per cent reduction in the risk of breast cancer in all women who exercise regularly, particularly in women younger than 45 years of age, for whom the risk was 62 per cent lower. In those who were lean, exercised approximately four hours per week and were pre-menopausal, the risk was reduced by 72 per cent. Similar findings have been found for lung cancer.

In post-menopausal women, brisk walking has been shown to reduce breast cancer risk.

EXERCISE AND CANCER SURVIVAL

Just as interesting are some of the studies of the effect of exercise after a cancer diagnosis. For example, a study of 2987 women with stage 1–3 breast cancer followed for up to 18 years found that the risk of death for those women who exercised for an amount approximately equivalent to walking three to five hours per week had half the chance of dying during that time. This was confirmed in another study over a nine-year follow-up on women with breast cancer, where regular exercise was associated with a 44 per cent reduction in death rates.

If you understand the benefits of exercise in cancer recovery, then hopefully you will be motivated to do it and sustain the program of exercise in the long term. Exercise simply has to be an essential part of your management plan for preventing or treating any type of cancer.

When you initiate an exercise program, you will need to carefully consider your age, previous exercise history, current medical treatment, and level of fitness. It is also wise to discuss your plans with your GP and, if necessary, you can be referred to an exercise physiologist or a physiotherapist with expertise in exercise.

DIARISE EXERCISE

To begin, keep a diary audit of the amount and type of exercise you do over a few weeks. That will give you a clear indication of what you are actually doing now on a regular basis.

There are also wristband devices that measure your activity levels and provide a computer record.

This audit might include walking the dog, playing a game of tennis or golf, dancing, swimming, gardening, a gym session, tai chi, or yoga or a Pilates class.

DAY	TYPE OF EXERCISE	TIME	INTENSITY
MONDAY			
TUESDAY			
WEDNESDAY			
THURSDAY			
FRIDAY			
SATURDAY			
SUNDAY			

If your audit shows that you are not exercising enough – or not at all! – then you should definitely consider making exercise a priority. One of the hardest things about changing entrenched habits, especially bad habits, is getting a start. You might need to try a few different types of activity before you find one or two you enjoy. Some cancer units have specially designed exercise programs to get you started.

You need to think of exercise in the same way as taking your medication on time or turning up for chemotherapy. Exercise matters, and is an essential part of your treatment and recovery program and beyond. Make exercise a priority and put it in your diary so that the time slot is quarantined from anything that might bump it out of the schedule.

THE RIGHT GUIDANCE

Exercise physiologists are allied health practitioners who specialise in using exercise as part of the treatment for patients with a medical condition. They complete a university degree and have wide knowledge about the workings of the human body and the physical and mental effects of exercise on it. They can prescribe a course of exercises for either fitness or rehabilitation.

They differ from personal trainers (PT), who would be more accurately described as fitness professionals. The education of personal trainers is very variable and their focus is on fitness, motivation, and the technical accuracy of exercises. I strongly advise you to check the qualifications of a PT before undertaking a training program with them.

If you are undergoing cancer treatment or you are in the early stages of recovery, or if you have another significant medical problem such as diabetes, heart disease, arthritis, back pain, asthma, osteoporosis, or you are recovering from an injury or illness, then I advise you to have your exercise program carefully worked out and supervised by an exercise physiologist or physiotherapist.

Getting Started

Getting started can be a bit overwhelming if you don't know where to go, what to expect, what gear you need, how to use it, and whether you are likely to do yourself any damage in the process. Proper form and instruction will reduce the chance of injuries, so I recommend taking lessons, even if you are not a complete beginner.

If there is a form of exercise you have enjoyed in the past, then that is a good place to start – unless that was something like school rugby. Gentler exercise forms are better to begin with. Regard this is an opportunity to try something new, like yoga or dance.

You might need an initial motivator to get started, a spark that ignites you to take on a different pattern of behaviour. A lot of the time in medical practice, I see that 'spark' coming in the form of a major health scare. Your cancer diagnosis can be the catalyst to focus your attention on your fitness as a priority.

Your choice of fitness program involves a risk assessment based on your medical history, your current level of activity and fitness, lifestyle factors and some measurements such as height and weight, waist measurement, lipids (including cholesterol and triglycerides), and blood sugar levels.

Start with a slow pace and light intensity. If treatment has left you with fatigue or weakness, then expect to need to take it slowly and gradually. Even a few five or 10 minute sessions a day are a start. The idea is to build towards moderate intensity, where your pulse and breathing rate increases as a response to exertion.

There are also opportunities throughout the day when you can take exercise opportunities, such as walking up the stairs instead of taking the escalator, or walking to the local shops instead of taking the car.

TYPES OF EXERCISE

There are three different types of exercise you will need to incorporate into your activity plan to make sure you get the most benefit. These are aerobic, resistance (weight training), and flexibility. Some forms of exercise, such as yoga, will incorporate all of these elements. Other forms are predominantly one or the other, and so you will need to work out combinations of exercise forms to achieve all three.

Aerobic exercise

Aerobic exercise is the sort of activity that makes you puff and sweat. Using the large muscle groups, it might involve walking, cycling, swimming, dancing, running or rowing. Ideally, it is performed at low intensity, building to moderate intensity over a period of time, working up to a combination of 50–60 minutes a day of aerobic and resistance exercise three days a week, and at least 30 minutes of aerobic exercise on other days. For the best benefits, you will be doing some form of aerobic exercise every day but try to make five days a week your minimum.

If you were exercising regularly before your cancer treatment, you will probably need to reduce the intensity and duration of exercise during treatment. On days when fatigue is particularly bad, ease back and do one of the gentle forms of exercise such as tai chi or a gentle hydrotherapy program.

Aerobic exercise seems to be the best type of exercise for protection against cancer, and the suggested reasons as to why exercise protects against cancer include:

- changes to prostaglandins and other modulators of inflammation
- antioxidant effects
- maintaining a regular bowel habit and reducing bowel transit time
- protecting against obesity and metabolic syndrome by contributing to better overall energy balance
- encouraging other healthy lifestyle changes, such as a better diet
- improvements in mental health and depression
- stimulation of melatonin production.
- improvements in immune function.

Boosting your immune system needs lower intensity and shorter duration of exercise than you need for cardiovascular training. About 20–30 minutes of brisk walking five days per week will help to maintain a healthy immune response.

You can do a single session of exercise in a day, or you can accumulate bouts of exercise – for example, a 10-minute walk several times a day.

Resistance training

Resistance training is characterised by short intense bursts of movement against the resistance of weights, elastic, or resistance machines. The amount of resistance is set so that the number of repetitions you are physically able to do in each set of exercises is 12 or less.

If you are able to do more than 12 repetitions in a set, the amount of resistance (or weight) needs to be increased to get the positive effects of strengthening your muscles, building your bones, and releasing hormones. To achieve the desired effect, the resistance program should be done regularly, two or three times a week.

The recommended resistance levels are 8–10 different strength-training exercises, with 8–12 repetitions of each exercise, repeated 3–4 times, three times a week. The amount of resistance you can manage will be determined by your strength. As your strength builds, so the amount of resistance (or weight) will be increased.

This form of exercise is important for overall wellbeing, and it is very helpful in increasing muscle bulk and strength and reducing body fat. Most research on exercise and cancer has focused on aerobic-type exercise, but resistance exercise contributes other benefits for cancer recovery.

Flexibility

Flexibility is a term that refers to the total range of motion of a joint, or group of joints. The degree of flexibility depends on the structure of the joint and the mechanics of the muscles and soft tissues around the joint. Holding a muscle in a position which places it on stretch and repeated over time causes the muscle to increase in length, which in turn increases the range of motion of the joint and helps to overcome joint stiffness.

Lack of flexibility is a common problem for people who lead a sedentary lifestyle, and it gets worse as you grow older. Flexibility naturally decreases with age unless you actively work to maintain it. On the whole, women tend to be more flexible than men at all ages. The benefits of flexibility training include reduced muscle soreness after exercise, improved posture, reduced injury, reduced low back pain, increased functional range of motion, delayed muscle fatigue, and better relaxation.

The goal of flexibility training is to optimise joint mobility while maintaining joint stability. Try to stretch 3–4 times a week. Complete 2–4 sets of 4–6 different stretches and hold each stretch for 15–30 seconds. Include stretches for arm, leg, and trunk flexibility.

The Cancer Council Victoria has a series of flexibility exercises on their website: www.cancervic.org.au/

Safety first

Because you have had cancer there may be limitations on your physical fitness for exercise. Your cancer care team in hospital may have supervised exercise programs to get you started and to help you to work around any limitations. Once you have left the cancer clinic environment, however, you can talk to your GP about referral to an exercise physiologist, a rehabilitation expert, or a physiotherapist who is experienced in devising exercise programs for people with medical conditions.

Don't try to go too hard if you have lost fitness and you are just starting up, or deciding to get fit again when you haven't done anything active for a long time. Getting exhausted or injured in the early phases of your fitness program will discourage you and may slow down your recovery rather than enhance it. Start slowly and build up time and intensity gradually as your fitness improves.

If you have recently undergone cancer treatment and you want to do your own exercise program, ask a friend or family member to accompany you initially, in case you start to feel faint or unwell or you find you are unsteady on your feet.

Pelvic floor exercises

These muscles support your bladder and lower bowel. In women they also support the uterus. They are important for normal sexual function, urinary and faecal continence, and stability of your lower spine.

This muscle group needs to be included in your exercise program, particularly if you have had recent abdominal or pelvic surgery, such as a hysterectomy or prostate cancer surgery. Even if you do not have symptoms of weak pelvic floor muscles, it is important to give them some attention.

Weak pelvic floor muscles can lead to difficulty controlling your bowel or bladder function, and you may experience leakage when you cough, laugh, sneeze, or lift heavy objects. You may experience an urgent need to rush to the toilet, or a dragging feeling or bulge in the vaginal area. There may also be a loss of sexual sensation.

There are specialist physiotherapists and continence advisers who can instruct you on how to do pelvic floor exercises, and I would advise that you get some expert one-on-one instruction.

Pelvic floor exercises can be done when standing, sitting or lying, and you can do them while you do your daily tasks. First you will need to identify your pelvic muscles. You can do this when you are urinating by trying to stop the flow of urine midstream. You can also try to stop yourself passing wind by squeezing your anal muscles. These are the muscles to locate.

Once you have identified the correct muscle groups, squeeze slowly and hold for 5–10 seconds while you breathe normally, then release slowly and relax for 5–10 seconds. Repeat this about 10 times, then do about 10 strong, short squeezes in quick succession.

Aim for 5–10 sessions of these exercises every day. If you have any weakness in your pelvic floor muscles, it can take weeks or months to notice an improvement, so you will need to persist.

OVEREXERCISING

When you are coping with the physical limitations of cancer and its treatment and aftermath, you will need to pace yourself gradually. Even when you are in reasonably good health there is a limit to the amount your body is able to adapt. Beyond this limit, your body does not have the chance to repair and recover. This is called 'overtraining'. While this is most likely to be seen in elite athletes, I also see it in people who have been unwell and who are overly ambitious about their exercise program before they are ready.

The signs of overtraining are almost the opposite of some of the benefits of well-planned exercise. They include excessive or persistent pain, sleep disruption, tiredness/fatigue, anaemia, recurrent infections, recurrent injury, decreased appetite and weight loss, persistent muscle soreness, increased resting heart rate, depression and irritability. To avoid overtraining:

- ask for professional advice on your training program as part of your cancer prehabilitation/rehabilitation plan
- start with a light program and gradually work up intensity
- limit most exercise sessions to less than 60 minutes
- set aside one day each week for light activity or very light recovery – walking, gentle aquafitness, tai chi
- mix up the types of exercise you do so you do not repeat the same program on consecutive days
- allow at least 48 hours between resistance training on the same muscle group
- measure your resting heart rate each morning on waking, to detect increases.

Nutrition

After decades of research we have increasingly been proving something that we have intuitively known for a very long time: that what you eat contributes to your risk of developing cancer and your chances of a long remission and recovery. There is a never-ending effort to establish not only the link between nutrition and cancer, but exactly what foods and components of foods protect you from cancer, which foods might increase your risk, and what dietary mix is optimal.

Although most studies look at just one food group or one type of cancer, the same principles are likely to hold for other cancers. There may be some individual foods that have a particularly important role for individual cancers, but as a general rule, if a food has been found to be protective against one cancer it is likely to be protective against other cancers as well, to a greater or lesser degree. The challenges in establishing the 'facts' about foods and cancer are:

- the effect of diet in any individual is long term (probably starting from your conception or before)

- any individual diet changes from time to time and day to day
- there are broad cultural and geographic generalisations about diet
- nutrition is only one element of the causes of cancer and why it takes a particular course.

Despite the challenges of research in this area, the link between what you eat and the risk of cancer, both as a cause and as a preventive measure is now very well established. Diet-related factors are thought to account for about 30 per cent of cancers in developed countries.

Almost every patient I see who has been diagnosed with cancer wants to know how they can change their diet to improve their recovery and chances of survival. It is not enough to just be told to 'eat a healthy diet'. Different people have different ideas about what constitutes a 'healthy diet' depending on their culture, food preferences, understanding of nutrition and objectives. Once you have been diagnosed with cancer, you need detailed information about what to include in your diet. Just as importantly, you also need detailed information about what to avoid.

The aim of this chapter is to provide you with some principles of an ideal diet as well as some practical solutions to nutrition challenges.

PROTECTIVE ELEMENTS IN FOOD

So far, evidence has not identified a single 'miracle' food to cure cancer, but many foods are known to significantly contribute to cancer prevention and treatment. These days it seems every time you blink there is a new, so-called 'superfood'. The upside of this information overload is that medical science is looking more closely than ever at foods for the quality of their nutrients and the way they function within your body to enhance the natural processes, such as energy production, the working of your immune system and protection from cancer. Some foods are better at this than others.

It is the consistent intake of a high-quality, balanced, varied, and healthy diet over the long term that provides the best protection. Eating well during and after cancer treatment helps to maintain your body weight, improve your strength and energy, decrease the risk of infection, and assist your body in healing and recovery.

CAN YOU GET EVERYTHING YOU NEED FROM FOOD?

I often hear an argument, and I have to say it is a glib and simplistic argument, that 'you can get all the nutrients you need from food'. I want to address this because it is nonsense.

There is a vast chasm of difference between knowing what you ought to be eating and what you actually do in practice, or what you are able to do within the limitations of your particular cancer and the treatment you are undertaking. There can also be food supply issues for some people and for people in some locations. For example, people who are unwell may not be able to manage to get to the shops regularly or prepare food if they live alone, and some forms of cancer and other medical conditions make it impossible to digest or absorb certain nutrients from food.

There are times during cancer-specific treatment, recovery and beyond when it is just not possible to eat all the nutrients your body needs, and you will have to complement the nutrition in your food with supplements. This will be for all sorts of reasons such as your appetite, whether your treatment has affected your digestion (such as surgery to remove parts of the gastrointestinal tract), and the practicality of you being able to eat the foods that are recommended. There will be some stages during treatment and some circumstances where you will need specialised advice from a dietitian.

Nutrition is integral to your cancer recovery. Healthy nutrition appropriate to your needs boosts your sense of wellbeing, helps you maintain your energy and physical strength, maintains your body weight, helps you tolerate the side effects of treatment, lowers your risk of infection, and aids healing.

YOUR FOOD AUDIT

It is possible that your usual dietary patterns change during the course of cancer treatment and recovery. Revisit your food diary from your health audit, page 28, and compare it to your current diet and eating patterns. Like most people, if your GP or dietitian asked you about your diet, you would most likely tell them about your usual patterns of eating or an idealised diet, what you know you should be saying, or you would like to eat on a 'perfect' day when all is well, leaving out the odd snacks and junk food and grazing.

So the best thing about accurately recording a food diary is that it will show you the diet you are actually eating and not the one you would tell your doctor about. It's an almost sure bet that it won't be the diet you know you should be eating to stay healthy or recover from illness, but from this honest recordkeeping you can properly evaluate your diet.

By assessing what you are eating and what you are not eating, you might realise you are manifestly deficient in a key nutritional area, like carbohydrates or protein or iron. Or perhaps you will see a pattern of skipping meals and snacking later in the day, or times in the day when your appetite is poor.

Once you have completed your food diary, take a good hard look at what it reveals:

- What patterns can you see?
- Do you tend to miss any meals?
- Are there times of the day when you find it more difficult to eat?
- Are there some types of food you cannot eat because of physical limitations or lack of appetite for them?
- How many pieces of fruit do you eat every day and how many varieties?
- How many serves of vegetables do you eat every day and what varieties?
- What are your sources of protein?
- Do you snack? What do you use for snacks, and what quantities?
- What processed or packaged foods do you eat?
- How much water do you drink? What about other types of drinks?
- How many shots of coffee or cups of tea do you drink each day?
- How much alcohol do you drink?

MINDFUL EATING

The value of this exercise is in recording what you actually eat and drink, but there is an additional benefit from keeping a food diary: it encourages what might be called 'mindful eating'. A food diary is as therapeutic as it is informative. Here's why. In writing down everything you eat and drink, you become really aware of your eating behaviours.

Patients tell me that when they know they have to write down what they eat, they feel accountable. They may initially feel accountable to me, or their dietitian, but before long they start to feel accountable to themselves. You become, literally, mindful of what you are doing. Once you have knowledge of healthy eating, then the food diary reminds you constantly to think about whether a particular choice is healthy for you because you know the aim of the exercise is to record it all.

Put simply, mindfulness is deliberately paying attention, non-judgementally, to what is going on in your internal and external environment. It is a technique used to help you overcome all sorts of automatic, habitual patterns of thinking, feeling and acting.

Learning 'mindful eating' involves a number of elements:

- deliberately paying attention to the positive elements of the experience of food preparation and eating
- choosing to eat food that you enjoy and which is nourishing to your body
- using all your senses to explore, savour and taste
- simply noting your responses to food – like/take-it-or-leave-it/dislike
- being aware of your mind and body cues that you are hungry and need to eat; or if your normal cues to eat are not present, reminding yourself to eat
- being aware of your mind and body cues that you have eaten enough and it is time to stop eating.

If your appetite is poor, then you will need to plan what you *need* to be eating, rather than what you *feel* like eating or relying on your usual cues like hunger.

MEALTIMES

When you are going through cancer treatment, it may be difficult for you to observe normal mealtimes. If this is a problem for you, you may need to work out what your total food requirement is for a day and spread it out over five or six smaller portions, eating your favourite foods when you feel like them. Once your treatment is finished, you can transition back to more regular mealtimes if that is possible for you.

Breakfast

Physical and mental energy, attention, concentration, memory, and work performance are optimised if you eat breakfast in the morning. And if you are inclined to unstable moods at all, then eating breakfast will contribute to a steadier mood state.

Make sure your pantry and fridge are kept stocked with food you like to eat in the morning so that you don't skip breakfast. If you are finding it difficult to get to the shops to buy food, accept help from friends or family to do the shopping for you until you feel up to doing it. The major supermarkets offer online shopping with delivery to your home, so you don't need to leave the house. There are also businesses that will pack and deliver healthy fresh food to you.

When you are planning your breakfast each day, think about including the fundamentals: a protein, whole grains, fruits and/ or vegetables and a source of healthy fat. Consider stocking up with wholegrain cereal, low-fat milk, fruit, low-fat yoghurt, wholegrain bread, eggs (boil them all in one go and store in the fridge for quick cold boiled eggs), and fruits in season. Most of these items last a week in the refrigerator or pantry, so weekly shopping would take care of these basic supplies.

Lunch

If you think about the recommended amount of vegetables then packing the five serves of raw chopped or peeled vegetables or homemade soups you are making sure you cover your vegetable intake by the middle of the day.

Another easy option is to make a little extra food the night before and keep some leftovers for lunch the next day. However, you should avoid leftovers if your immunity is compromised.

Dinner

Most people use their evening meal as the main meal of the day. It is often the time when all of the household members are home. At some stages of cancer treatment you may not be able to eat a large evening meal. Focus on quality of nutrients rather than quantity and spread out your kilojoue and nutrient intake across the day when your appetite is at its best.

Mindful snacking

If you go through periods of time when your appetite is affected by your cancer treatment, healthy mindful snacking takes on a new significance because this is when snacks are the opportunities to eat small amounts of nutrient-dense foods. There are smart choices and not-so-smart choices for snacks.

Smart choices are portions of fruit, low-fat yoghurt, nuts, hummus with rice crackers or fresh chopped vegetables, a fruit smoothie or crackers with some avocado. If your appetite is poor, juicing can help you to get the nutrients you need in liquid form, which is easily digestible.

If you need to increase your calorie/kilojoule content (energy density), look for nutrient-dense, high-calorie foods such as nuts, seeds, nut and seed pastes like tahini or peanut butter, olive oil, avocado and chia seeds, rather than foods with low nutrient quality, like packets of crisps, lollies, packaged biscuits or donuts.

For drinks, filtered water is a much better choice than soft drink, sodas or fruit juice.

NUTRITION BASICS

When you have been diagnosed with a significant medical problem like cancer, it is likely that you will be asking more detailed questions about the effect of nutrition on your cancer recovery and general health, what foods to include or avoid, and whether supplements are necessary for you. It is also important for you to develop a growing awareness of the role of micronutrients, food safety, and food quality in health.

Before I get to the finer details of foods that are known to benefit cancer recovery or not, we need to cover the basics of nutrition, because that is where I see most of the problems occurring, and most of the benefits to be gained.

OVERWEIGHT AND OBESITY

There is an epidemic of obesity in many countries in the world. The World Health Organization estimates the rate of obesity at up to 60 per cent of people in Western countries and an estimated 15 per cent of the total world population. Being overweight or obese is clearly associated with a greater incidence of developing cancers of the oesophagus, breast (after menopause), endometrium (the lining of the uterus), colon and rectum, kidney and pancreas. There is also a possible association between obesity and other cancers, including liver, gallbladder, non-Hodgkin lymphoma, multiple myeloma, cervix, ovary and the more aggressive forms of prostate cancer.

The exact mechanism that explains how excess body weight relates to cancer risk is a complicated interaction of cell biochemistry, genetics, immune function, hormones, inflammation and environmental factors. The links between obesity and cancer are not yet fully understood. For example, overweight is linked to an increased risk of breast cancer after menopause but does not seem to increase the risk of breast cancer before menopause.

WAIST MEASUREMENT

There is a direct link between excess waist measurement and increased risk of several types of cancer, in particular cancer of the colon, post-menopausal breast cancer, and cancers of the endometrium, kidney and oesophagus.

Checking your waist circumference is as easy as putting a tape measure around your waist at the level of your belly button. If you are a man with a waist measurement over 100 cm or a woman with a waist measurement over 85 cm then your risk for various cancers increases.

For women, a waist measurement above 85 cm means you have a moderately increased risk of the following cancers: kidney, breast (after menopause), colon and rectum. If your waist measurement is above 85 cm, then you have a *significantly increased risk* of some cancers of the oesophagus, cancer of the uterus and myeloid leukaemia.

For men, if your waist measurement is above 100 cm then you have a *moderately increased* risk of cancer of the kidney and rectum. If your waist measure is above 100 cm, then you have a *significantly increased* risk of some cancers of the oesophagus, colon cancer, aggressive prostate cancer and myeloid leukaemia.

Waist measurement has also been linked with other health risks such as type 2 diabetes and cardiovascular disease.

If you are overweight or obese, making the decision to take off weight is a crucial element in your plan to recover from cancer and gain a sense of wellness.

ACHIEVING HEALTHY WEIGHT LOSS

If you are overweight or obese, lowering your total energy intake (also known as kilojoule or calorie restriction) helps to reduce the risk not only of cancer but also of a range of other illnesses, and significantly increases the potential for the length of time you live. Once you have been diagnosed with cancer, being overweight or obese is thought to increase the risk of the cancer coming back after treatment. Being overweight may also affect the overall chances of survival for many types of cancer.

Timing will be important. For example, if you have been diagnosed with prostate cancer and you have been advised that active surveillance is the best approach for you, then a long-term weight management program will be a central part of your health plan. On the other hand, if you need urgent chemotherapy for a disease like leukaemia, then quality of nutrition will be the main consideration, and achieving weight targets will be a secondary issue once your initial treatment cycles are completed. Having a few extra 'insurance kilos' also isn't a bad idea at this time as significant weight loss is common during some types of chemotherapy, mainly because of nausea and reduced appetite.

If you are very obese, the task of reaching your healthy weight range may seem too high a mountain to climb. Even a relatively small intentional weight loss (say, just 10 per cent of your current weight) will help to lower your risk of surviving this cancer or developing obesity-related diseases in future.

If you need to lose weight, then you will need to do it safely and in stages, setting progressive goals under the supervision of your GP, oncologist and a qualified dietitian. You may need to get advice on appropriate increases in physical activity from an exercise physiologist or a physiotherapist with experience in setting exercise programs for people at various stages of cancer treatment and recovery.

UNDERWEIGHT AND CANCER

You may have started out underweight, or cancer and its treatment may be the cause of losing weight unintentionally. Being significantly underweight has its own attendant general health risks, including a higher likelihood of infection, loss of muscle mass, hair loss, osteoporosis and disturbed hormonal function.

The problem is not just about insufficient energy intake (calories or kilojoules) for your body's needs. Low body weight can be a marker for malnutrition, literally a deficiency of nutrients. Malnutrition will impair the efficient operation of all your body's processes, including your immune system. Without the right balance of all the nutrients your body needs, your major organs will not function efficiently. Wound healing will be delayed and you will have increased susceptibility to infections. This obviously takes on extreme significance when you are undergoing treatment for cancer, or in the recovery stages after treatment.

Unplanned or unexpected weight loss can be one of the presenting symptoms of cancer, and may have been one of the reasons you and your GP embarked on a search for the answer to why your weight mysteriously dropped. Weight loss can also be a result of reduced appetite or nausea caused by some forms of chemotherapy, and can also be a side effect of some of the prescribed medications.

Taste or smell can also be affected by some cancers and by chemotherapy, and this will affect your enjoyment of food. Some forms of cancer affect the digestion and absorption of food. This is particularly the case with cancers of the oesophagus, stomach, liver and colon.

If you are significantly underweight, you will need to focus on increasing your body weight with high-quality, high-energy foods. This does not mean any old high-calorie/kilojoule food. The principles of fresh high-quality ingredients still apply.

Exercise lightly before meals to increase your appetite. Drink high-calorie, high-protein shakes *away* from main meals to increase your calorie/kilojoule intake. Drinking fluids with your meals can make your stomach feel more full, so drink most of your fluids between meals instead.

There are some simple steps you can take to gain weight mindfully:

- Eat nutritious foods, organic where possible.
- Focus on fresh vegetables and fruits. Think of the 'rainbow' of different colours representing different essential phytonutrients (see page 336).
- Include quality sources of protein such as organic eggs and chicken, fish, beans and legumes, soy foods, and lean meat.
- Increase quality sources of carbohydrate such as whole grains and sweet potato.
- Include healthy fats such as omega-3 fatty acids in fish and fish oil supplements, olive oil, and nuts.
- Avoid all 'bad' fats such as animal (saturated) fats and trans fats.
- Eat five or six meals a day, rather than two or three meals, and try to increase your portion sizes.
- If you are put off by the smell of cooked food, try to eat raw, juiced, or cooled foods, or combine foods with foods you like and enjoy.
- If anxiety is affecting your appetite, try relaxation exercises or meditation before meals.

Focus exercise sessions on building lean muscle mass through weight/resistance training and light aerobic workouts. If you are weak or unwell, an exercise physiologist will devise a suitable program that you can do in a bed or a chair or wheelchair, or be adapted to your current ability level.

You may need more nutrient intake than you can manage to eat and drink, so you will need advice on nutrition supplementation, feeding tubes or vitamin and mineral supplements to increase your energy and nutrient intake. Aim for gradual weight gain of 0.5 to 1 kg per week.

The aim is to keep your weight in the healthy weight range for your height. If it proves to be too difficult to gain weight, it is still important to have that focus on nutritional quality to improve your general wellbeing and energy levels. Again, this is best achieved under supervision of your GP, oncologist, and a qualified dietitian.

COMPONENTS OF A HEALTHY DIET

We have looked at your food diary and the timing of your meals and snacks, so now let's consider nutritional quality. If you look at any guide to balanced nutrition, you will find the same basic list of foods to include:

A variety of plant-based foods.

Protein: lean meat, fish, poultry, eggs, nuts and seeds, legumes and tofu – these all provide protein. It's easy to include a mixture of protein into snacks and meals.

Bread, cereals, rice, pasta and noodles – grains and cereals come from a wide variety of sources including breakfast cereals (oats, muesli, and wholegrain flakes), wholemeal breads and crackers, rice, barley, and varieties of pasta.

Milk, yoghurt and cheese – a diverse range of low-fat dairy foods including milk, yoghurt, cottage cheese and other types of cheese.

Breaking your diet down into nutritional categories, you need to find a balance of carbohydrates, protein, fibre and micronutrients.

EAT A 'RAINBOW DIET'

Different colours in fruits and vegetables indicate different 'phyto-nutrients'. This means, literally, the nutrients you get from plants that affect human health.

Phytonutrients have official names: antioxidants, flavonoids, flavanols, flavanones, isoflavones, catechins, epicatechins, anthocyanins, anthocyanidins, proanthocyanidins, isothiocyanates, carotenoids, allyl sulfides, polyphenols and phenolic acids. The more variety of natural colour you eat, the more likely it is that you are getting enough of these important nutrients. The ideal sources are foods, specifically plant foods such as fruit, vegetables, legumes, and grain and cereals.

As an exercise, think of the colours in your food on an average day. If you had white bread toast for breakfast, pasta for lunch, and meat and potatoes for dinner, with this beige diet you are missing out on the nutrients you need from eating a variety of plant-based foods.

Colour variety is a marker for the multitude of phytonutrients your body needs.

CARBOHYDRATES

Carbohydrates or 'carbs' are not the demons they are made out to be. You need carbohydrates for energy to carry out all your body processes, including physical and mental activity and the functioning of your body organs.

What all carbohydrates have in common is that they provide glucose for your body's essential energy needs. There is a hierarchy of carbohydrates from healthy to unhealthy.

Healthy sources of carbohydrates are whole grains, fruit, vegetables and legumes. These foods come with the added bonus of essential vitamins, minerals and phytonutrients (nutrients from plants).

Unhealthy carbs are the 'refined' foods you need to steer away from. These are 'white foods', like white flour, white bread and refined sugar, which provide lots of kilojoules for little nutrient value.

What is 'GI'?

GI stands for 'glycemic index'. This refers to the effect that a carbohydrate food has on blood sugar levels, but does not refer to the amount of food you consume. Glycemic load refers to the quantity of food you consume. High GI foods are absorbed rapidly into the bloodstream, converted into glucose and increase blood glucose levels. Low GI foods take longer to absorb and cause a lower peak of blood sugar levels.

Cancer survivors wanting to prevent a recurrence need to consider a low GI diet according to research by the Dana Farber Cancer Institute in Boston. A low GI diet has been associated with a lower risk of some cancers. A mainly low GI diet followed over many years has also been shown to be associated with a lower risk of type 2 diabetes, heart disease, and age-related macular degeneration.

A healthy diet will emphasise a balance in favour of low GI rather than high GI foods.

PROTEIN

Protein deficiency is a significant problem for many people with cancer. You need protein for growth, healing, repair of damaged tissues, and maintenance of your immune system.

When your body has been through a time of physical stress or illness, you may break down muscle to get the protein your body needs to heal. You need to concentrate on getting more protein than usual when you are going through cancer treatment and recovery.

Protein deficiency is surprisingly common, particularly in vegetarians, the elderly, and during periods of illness, following surgery, chemotherapy and radiotherapy. Signs of protein deficiency include muscle wasting and weakness, ankle swelling and anaemia.

Very high protein diets are dangerous to your health because they often do not allow for enough carbohydrate to give you energy, or enough fibre to keep your bowels moving normally. High protein diets can also increase the risk of liver and kidney problems, gout, gallbladder disease and the long-term risk of osteoporosis.

Food sources include fish, poultry, lean meat, eggs, low-fat dairy products, soy foods, nuts, beans, peas and lentils.

Protein supplements

You may find it difficult to digest protein at times of illness, so a protein supplement is often recommended. Balance is important. High-protein, low-carbohydrate diets have had a lot of attention and gained popularity as an option for weight loss. Two studies have shown that this type of diet leads to a shorter lifespan and poor cardiometabolic health, along with an increased risk of cancer and diabetes.

'Balance' in this context means including in your diet moderate amounts of high-quality protein that is low in unhealthy saturated fat.

A note to vegetarians

Plant-based foods have varying amounts of the components of protein. Proteins that come from vegetable sources tend to be low in one or more of the amino acids essential for health. For example, the limiting amino acid in grains is usually lysine; in legumes it can be methionine and tryptophan.

So to avoid deficiency on a vegetarian diet, you will need to focus on food-combining to get your daily protein needs. The amino acids in one type of food will balance the amino acid found in other foods across the day, provided that you eat combinations of the different groups. To give an example, grains, nuts and seeds complement legumes. For vegetarians (not vegans), milk products and eggs are other non-meat sources of protein.

Plant-based protein sources:
- legumes (beans, legumes, chick peas)
- whole grains (rye, wheat, oats, rice, buckwheat, barley)
- nuts and seeds
- tofu, tempeh and other soy products.

I advise you to see a qualified dietitian to analyse your vegetarian diet and ensure you are getting the right balance of nutrients.

FIBRE

If you are feeling bloated or constipated or your bowel is sluggish, you need to look at the amount of fibre in your diet. If you don't have enough fibre in your diet (and most people don't), it can contribute to constipation, irritable bowel syndrome, bowel cancer, cardiovascular disease, haemorrhoids and diverticulitis.

Dietary fibre is found in all plant foods. There are two types of fibre, soluble and insoluble. Soluble fibre softens faeces making it easier to pass through your gut. Sources include fruit, vegetables, oat bran, barley, seed husks, flaxseed, psyllium husks, cooked dried beans, lentils, peas and soy products.

Insoluble fibre acts as a natural laxative, which speeds up the transit of foods through the gut, bulks up stools, and prevents constipation. Sources include wheat bran, corn bran, rice bran, fruit and vegetable skins, nuts, seeds and wholegrain foods.

If you have been eating a low fibre diet and you decide to switch to a high fibre diet, you might find your bowels object at first. If you increase fibre content suddenly, you can get flatulence and abdominal cramps. Introduce fibre gradually by increasing fruits and vegetables and other wholefoods into your diet.

If you have had bowel surgery and lost some of your bowel, you may be advised to decrease your fibre content.

HERBS AND SEASONINGS

Seasonings and herbs such as turmeric, parsley, thyme, mint and capers have been found to have inhibitory activity on the growth of cancer cells, as well as preventing the development of tumours. These can all be safely incorporated into your cooking.

DARK CHOCOLATE

Good-quality dark chocolate that contains a minimum 70 per cent cocoa mass (plenty of cocoa but not too much fat or sugar) contains polyphenols. Eating two 20 g squares a day is enough. Any anti-cancer effect is likely to be very subtle, but subtle on the positive side.

OMEGA-3 FATTY ACIDS

Omega-3 fatty acids are found in sardines, mackerel, salmon, flax seed, soy, and nuts, especially walnuts. Studies have shown that consuming fish rich in omega-3s decreases the risk of developing breast, prostate or colon cancer.

Seafood contains both EPA and DHA: preferably oily fish like sardines, salmon, swordfish, tuna, mackerel, as well as mussels, oysters and squid.

HEALTHY OILS

The healthiest oils are high in mono-unsaturated and polyunsaturated fats, such as vegetable oil, olive oil, nuts, avocado, safflower, sunflower, grapeseeed and macadamia.

ORGANICS

The question of whether to 'go organic' often comes up in consultations after a diagnosis of cancer. A lot of people who speak to me about this have done their reading and decided to play it safe by reducing their exposure to environmental chemicals and toxins in any way they can.

The term 'organic food' is usually taken to mean a food that has been produced without artificial fertilisers and that has not been treated with synthetic pesticide chemicals or growth promoters of any type, including hormones and antibiotics. Apart from the cancer-causing potential, exposure to agricultural pesticides has been linked to hyperactivity, learning disabilities and behaviour disorders, memory problems and mood disorders. Recent US studies found that in blood samples of children aged two to four, concentrations of pesticides were six times higher in children eating conventionally farmed fruits and vegetables compared with those eating organic food.

Eating certified organic fruits and vegetables is probably advisable, because of their higher concentrations of some important vitamins, minerals and antioxidants, and the lower exposure to agricultural chemicals. Organic varieties have been demonstrated in a number of studies to provide significantly greater levels of vitamin C, iron, magnesium and phosphorus than non-organic varieties of the same foods.

On a decision level, the question of whether to spend the extra time and money sourcing organic foods to reduce your exposure to environmental chemicals is a personal one.

Availability is a key issue. Check your local area for growers' markets or stores that stock organic products. The major supermarkets sensing the meme of the time and the commercial opportunity, have an organic food section. You may find it difficult to stay totally organic and still have wide variety in your foods, but buy organic where you can and as much as you can to reduce your overall chemical exposure. I would like to stress the point that if organic produce is not available or affordable, then you still need to ensure adequate fruit and vegetable intake from regular sources.

WATER

Your body needs water for every single function in every cell, and maintaining hydration is essential to your wellbeing. Not all water supplies are reliable or free of contaminants and pathogens (disease-causing micro-organisms). If you have any immune problems or you are concerned about the quality or consistency of your tap water, then you can have a high quality water filter installed on your tap.

There will be times when your immunity is low and your resistance to infection impaired, so I would suggest drinking only water that is filtered or bottled at these times.

CANCER-PROTECTIVE DIET: SPECIFIC ELEMENTS

The American Institute of Cancer Research estimates that if the only dietary change the general population made was to increase the daily intake of fruits and vegetables to five servings per day, cancer rates could decline significantly.

Fruits and vegetables

According to the Australian Bureau of Statistics, only 5.5 per cent of Australian adults have an adequate usual daily intake of fruit and vegetables. Regularly eating fruit reduces your risk of heart disease, type 2 diabetes, some cancers, and macular degeneration. With that in mind, we can take a look at what research has shown us about some specific fruits and vegetables.

Cruciferous vegetables such as cabbage, broccoli, Brussels sprouts, kale, watercress, bok choy, turnip and cauliflower are part of the cabbage or cruciferous family. They may not all be your favourite vegetables but they are very important in your eating plan for cancer management, especially for their role in slowing the spread of cancer. In a study involving 47,909 people over a 10-year period, eating five or more weekly servings of cruciferous vegetables, especially broccoli and cabbage, was associated with half the risk of developing cancer compared to people consuming one or less servings per week.

The cooking technique is also important. For example, the cancer-protective effects of broccoli are significantly diminished when it is over-cooked. Kale can be eaten raw or lightly steamed.

Garlic and onions are allium vegetables and they may help in the prevention of prostate, ovary, stomach, colon, oral, larynx, and oesophageal cancers, and possibly breast cancer. Freshly crushed garlic is the best nutritionally.

Citrus fruits such as oranges, grapefruits, mandarins and lemons are important foods in cancer prevention. One of the important ingredients in citrus fruits is vitamin C, or ascorbic acid. According to the US National Cancer Institute, vitamin C may protect against cancer of the oral cavity, stomach and oesophagus, and may also reduce the risk of developing cancers of the rectum, pancreas and cervix, as well as breast and lung cancer.

Red grapes contain a compound in their seeds and skins called resveratrol. It is the presence of resveratrol in red wine that has prompted a lot of speculation about wine being 'good for you'. But the amount of resveratrol in wine is extremely small and this has to be balanced against the potential cancer-promoting properties of alcohol.

Resveratrol can be taken in supplement form. Because it has some oestrogen-like properties, resveratrol in supplement form should be used with caution if you have a hormone-sensitive cancer such as breast cancer or prostate cancer.

Carotenoids

Carotenoids are the yellow, orange, and red pigments found in vegetables such as pumpkin, carrots and tomatoes. For dietary carotenoids to be absorbed through the gut, there must be presence of fat in a meal. Just 3–5 grams of healthy fat in a meal appears to be enough to assist carotenoid absorption.

Women with breast cancer are significantly less likely to have recurrences if they eat five or more vegetable servings per day. A study found that women with breast cancer who had a high intake of fruit and vegetables – indicated by a high blood carotenoid concentration – had a 43 per cent reduced risk for breast cancer recurrence.

The research findings for carotenoids from food do not translate to high dose supplements and some caution does need to be applied. For example, while carotenoid levels from dietary sources appear to be protective against lung cancer, two randomised controlled trials found that high-dose betacarotene from supplements increased the risk of lung cancer in smokers and former asbestos workers (but not in non-smokers).

If you consume too much you may notice a yellow/orange discoloration of your skin (carotenemia) which is benign and reversible once you reduce the high amounts of dietary carotenoids.

Lycopenes

I mention lycopenes specifically because there has been a lot of scientific attention paid to its potential role, particularly in prostate cancer prevention and recovery.

Tomatoes have high levels of lycopene, a pigment that gives them and other foods their bright red colour and their anti-cancer potential. Lycopene's anti-cancer effect is increased by cooking tomatoes in the presence of vegetable fats such as olive oil.

Several population studies have found that men with high intakes of lycopene from tomatoes and tomato products were less likely to develop prostate cancer than men with low intakes, but we do not know whether lycopene supplements will decrease the incidence or severity of prostate cancer. There is a lot of interest in the potential for lycopene to help prevent prostate cancer, but it is not yet clear whether the prostate cancer risk reduction observed in some of these studies is related to lycopene itself, or to other compounds in tomatoes, or indeed other factors associated with lycopene-rich diets.

Soy

There are great differences in the rates of hormone-dependent cancers (breast and prostate) between Eastern and Western countries. It is thought that this may be related to the protective effects of consumption of soy-based foods in Asian countries, especially when consumption begins before puberty.

Soy foods include soybeans, soy flour, miso, tofu and soy milk. Studies have shown that to benefit from the anti-cancer effects of soy, you need to consume about 50 g per day of soy-based food. Only whole soy foods are considered cancer protective. Supplements containing soy isoflavones are not thought to have the same effectiveness.

Soy foods have also been found to be protective against colorectal cancer and gastric cancer.

Berries

Strawberries, raspberries, blueberries, goji berries and cranberries are rich in antioxidants and phytochemicals with the potential to limit the development and severity of some types of cancer. There are many mechanisms that are believed to work together to give whole berries their anti-cancer activity.

Pomegranate (*Punica granatum l.*)

Pomegranate has been used medicinally for hundreds of years. Pomegranate juice is a natural juice isolated from the fruit of the plant *Punica granatum*. It has known anti-cancer and anti-oxidant properties. Pomegranate juice and extract has been shown to slow the growth of prostate cancer cells.

Mushrooms

Mushrooms are not vegetables, rather, they are a type of edible fungus. Many different types of mushrooms are being investigated for their anti-cancer effects. Most medical studies have focused on three main varieties: reishi (*Ganoderma lucidum*), maitake (*Grifola frondosa*), and shiitake (*Lentinus edodes*).

Reishi has been used in Traditional Chinese Medicine for thousands of years for longevity and as a cancer treatment, and we are still unlocking its potential. It is also popular in other Asian countries. It has been shown in vitro to have anti-cancer effects on prostate and breast cancer cells, and to stimulate the immune system, and it has also been shown to have some potential in prevention of metastatic disease.

Maitake mushroom is known to be able to stimulate the immune system and activate certain cells that attack cancer, including macrophages, T-cells, and natural killer cells. According to the US National Cancer Institute, maitake mushrooms appear to have significant anti-cancer activity. One recent study found that maitake mushroom modified the gene expression of over 4000 genes in breast cancer cells.

The shiitake mushroom is popular in Japan. Lentinan (1,3 beta-D-glucan), a polysaccharide isolated from shiitake, has been well studied and is thought responsible for the mushroom's beneficial effects. It was shown to have anti-cancer effects in colon cancer cells.

Green tea

Green tea contains large amounts of antioxidant flavonoids and catechins (polyphenol compounds), which have been found to have many anti-cancer properties via several different mechanisms, most notably in prostate cancer.

'Juicing'

Juicing involves the extraction of juice from fruit and vegetables without the pulp or fibre. It is not healthier than eating an equivalent number of fruit and vegetables, but it does have some advantages.

If you are trying to gain body weight or maintain your current weight without losing more, then juicing fresh fruit and vegetables can be an effective way to gain the readily available and digestible phytonutrients and to help you to manage a poor appetite. Juicing is also a useful way of lifting your intake of fruit and vegetables if you have a gut problem that makes it uncomfortable for you to digest fibre.

If you know there are fruits or vegetables that would be healthy for you to include in your diet but you don't really like eating them, juicing can be a good way to disguise them.

Many vegetables lose some of their nutrient content through heat in the cooking process, so juicing them is an effective way to maintain the nutrient value. Avoid overdoing fruit juicing because of the high sugar content of fruits.

Antioxidants and cancer

Oxidation is part of the ageing process and is largely mediated by 'free radicals'. Antioxidants help to 'mop up' excess free radicals and slow the ageing process. Principally, dietary antioxidants reduce cancer risk, and a healthy diet with nutritious whole food prepared in a way that preserves its nutritional value is most protective. There are multiple protective elements in a cancer-preventive diet including selenium, folic acid, vitamin B_{12}, vitamin D, chlorophyll and antioxidants.

If your diet is deficient in any of these elements, then nutritional correction through the foods you eat will generally be preferable to a supplement. This point is illustrated by a study on breast cancer, which concluded that vegetable and, particularly, fruit consumption contributed to the decreased risk indicating the importance of diet, rather than supplement use in the reduction of breast cancer risk.' Antioxidant supplementation may be necessary where it is not possible to eat sufficient nutrients in food, or where higher doses are recommended for their therapeutic effect rather than just correcting a deficiency. An example is in providing protection against the adverse effects of radiotherapy.

CARCINOGENIC FACTORS IN FOOD

Unhealthy fats

It is not the total amount of fat in your diet that is related to an increased risk of disease, but rather the type of fat and the total energy intake (measured in calories or kilojoules). 'Healthy fats' are mono-unsaturated and polyunsaturated fats. 'Unhealthy fats' are trans and saturated fats. The main sources of saturated fats are red meat and full-fat dairy products.

Trans fats are mostly found in commercially prepared baked goods (biscuits, pies, donuts), snack foods and processed foods.

There is a link between dietary trans fats and obesity, insulin resistance, diabetes and heart disease.

The World Cancer Research Fund advocates a diet low in saturated fats. A trial on nearly 2500 women with breast cancer found that a low-fat diet was associated with a 24 per cent reduction in recurrence and 19 per cent improvement in survival after 5 years. There is also a possible association between dietary trans fats and colon cancer.

Red meat

We know that people who eat red meat (beef, veal, lamb, pork) have a higher risk of developing bowel cancer, heart disease and diabetes, and a higher risk of dying from heart disease, cancer or for that matter from any cause. Replacing red meat with fish, poultry, beans, or nuts, could help prevent heart disease and diabetes, and could lower the risk of early death. But that needs to be balanced against your need for vitamin B_{12} and iron. It is difficult to get enough of those nutrients without eating two to three serves of red meat a week.

If you do eat red meat, where possible, buy certified organic and free range to avoid added hormones, antibiotics, and chemicals used by many commercial meat producers, and keep to less than 500 g in total per week. Trim any visible fat off meat and do not overcook it. Research suggests that overcooked meat may increase the risk of cancer because carcinogenic substances called heterocyclic amines are formed in foods that are cooked and charred or blackened at high temperatures.

Processed meats

The World Cancer Research Fund recommendation is that there is no amount of processed meat (bacon, ham, salami, corned beef and some processed sausages) that can be confidently shown not to increase cancer risk, particularly for bowel cancer. Bacon, hot dogs and processed meats are known to increase your risk of cancer, heart disease and diabetes. These foods are best avoided.

Processed juices, soft drinks, sweet drinks

A lot of people think that fruit juice is healthier than soft drink because it's full of 'natural sugars'. Fruit juice does contain natural sugar – fructose, sucrose and glucose – but the amount of sugar and kilojoules is on par with soft drinks. One fruit juice might contain the sugar of up to five or six pieces of fruit but without the fibre.

I would advise you to avoid soft drinks for their high sugar/low nutrition when recovering from cancer, trying to lose weight or wanting to improve your overall wellbeing.

Alcohol

I discussed the relationship between alcohol and cancer in the chapter on alcohol (see page 295).

Artificial sweeteners

For decades there has been a debate about the potential of the artificial sweeteners saccharin and aspartame to cause cancer. While some animal studies have suggested there is a link, the official view from the US National Cancer Institute is that the current state of the evidence fails to show a convincing association between saccharin, aspartame and other sweeteners and the risk of several common cancers. This could not be considered a resounding endorsement of safety, so I would advise you to avoid artificial sweeteners. There are natural low-kilojoule sweeteners such as stevia which can be used as sugar substitutes.

Processed foods

The way food is grown, harvested, stored, processed and cooked will affect its nutritional value. The refining of grains reduces their nutrient quality. For example, if you remove the husks from cereals and grains in processing, you remove most of the fibre, B vitamins, and other phytonutrients. That is why wholegrain breads and cereals are recommended for you instead of the more refined and processed products.

Some nutrients are lost in the processes of freezing or canning, but the benefit of having more vegetables in your diet outweighs that loss. In general, focus on eating fresh, unprocessed or minimally processed foods where possible.

'Dieting'

I have a problem with most fad diets because they encourage an unhealthy obsession with one element of nutrition, usually weight loss, and many of the fad diets that are promoted by celebrities or the media are not nutritionally balanced or sustainable in the long term. It's time to get away from the notion of 'dieting' as something special or different and transition to a carefully planned, personalised eating plan that incorporates all the nutrients your body needs to recover from cancer and cancer-specific treatment and helps give you the best possible chance of a long, cancer-free life.

The only constructive outcome of short-term 'dieting' is as an exercise in mindfulness. By this I mean that for the few weeks you are on the fad diet, it forces you to prioritise thinking about the food you eat. It can also force you to get out of the rut of any bad eating habits you may have and establish healthy, long-term eating patterns. In other words, eating the right combination, quality, and balance of foods needs to become your usual pattern.

The 5-2 diet of intermittent fasting, where you eat normally and healthily for five days a week and then severely restrict kilojoule intake on two days a week, does have research evidence to support its effectiveness in weight loss and improving cholesterol levels and insulin sensitivity. However there is no evidence that it reduces the risk of cancer. It may not be suitable for you if you need to maintain steady blood glucose levels. In fact you may find it difficult to just do your normal activities on days of a restricted energy intake. Discuss this with your doctor or dietitian.

All about balance

Some years ago the food pyramid was used as a guide to healthy eating. This has now been superseded.

The Harvard School of Public Health developed a more updated and practical guide called the Healthy Eating Plate to illustrate the most appropriate balance of nutrients for your diet:

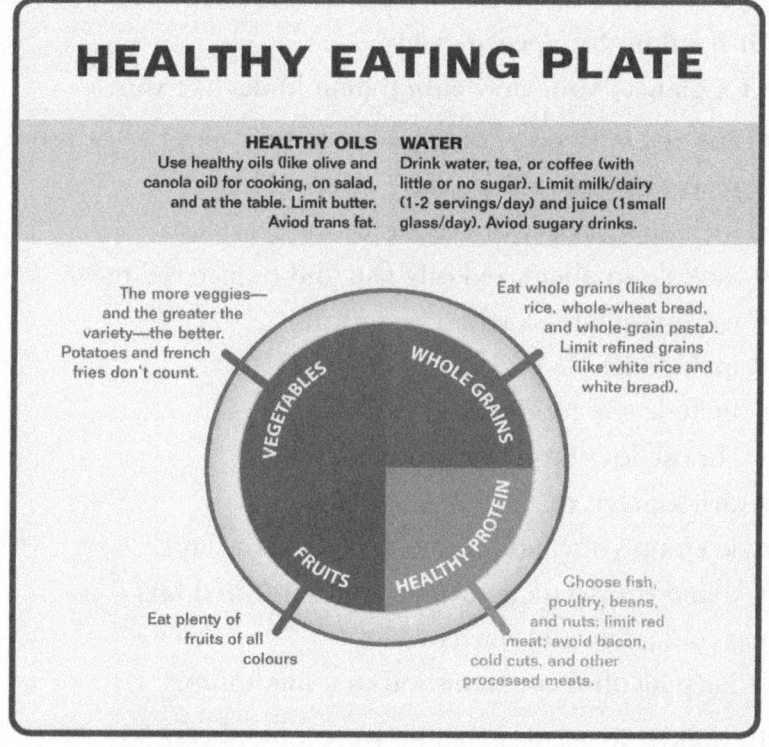

HEALTHY EATING PLATE

HEALTHY OILS
Use healthy oils (like olive and canola oil) for cooking, on salad, and at the table. Limit butter. Aviod trans fat.

WATER
Drink water, tea, or coffee (with little or no sugar). Limit milk/dairy (1-2 servings/day) and juice (1small glass/day). Avoid sugary drinks.

The more veggies—and the greater the variety—the better. Potatoes and french fries don't count.

Eat whole grains (like brown rice, whole-wheat bread, and whole-grain pasta). Limit refined grains (like white rice and white bread).

VEGETABLES

WHOLE GRAINS

HEALTHY PROTEIN

FRUITS

Eat plenty of fruits of all colours

Choose fish, poultry, beans, and nuts; limit red meat; avoid bacon, cold cuts, and other processed meats.

Nutritional supplements

See the chapter on herbs and supplements (page 188).

YOUR NEW EATING PLAN

The goal from this point on is to adapt your diet to optimise your energy levels, facilitate a rapid recovery from cancer treatment, and ultimately to maximise your chances of long-term cancer-free survival. Sound, healthy nutrition is about ensuring that you create a lifelong pattern of healthy eating.

You may have some special dietary needs, particularly if your cancer or its treatment has affected any part of your digestive system. If this is the case, I would advise you to see a qualified dietitian experienced in advising people with cancer.

You can personalise a new eating plan that satisfies your hunger, energy needs, food tastes, social life, any cultural issues and your particular health needs. You can also allow yourself a bit of freedom for special events.

At a glance, your new eating plan looks like this:

- aim to eat two or more pieces of fruit and five or more serves of vegetables a day. Think colours!
- include a variety of cruciferous vegetables
- include smaller-sized oily fish and reduce red meat
- eat organic food where practical
- include whole grains and cereals
- include soy foods
- choose low-fat dairy products
- drink green tea
- keep up your fluid intake (1–2 litres a day)
- avoid trans-fats, hydrogenated saturated fats
- avoid artificial sweeteners
- keep alcohol consumption to a minimum.

With thanks to dietitian Jaime Rose Chambers.

Immunity

If you have been diagnosed with cancer, there has already been a malfunction of your immune system. Cancer treatments such as chemotherapy and radiotherapy will cause significant damage to your immune system and so a vital part of your recovery will be to rehabilitate your immune system.

Like all other aspects of your health and wellbeing, rehabilitating your immune system is about adopting a total approach to your lifestyle rather than drinking a juice or taking a pill or going on a fad diet. Your immune system is incredibly complex and the state of your immunity depends on intricate interactions between your gut, hormones, bone marrow and blood system, respiratory tract and other body systems. Maintaining a healthy immune system requires certain raw materials to be available to the body, as well as efficiently functioning immune cells.

There are two types of immunity: innate immunity involving your body's barriers to the outside world – including the skin and the lining of the gut and respiratory tract – and your body's responses to inflammation. Overactivity of the inflammatory response causes the immune system to wrongly recognise itself as foreign and mount a counterattack, resulting in 'autoimmune' disease. Underactivity of your inflammatory response results in immune deficiency. If the immune system is under-performing, the result could be recurrent or unresolved infections, or the development of a cancer.

As our knowledge of the immune system grows, we are recognising more and more links between immune dysfunction and dysfunction of the gut.

YOUR GUT

The state of your digestive system is critical to your immune responses. The lining of the gut is populated by billions of bacteria that constantly communicate with the cells in your immune system. The immune system in the gut is constantly trying to discern what is harmful or harmless. Immune cells of different types are able to turn the inflammatory response of the immune system up or down. Specifically prescribed probiotics can help restore the balance of microflora in your gut to enhance immunity.

THE FUNDAMENTALS

My advice is always to check the fundamentals first. You might be surprised at how simple changes can give your immune system a lift:

- Get your sleep quota every night.
- Get to a healthy weight and stay there.
- Drink plenty of water.
- Keep alcohol to a minimum.
- Stop smoking.
- Eat two serves of fruit and five serves of vegetables a day. Raw or lightly cooked is best. Dark colours – for example in berries and broccoli – tend to be higher in antioxidants.

- Eliminate junk foods that are high in calories and harmful ingredients such as trans fats, but low in nutritional value.

FOODS TO INCLUDE

Foods that enhance your immune function include fruit and vegetables, low GI foods, omega-3 rich foods such as fish, mono-unsaturated fats, nuts, green tea, small doses of alcohol, antioxidant-rich foods, and herbs (for example, garlic, ginger and cumin).

FOODS TO AVOID

Foods that increase inflammation include excess kilojoules; high-GI foods; trans fats; saturated fats; salt; excessive alcohol; refined carbohydrates; artificial colours, flavours and preservatives; and gluten if you are gluten intolerant.

SPEND TIME IN THE OUTDOORS

Vitamin D is an essential regulator of the immune system, yet it is one of the most common deficiencies I see. Vitamin D deficiency is strongly associated with an increased risk of 17 common cancers. The simple antidote is regular time spent outdoors without over-doing the sun protection. That means sunshine without sunburn, ideally 20 minutes a day on average, with your limbs exposed.

EXERCISE WITHOUT OVEREXERCISING

Regular moderate aerobic and resistance activity enhances immunity and reduces inflammation, whereas overtraining makes you more susceptible to infections and chronic fatigue.

SORT OUT STRESS

The immune system responds to the biochemical effects of emotions on your body. Excessive and unmanaged chronic stress leads to increased cortisol and suppressed immunity, increasing the likelihood of infections and cancer. Make sure you take time out for yourself, spend some time with friends who make you feel good about yourself, and indulge in the things that bring you joy. Fix or eliminate toxic relationships. You may find you benefit from seeing a psychologist for help with managing your responses to stress.

FIND TIME FOR STILLNESS

Mindfulness meditation, yoga and tai chi are ways of helping achieve stillness, helping you to overcome anxiety and to give yourself a break from intrusive thoughts. Hypnosis, relaxation and guided imagery have been shown to be effective in cases of breast cancer, viral illnesses including chronic herpes simplex, and the common cold.

YOUR ENVIRONMENT

Check your house for chemicals that you can eliminate from your environment. This might include household cleaning agents, paints and solvents, passive smoking, unnecessary pharmaceutical drugs (check with your GP first), plastic containers with BPA. Turn off home appliances at the power point when not in use.

Investigate whether there are any sources of mould in your environment and take steps to remove it wherever possible.

Also check around your workplace for sources of chemicals and see whether some can be changed to less toxic agents.

SUPPLEMENTS

The best way to correct nutritional deficiencies is by correcting dietary inadequacies with a balanced diet containing as much raw, whole and organic components as possible. See a dietitian for an analysis of what you might be missing.

Some people will need supplements to quickly correct significant deficiencies such as iron or zinc. Vitamins A, B_6, B_{12}, C, D, E, folic acid and the trace elements iron, zinc, copper and selenium all work synergistically to support the protective activities of the immune cells. A multivitamin can assist with this.

The mineral zinc is especially important for the healthy functioning of the immune system. Even mild zinc deficiency can result in impairment of your immune system.

Vitamin C has long been known to help immunity. It is also necessary for iron absorption. Your body is not able to store vitamin C, so you need to eat or drink something with vitamin C and, if you exercise heavily, also take a supplement every day to maintain adequate levels.

Probiotics taken during pregnancy, when taking antibiotics, and at times of illness will enhance your immunity. Different probiotics have different actions and so the correct one to take would depend on what you are trying to achieve.

Herbs known to enhance immunity include echinacea, garlic, astragalus and andrographis. See the section on herbs (see page 188). Professional advice is important in deciding doses, combinations and timing of these herbs.

Sleep

Sleep problems such as difficulty falling asleep, trouble staying asleep, restlessness, early waking and daytime sleepiness are all common in the general population, but they are estimated to affect up to 50 per cent of people with cancer. Some of the causes will be obvious, such as anxiety or depression over your diagnosis, but there may be less obvious reasons for why you are having sleep problems, including the biochemical or physiological activity of the cancer, the adverse effects of cancer-specific treatments, or poorly managed pain.

It is a well-known fact that sleep deprivation is bad for you, both emotionally and physically. Lack of sleep makes it much harder to cope with day-to-day life. Your body needs sleep to replenish you for each day. Aside from the fatigue and mood disturbance it can bring, insomnia can be responsible for suppression of your immune system.

One of the most common prescriptions written for patients with cancer is for hypnotic (sleep-inducing) sedatives. Medication might be a temporary part of the solution but it is not the long-term answer.

Some people need very little sleep, but most of us need six to eight hours, mostly uninterrupted. Have a look at your own habits that could be affecting your sleep. For example, do you drink coffee in the evening? Do you head to bed early enough to give yourself a chance to go to sleep and get enough hours of quality sleep time?

You may have had a problem with sleep before your cancer diagnosis and it has become worse. Or it may be a new problem that has come as a part of the disease or its treatment. In some cases, sleep remains a long-term problem well after treatment for cancer has been completed. If sleep is a problem for you, it needs to be addressed.

So knowing that sleeping is important for your health now and into the future, how do you get enough of it? First we are going to look at the physiology and the nature of normal sleep patterns, and some of the common mistakes people make which lead them to lose sleep. Then we will look at ways of improving your chances of correcting unhealthy sleep patterns.

It can be helpful to anticipate that insomnia could become an issue during your treatment and make some plans to prevent it. Trying to identify any underlying cause for a sleep problem (such as pain) that can be treated is also important. If you have a sleeping partner who is a loud snorer, the reason for your insomnia is obvious. But there are many other causes.

It is almost impossible to accurately judge your own sleep quality, and it is common to think you are getting more or less sleep than you actually are.

WHAT IS NORMAL SLEEP TIME?

Everyone needs sleep. How much sleep varies from person to person and changes with age. Some people naturally need less sleep (five or six hours), while some show signs of sleep deprivation if they do not get at least eight or nine hours. Elderly people might only sleep an average of six hours a night, but may need a nap during the day.

Virtually all our body functions operate on rhythms that are governed by the brain and the activity of hormones and other chemical messengers in the body. The hormone most involved in the rhythm of sleep is melatonin. It is produced by a small gland in the brain called the pineal gland, and secreted from about 9 pm until about 4 am. Maximum sleepiness occurs at around 4 am to 5 am. The main signal for sleep rhythm is exposure of the brain to light via the retina and the optic nerve from the retina to your brain.

The timing of your sleep rhythm is important. For most people, the optimum window for sleep is between 11 pm and 7 am. Going to bed too early or too late may disturb the rhythm.

CANCER AND SLEEP PROBLEMS

Cancer-specific causes of insomnia might include pain, fever, cough, breathing problems, itch, pressure from a tumour, gut problems (nausea, constipation, diarrhoea, reflux), and many other symptoms. Any symptoms need to be carefully managed by you in conjunction with your medical oncologist or palliative care team.

Medications used to treat cancer and manage symptoms can also contribute to sleeping problems. Some of these include chemotherapy, hormone treatments, corticosteroids (for example, prednisone or dexamethasone), some antidepressants, and anti-convulsant drugs. If you are prescribed these drugs, ask your doctor whether the medication is likely to be causing or contributing to your insomnia. Always remember it is important not to adjust the dosage or cease taking these medications without medical advice and supervision.

IDENTIFYING A SLEEP PROBLEM

You have a sleep problem if:

- it takes you longer than half an hour to get to sleep
- you wake frequently during the night
- you have difficulty staying asleep
- you wake up in the early hours of the morning and have trouble getting back to sleep
- you wake feeling unrefreshed.

Having a problem getting to sleep or staying asleep may be a short-term issue. Where a sleep disorder is the fundamental problem, regardless of the type of the disorder, the signs and symptoms of longer term sleep deprivation have a big impact on your health-related quality of life.

Sleep disorders are associated with daytime fatigue; impaired memory, alertness and concentration; poor coordination; irritability and depressed mood; high blood pressure; obesity; diabetes; increased risk of stroke; heart, immune system, and endocrine dysfunction; and an increased number of accidents.

Serious sleep disorders call for medical diagnosis and intervention. Here is a sample of a few that will need advice from your GP, and will quite possibly trigger a referral for specialist treatment:

- stopping breathing during sleep, with gasping, choking sounds or heavy snoring. This could indicate obstructive sleep apnoea (OSA)
- daytime fatigue and nodding off
- sudden attacks of sleep
- kicking about in sleep
- aching, jumpy restless feeling in legs at night
- sleepwalking

- night terrors with screaming and apparently terrified
- teeth grinding.

MANAGING INSOMNIA

If you have identified that lack of sleep or interrupted sleep are creating health issues for you, then you will need to take a rational approach to managing your insomnia. In this next section I will give you some practical suggestions for getting a good night's sleep.

FIX MEDICAL PROBLEMS

Maybe you are restless because you are in pain, perhaps from arthritis. There are many medical reasons for poor sleep, so ask your GP for help. It is possible that effective treatment is available to relieve your discomfort.

Check all your medications and supplements for side effects that mention insomnia. For example, some people are sensitive to high doses of vitamin B, which will keep them awake. Medications such as steroids, beta-blockers, some antidepressants, appetite suppressants, asthma medications and many others can hype you up or affect sleep quality. Some sleep disorders will need to be referred to a specialist sleep clinic for more advanced treatment techniques.

SLEEP HYGIENE

Let's start with the fundamentals for a good night's sleep. Experts call this 'sleep hygiene'. We can just call it the good habits for successful sleep.

Establish a comfort zone

Many people complain of sleep problems when their sleeping environment is not conducive to uninterrupted rest. Check your bedroom environment and make it as quiet and comfortable as possible. If your bed is not comfortable, toss out your old pillows and mattress and replace them with new ones. Make sure your bed linen is clean and fresh and the covers are suitable to the weather, so that you are not too hot or too cold.

Then check the bedroom itself. Is it too light or too noisy? If the room is noisy, is it possible to move your bed to another part of the house that is quieter, perhaps away from the busy street or noisy neighbours? Wearing earplugs is another possible solution.

If your room seems too light, that can affect sleep. Can you hang some dark curtains to block out as much light as possible? Alternatively, wearing a sleeping mask may work for you.

If you are lacking sleep because your partner snores, you have two choices: either fix the snoring or move out of the room to get some sleep. It can be a toss-up as to which is worse for the relationship . . . being a tired, sick, over-it grumpy partner or sleeping solo.

The noise in the bedroom could be coming from a pet. If you share your bedroom with a dog that snorts and snuffles and scratches, and barks at every movement, then you might have to make other sleeping arrangements for the dog.

Exercise and sleep

Exercise helps to relieve stress, improve daytime alertness and night-time sleep quality. Timing of the exercise is important, however. It is best to exercise early in the day. Exercising in the afternoon is fine, but get the session finished several hours before your scheduled bedtime.

If you exercise later than early evening it can affect your sleep rhythm, delaying the release of the hormone melatonin, which starts the sleep cycle. It also increases your body temperature, and your body needs to cool down in preparation for falling asleep.

Forms of exercise that incorporate relaxation, such as yoga or tai chi are also beneficial for sleep quality.

Bedtime ritual

Set up a bedtime ritual to start the wind-down process. Dim the lights about an hour before you go to bed. Turn off computers, electronic devices, televisions, and other sources of light and stimulation. You might like to run a hot bath with a few drops of lavender oil, and relax and soak in the warmth. Head off to bed when you feel sleepy.

Try not to start any difficult conversations where you are likely to have disagreements or arguments just before bedtime.

Regardless of the time you go to bed, set a regular time to wake up and go outside soon after waking to expose yourself to daylight. Gradually you will find that you feel tired in the evenings at an appropriate time to get enough sleep.

Nutrition

You can get better sleep if you are in a healthy weight range and you restrict kilojoule intake. Limit fatty foods, spicy foods, and refined carbohydrates. Avoid eating large meals too close to bedtime.

Include foods rich in tryptophan, an essential amino acid that encourages sleepiness. Tryptophan is a precursor to melatonin, which helps sleep rhythm, and is found in yogurt, milk, oats, bananas, poultry, eggs, peanuts and tuna. Also increase foods rich in calcium, magnesium, vitamin B_6 and niacinamide (vitamin B_3).

Alcohol

Alcohol disrupts normal sleep patterns and worsens snoring and obstructive sleep apnoea. If sleep is a problem for you, then you will need to stay off alcohol or minimise it.

Caffeine

You probably already know that caffeine is a stimulant that can keep you awake. If you drink a lot of coffee or tea, then consider cutting back. You might suffer from withdrawal headaches if you go cold turkey, so start reducing your intake by cutting out all sources of caffeine (medicinal, coffee, tea, cola drinks, chocolate) after about 3 pm then work backwards in the day from there, down to an average of zero to two coffees or the equivalent a day, drunk early in the day.

Nicotine

Avoid exposure to tobacco smoke. Nicotine is a stimulant that impairs your ability to go into a deep sleep.

Resolve worries of the day

If your cancer or some other important issue is on your mind and stopping you from getting to sleep, try to address it with a family member, a friend, or a work colleague early in the evening and then put it on the 'to do' list for tomorrow.

Consider whether you can constructively do something about this concern right now, or even before morning. If not, write yourself a note and put the thought aside until the morning or the next day.

If you are wide awake, try putting a mental shield between you and your worries. Then imagine yourself in the place where you have felt most relaxed. Maybe it is on a beach, on a ski slope, or somewhere you once had a relaxing holiday.

Stressful life events can increase your body's production of stress hormones like cortisol and adrenaline. Counselling may help you to manage your stress. Anxiety and depression can also show up as sleep problems. Conversely, sleep problems can create or exacerbate depression.

SEE THE LIGHT!

Well-timed light stimulation in combination with other measures to improve your sleep patterns can help reset your body rhythms. Trouble getting to sleep may be helped by exposure to bright morning light (between 7 am and 9 am).

People who get sleepy early in the evening but wake up very early may benefit from exposure to light in the early evening along with some gentle exercise.

ADDITIONAL SLEEP ASSISTANCE

You may find that altering your sleep habits and your sleeping environment still does not work sufficiently for you. There are some additional interventions you can try.

Acupuncture

Acupuncture works for a lot of people with insomnia and can be an effective alternative to sedative medication. The evidence is not overwhelming, but individuals do report success with it. If you would like to try acupuncture ask your GP to recommend a practitioner.

Melatonin

Melatonin is the hormone secreted at night by the pineal gland near the brain, which gives the signal to the body to sleep. Melatonin is commonly used to help people get over the effects of jet lag and to regulate sleep cycles. Bright light, whether natural or artificial, directly inhibits the release of melatonin. Natural production of melatonin in the body declines with age, and this may partly explain why older people can find it more difficult to sleep.

There are two distinct but related reasons for considering melatonin supplementation when you have been diagnosed with cancer. The first is to encourage a regular pattern of night-time sleep, the second is to harness the purported cancer-inhibiting properties of melatonin.

Melatonin is thought to inhibit cancer development and growth, and to enhance immune function. It may also help to reduce the toxic effects of chemotherapy and radiotherapy. Additionally, melatonin has been shown to increase survival at one year after cancer diagnosis.

We know that night-shift workers have a shift in their body's biorhythms, suppression of the night-time release of melatonin, and sleep disturbances. These people not only have a suppressed immune system, but also an increased risk of developing a number of different types of cancer. In particular, research has shown an increased risk of breast cancer in women who are exposed to light at night, either as a result of bright bedrooms or night-shift work. Despite this finding, it does not necessarily follow that melatonin supplements would result in a lower cancer risk.

Melatonin secretion is impaired in patients who have already been diagnosed with breast cancer, endometrial cancer, or colorectal cancer so supplementation may be helpful.

The safest approach is to ask for medical advice about the timing and doses of melatonin supplements. One of the main mistakes people make in self-prescribing is taking homeopathic rather than therapeutic doses, or doses too low to be clinically effective, or at the wrong time. For example, if you have trouble getting to sleep, a dose of around 2–5 mg of melatonin can be taken in the early evening to help you fall to sleep earlier.

Melatonin is generally very well tolerated. Some people have reported headaches or drowsiness after taking it. For more detail on precautions and potential interactions, see page 224.

Tryptophan is a precursor to melatonin, so tryptophan-rich food such as warm milk can boost melatonin levels.

HERBAL THERAPIES

Common herbal treatments for insomnia include valerian, lavender, lemon balm, and chamomile tea. These herbs and herbal combinations are generally available over the counter and are generally considered to be safe, but ask professional advice to be sure of your individual circumstances.

MEDICATION

Realistically, there are times when even the best of sleep habits and non-pharmaceutical treatments won't cut it and you desperately need to get some sleep. This is when you will need to plan medication carefully.

There is no one-size-fits-all approach. You need to have a detailed conversation with your GP to figure out the best medication or combination for you. The choice will depend on the suspected cause for your sleep problem, the nature of the sleep problem (such as trouble getting to sleep or early waking), what treatments you have tried previously, and possible interactions with other medications you are on.

The most common medications prescribed for sleep problems are the benzodiazepines, often referred to as 'benzos'. The best approach will be to start with one of the less potent, shorter acting benzos.

A warning about medications for insomnia

A sedative taken for few days or weeks here and there can be part of a short-term solution to a temporary problem, but it is not the comprehensive solution you need. It is likely that you will need some medication to help you sleep at some stages of your treatment.

Very few people who use 'sleeping pills' regularly will experience an improvement in their sleep problem in the long term, and in fact many find their sleeping problem gets worse with time. Sooner or later, tolerance to the drugs can develop so that increased doses or stronger drugs are needed to get the same effect.

There have been multiple media reports of one sleeping pill, zolpidem, causing bizarre night-time behaviours that the person is completely unable to recall. Such is the dependence on these sorts of medications that even these known side effects do not deter people from seeking a prescription for it. Also concerning is that the inappropriate use of sedatives like benzodiazepines commonly leads to dependence, depression, mental dullness and worsening of fatigue.

Taking these medications can be particularly dangerous if you are elderly as you are more likely to have a fall if you have to get up at night to go to the bathroom while you are under the influence of medication. Sedatives can also exaggerate any decline in cognitive ability.

CHECKLIST FOR A BETTER NIGHT'S SLEEP
- Arrange medical assessment and treatment for conditions that might affect sleep, such as chronic pain.
- Check you have a comfortable, supportive mattress that is not too old.
- Make sure you have a comfortable pillow that supports your neck.
- Make sure your bedroom is a comfortable temperature.
- Exercise within your ability, early in the day, finishing at least a few hours before bedtime.
- Avoid daytime naps of longer than 20 minutes.
- Reduce sources of noise in and around your bedroom, or wear earplugs.
- Do not sleep with pets in the room if they disturb you.

- Darken your bedroom, or wear a sleeping mask.
- Develop a bedtime ritual.
- Dim the lights in the house an hour before bedtime.
- Set the alarm so you get up at a regular time.
- Avoid drinking alcohol.
- Do not drink anything containing caffeine after mid-afternoon.
- Do not smoke. Nicotine is a stimulant, which affects sleep quality, so this includes all forms of nicotine replacement.
- Minimise the use of pharmaceutical sedatives or other medications except as a short-term measure. Have a plan for tapering down and ceasing them.
- Plan your next day and talk through any problems or issues long before you go to bed . . . and try not to go to bed angry or upset.
- Manage your time to give yourself enough hours in bed to get the sleep you need.
- Do not be too rigid about your bedtime, but avoid going to bed way too early or very late.

Detoxing

The aim of the detox process during cancer recovery is to minimise your exposure to carcinogens and other toxins through the choices you make in what you eat and drink and the products you use. Medical supervision and professional advice is very important if you are undergoing treatment for cancer, and particularly if you have another chronic medical condition such as diabetes, heart disease or kidney disease. Visit your doctor and consult with your healthcare team before you undertake any form of detox during your cancer journey.

I think my view of detoxing is particularly conservative, but it is fair to say that within the medical profession and the broader healthcare disciplines there is a range of views about what is conservative and what is not. Some of the more extreme detox processes have been studied and shown to be either ineffective, dangerous, or even reduce survival, so this is why I recommend caution with the type of detox process you plan to undertake. It is important for you to ask questions about whether a particular method has been studied for its safety and effectiveness. In particular, be cautious about products that are marketed as 'detox' products. They may be harmful to you, particularly if your health status is fragile.

TOXIN EXPOSURE

There are some toxins for which there is no safe level of exposure. The most obvious and well-publicised toxin–cancer link is the risk of lung cancer and cigarette smoking. The cancer risk related to other environmental carcinogens depends on dose. For example, excessive exposure to sunshine increases the risk of skin cancer, yet too little exposure to sunshine causes vitamin D deficiency, which in turn is related to the risk of developing some cancers.

You will read in the chapter on alcohol (see page 295) that there is growing understanding of the role of excessive alcohol as a carcinogen. Infectious agents such as some bacteria and viruses can cause the cell changes that lead to cancer. You may have the potential to change your chance of recovery from this cancer, the risk of recurrence of this cancer or developing other future cancers, and the prevention or better management of chronic diseases related to toxin exposure by doing a sensible and careful detoxing process.

Your body has natural mechanisms to deal with a certain level of some, but not all, toxins. There are three particular types of chemical toxins in use which cause concern for human health:

- persistent and bioaccumulative chemicals that do not break down, or that break down very slowly in the human body
- endocrine-disrupting chemicals that interfere with the endocrine (hormonal) systems
- chemicals that are carcinogenic, cause reproductive problems or damage DNA.

Modern lifestyles in the developed world, and the increase in environmental pollutants through industrialisation can combine to overwhelm your body's capacity to clear toxins, and they can accumulate in body fluids and tissues, particularly in adipose, or fat, tissue. We are increasingly recognising the link between environmental and dietary toxins and a range of diseases. We are also recognising that toxins can be passed on to the developing foetus through the umbilical cord during pregnancy, and to a baby during breastfeeding.

Some toxins are produced by your body processes. They include:

- the biochemical end products of stress and negative emotions
- some hormones
- free radicals from oxidative stress which are associated with diseases such as arthritis and cancer, and immune system disorders.

The bulk of toxins in the body are related to environmental or dietary exposure. The organs responsible for processing and eliminating toxins are the liver, gut, lungs, skin and kidneys. Some toxins are easily eliminated, while others are beyond your immediate control. They include:

- artificial food additives such as some food colourings, flavouring agents and preservatives
- pharmaceuticals
- lifestyle-related toxins, such as cigarette smoke, alcohol, caffeine and recreational drugs
- toxins produced by bacteria
- heavy metals, such as lead, mercury, cadmium, aluminium
- vehicle exhaust fumes
- pesticides used in agriculture and in the home and garden
- plasticisers used in packaging, such as phthalates, bisphenol A

- industrial chemicals
- household cleaning chemicals.

THE DETOX PROCESS

There are a number of different detox protocols or processes. Generally speaking, detoxing has three stages: identifying the toxins, eliminating them, and restoring balance.

IDENTIFYING TOXINS

The first step in any detox process is to identify the sources of toxins that might be affecting you.

- Do you smoke cigarettes or cannabis?
- Are you taking any prescribed pharmaceutical drugs?
- Are you taking any over-the-counter pharmaceutical preparations?
- Are you using any recreational drugs?
- Do you drink alcohol?
- If so, how often do you drink and how much?
- Have you been exposed to any toxic chemicals in the workplace? This might include a wide variety of industries, including hairdressing, nail technician, gardener, cleaner, construction worker, painter, farmer etc.
- Do you use any pesticides in your house or at work? This would include domestic fly sprays and surface insect sprays, garden pesticides and agricultural chemicals.
- Do you eat meat or chicken that is not organically farmed?
- What foods do you eat that are processed and contain preservatives and other additives? Check labels for chemical content of packaged or processed foods.
- Do you eat processed fast foods?
- Which household cleaning products do you use? Are there less toxic choices?

- Do you store food in plastic food or drink storage containers, particularly ones containing bisphenol A?
- Which cosmetic products do you use, including nail polish, shampoo, perfumes, moisturisers (especially those containing parabens).
- Have you had any dental work involving mercury amalgam?
- Do you live in an area with high pollution levels?
- Does your home have an attached garage?
- If yes, do you run the car, lawn mower or other machinery in the garage?
- Are there adequate seals between the garage and the interior of the house?
- Is there adequate ventilation?
- Are potentially toxic items stored in the garage?
- Are they kept in containers with tightly sealed lids?
- Is your bowel function regular or are you constipated? (Optimal gut function is necessary for effective detoxing.)
- Do you have unchecked sources of stress in your life?

You can have laboratory tests done on your blood, urine, faeces, or hair to assess the levels of some specific toxins. Laboratory tests can be used to measure the levels of some toxins, assess your physiological detoxification pathways, and help in coming to the right conclusions. You need to think carefully when making the decision about which, if any, tests to have, because some of the investigations are expensive and are only performed by a small number of laboratories. In addition, you could find that many of the tests are not refundable through government or private health insurance.

THE ELIMINATION PROCESS

Eliminating potential toxins from your environment starts at home.

The first place to search is your kitchen. Check the nutrition panels on packaged food for artificial colourings, flavourings and preservatives. Throw these out. While you're at it, throw out any foods that have passed their use-by date.

A list of the codes for these food additives can be found here: www.foodstandards.gov.au/consumer/additives/additiveoverview/Pages/default.aspx

Look at your storage containers. It is preferable to store food in glass, but if you do use plastic, check that it is free of bisphenol A (BPA), which can increase the risk of prostate and breast cancer.

Avoid drink bottles that have the recycling codes of 3 or 7, particularly for children. Plastic bottles with BPA are usually marked with a number 7 recycling code. The best bottles to use and reuse are those with the recycling codes 2, 4 and 5. Those marked with 2 and 4 are made from polyethylene and 5 is made from polypropylene. Some reusable plastic bottles and containers will be marked 'BPA-free', which makes your task very simple indeed. But it is even better if you can avoid plastic altogether.

Avoid heating any food in plastic containers, and do not use plastic cling-wrap when you are heating or cooking food in the microwave.

Next, check the ingredients of your household cleaning products. Replace them with less toxic, more environmentally friendly products where possible.

Take out all your cosmetics, perfumes, toothpastes, and other toiletries. Check the labels for ingredients, especially parabens.

Use unbleached toilet paper and sanitary products.

If you have an attached garage, you can make sure the garage is well ventilated. Turn off your car engine before closing the garage door and open the garage door before turning on the ignition. Make sure there is an effective seal around the door leading into the house. Also avoid running any petrol or diesel driven machinery in the garage unless the garage door is wide open.

If your house has air-conditioning, make sure to have it regularly serviced and cleaned by a professional. If you have a slow-combustion heater or an un-flued gas heater, consider replacing it to reduce your exposure to carbon monoxide.

VOLATILE ORGANIC COMPOUNDS

Volatile organic compounds (VOCs) are organic chemicals that have a high vapour pressure at ordinary room temperature. VOCs are emitted by thousands of different products, including cleaning products, disinfectants, floor coverings, office equipment, pesticides, building materials, furnishings, glues, adhesives, permanent markers, paints and lacquers.

VOCs in the air are up to 10 times higher indoors than outdoors. Some VOCs, such as benzene, are known to be carcinogenic.

You can reduce the VOC load in your home by making sure your home is regularly ventilated with fresh air and only using VOC-containing products such as marker pens in a well-ventilated room. Replace whatever products you can that contain VOCs with environmentally friendly products. This can be as simple as choosing non-scented garbage bin liners and thinking about buying non-VOC-containing furnishings. Do not store VOC-containing products in your home.

Buy clothes that are macine washable and avoid dry-cleaning where possible.

DO I NEED TO ELIMINATE CAFFEINE?

In general, a couple of cups of coffee a day is fine, but while you are detoxing it is worthwhile reducing your caffeine intake to zero for a few weeks.

Stopping your caffeine intake abruptly can be harsh on your body, because the withdrawal from caffeine can cause headaches and make you feel tired and flat for several days. The more coffee you drink, the more gradually you will need to wean yourself off it. To cut down, start by reducing your total daily intake by one, then after four or five days reduce again until you get to zero. After a few weeks, if you start back on caffeine drinks, try to keep your daily quantities to one or two coffees a day, at a level where you are unlikely to experience withdrawal effects.

ALCOHOL

My advice is to avoid alcohol completely during chemotherapy and radiotherapy and for at least three months after completion of cancer-specific treatment, or longer if your liver function tests are abnormal – at least until the tests return to normal levels.

After that you can make a decision about what level of alcohol you want to resume, ranging from keeping it at zero, and hopefully not increasing it past the generally agreed 'safe' maximum level of two standard drinks in a 24-hour period no more than five days a week.

This is an important decision. In the chapter on alcohol (see page 295), you will see that alcohol is listed as a Group 1 carcinogen. It follows that avoiding carcinogens, including alcohol, will improve your chance of long-term remission.

ILLICIT DRUGS

You might not tell your doctors if you use illicit recreational drugs, but we know their use is common. The primary and immediate concern is that illicit drug use could interfere with the effectiveness of your cancer treatment. Some illicit drugs also interact with the medications used to relieve pain and other symptoms of cancer, and the side effects of treatment.

Cannabis is sometimes used by people who have cancer to relieve nausea and cancer pain, and to stimulate appetite and prevent weight loss (see page 230). It is also used to reduce anxiety and aid sleep. If you have been using a cannabis product during your cancer treatment and you want to do a comprehensive detox, then I would advise you to stop using it if you have other ways of effectively managing your symptoms.

TOXINS IN YOUR WORKPLACE

While it will be possible to eliminate some of the toxins in your workplace, others are an inherent part of the job. If you have an Occupational Health and Safety committee or officer, then it may be possible to ask him or her to deal with this. Obviously if there is protective clothing or breathing apparatus you will be using them. You may be able to suggest some simple solutions to reduce workplace toxin exposure, such as improving ventilation or having air-conditioners serviced regularly, or choosing less toxic cleaning products.

SUPPLEMENTS TO SUPPORT THE DETOX PHASE

A number of herbs and vitamin supplements can assist the detox process, but I would urge you not to self-prescribe. Rather, get expert professional advice first because planning of timing, combinations, and dosage details is important.

St Mary's thistle or 'milk thistle', probiotics, iodine, chlorophyll or chlorella, and dietary fibre and fibre supplements are all helpful.

EXERCISE

Exercise is essential to a detox process. Exercise stimulates your circulation and lymphatic system and boosts the physiological processes that help rid your body of toxins through your excretory organs. Make sure you don't overdo it at first, especially if you are suffering any withdrawal effects from alcohol, caffeine or illicit drugs. Gentle exercise such as walking, light yoga, stretching, and tai chi are fine no matter what type of detox you choose to do. If you have any physical limitations related to your cancer or its treatment, then you may need individual attention to your exercise program with instruction from a yoga teacher or exercise physiologist to adapt the program to suit you. You can increase the time and intensity of your exercise as your energy levels improve.

DETOX YOUR MIND

Stress is an internal toxin that generates potentially harmful chemical by-products in your body. Negative emotions affect your mood and also change your body's physiology through hormones, brain chemicals, and the functioning of your immune system.

To reduce the impact of stress and negative emotional states, your detox program should include some stress-management techniques such as simple relaxation and breathing exercises, meditation, tai chi, or yoga (see page 239). You may find that you unearth the need for individual counselling or joining a support group, or decide to make some major decisions about changing the way you live and work.

MERCURY FILLINGS

Your doctor can arrange a blood test to assess your mercury levels. Some people have their old mercury amalgam fillings removed as part of a detoxification process. Most dentists would advise you to leave stable amalgam fillings in place, and replace them with non-mercury fillings only if you have a problem with that tooth. I don't necessarily agree. There is some evidence that old mercury fillings do leach small amounts of mercury into your body, and there is a real question about the extent to which that might affect your health. Exposure to mercury vapour can greatly increase as a result of tooth grinding, chewing gum and drinking carbonated drinks.

If you decide to have mercury fillings replaced for any reason, make sure the dentist has systems in place to remove the amalgam safely, including dental dams and vapour suction.

The other possible source of mercury is from eating large fish varieties such as swordfish.

COLONIC IRRIGATION

There is no scientific evidence that colonic irrigation reduces the incidence of cancer or enhances wellbeing or other outcomes after a cancer diagnosis.

Potential complications include perforation of the bowel wall and dangerous electrolyte imbalances. You are at particular risk of electrolyte imbalances if you are elderly or physically frail, especially if you have kidney or heart disease.

STAYING THE COURSE

The duration of a detox depends on your current toxin load and what type of individual detox program you are planning. Every part of your daily life involves a risk of exposure to chemicals, many of which are potentially harmful to health. At the very least, a detox process serves as a consciousness-raising exercise to show you how many ways you are exposed to toxins. Yet many of these toxins can be easily eliminated or replaced with safer habits or alternatives.

Part of your strategy to elevate your health to its best level is to identify the toxins you are able to permanently remove from your life and reduce your overall toxin load. This is not just an occasional, once a year fad; it can be the plan for your long-term future.

Once you have completed the cleansing process, you can decide what you want to reintroduce. For example, you might resume drinking alcohol but at a lower level than before, and decide you will not take up smoking again.

THE DETOX PHASES

- Begin by seeing your GP for a comprehensive medical history and examination, appropriate investigations, accurate diagnosis and medical advice.
- Speak to your GP and your oncologist about your plan.
- Do a personal toxin audit of your home, workplace and other environments you visit frequently.
- Assess what you will eliminate from your lifestyle and what you will add in.
- Do a household clean-out.
- Plan your exercise program.
- Decide on your relaxation components.
- Work out a long-term plan for lower toxin exposure that you can sustain for long-term cancer recovery.

Smoking

For a lot of people who smoke, a cancer diagnosis is a strong stimulus to quit so that they improve their chances of recovery.

Cigarettes are loaded with carcinogenic chemicals. Smoking is considered to be the most important preventable cause of cancer, and quitting is one of the most effective strategies for improving your chances of survival.

Lung cancer is the most obvious cancer to be linked to smoking, but according to the World Health Organization, the risk of many other cancers is also increased by smoking. These include cancers of the head and neck (including cancers of the oesophagus, larynx, tongue, salivary glands, lip, mouth and pharynx), bladder, kidneys, cervix, breast, pancreas and colon. Even if your particular cancer is not on this list, common sense will tell you that quitting smoking may well increase your chances of surviving the cancer but will certainly improve your general health as well.

I have helped a lot of patients through the process of quitting smoking, so I know how difficult it can be. This is because nicotine has such a powerful addictive potential. Some people are more physically or psychologically addicted than others, so they can have a harder time quitting.

From my clinical experience though, the best prediction as to whether you are going to be able to quit smoking is how strongly motivated you are. If you have been diagnosed with cancer and you know that smoking increases the risk of cancer and other health problems, then that should be all the motivation you need.

Unfortunately it is not always the case. I have seen people who have to breathe through a tracheostomy hole in their neck because they have had surgery for a tobacco-related throat cancer sitting in a wheelchair outside the hospital and smoking through the tracheostomy.

If you are going to give yourself the best chance of recovery from your cancer and its treatment, you will need to avoid tobacco smoking. Forever.

So you think the horse has bolted? Not so. Even after you have been diagnosed with cancer, your risk of dying will be reduced if you quit smoking.

The benefits of quitting go far beyond survival from your cancer. There is also the benefit to your heart, lungs, blood vessels, bones, and all other organs of your body.

QUITTING

Once you have the motivation, the next thing is to make a plan.

What are my health priorities? You have been diagnosed with cancer so that will almost certainly be one of your highest priorities for the foreseeable future. Your full recovery will depend on you making quitting smoking a permanent high priority issue. As time goes by, it does get easier.

What can I change? It helps to look at the patterns of your life and where smoking fits into that pattern. You can try keeping the same patterns and just not smoking, but if you find that too difficult, then you may need to change what you do that is linked to smoking. I will give you an example. Some years ago I was helping a woman to quit smoking. She had a strong family history of heart disease and her blood pressure had started to increase. She worked in a non-smoking environment so she was mainly an evenings-and-weekends smoker. Her daily weekday pattern involved coming home tired from an intense day in the office and sitting in the back garden smoking. As we talked it through, she figured out that what she enjoyed was the moment of solitude and quiet, and just being able to stop for a while before she got into her evening routine of supervising the children's homework, making dinner, and getting the children off to bed. So we decided on a strategy where she would come home and make a pot of green tea or other herbal tea, and take that into the back garden. She also learned some yoga breathing techniques for relaxation. That was all she needed to be able to quit. Although she maintained the same pattern, she replaced the harmful part of that habit with a beneficial one.

On the other hand, I recall trying to help a man in his forties quit smoking. The problem for him was that all his social contacts were smokers. He would go well for most of the week, but from Friday night and across the weekend, his friends would pass around the cigarettes and encourage him to go outside to smoke with them. Once he had a couple of drinks he found his resistance was down and he would start smoking again. Over the course of a week he was smoking less, but he still had not quit. So he changed his social pattern to seeing friends over dinner at a restaurant but not in smoking environments for several months. That strategy worked for him. Once he became accustomed to socialising without smoking, he was able to go back into groups of smokers without taking it up again.

How committed am I to the change? Even if every neurone

in your brain tells you that it is a good idea to stop smoking, no strategy will work if you are not committed to the end result. If you don't really want to quit, even if continuing to smoke means less chance of surviving your cancer, then try by all means, but you are not likely to succeed unless you are committed. Remind yourself of the reason you need to quit, even if you don't really want to quit right now. It is important that the people close to you understand and support your decision to quit, but you need to avoid making it 'their problem' or their responsibility.

What are the likely/real obstacles and what are the practical ways to get around them? Some obstacles are very predictable. For example, if you have a partner who smokes at home and you are used to smoking together, then unless you both commit to quitting, you are less likely to succeed. If you do both quit, it is a win–win situation.

Spend some time thinking about the likely obstacles for you and then plan your way around them. An example of this is the potential for weight gain when you quit smoking. Some people will put on weight. A weight gain of three or four kilos in the months after you quit is common, but again, not inevitable. You will need to plan a comprehensive strategy involving careful attention to what you are eating and regular exercise. It may help to see a dietitian for an eating plan in preparation for quitting.

The key to successful quitting is to change the patterns and routines you associate with smoking. Stop weighing yourself for a while, plan to take up a new activity routine, adopt a healthy low-fat diet, change your social patterns associated with smoking.

Having the determination to overcome such a powerful addiction as nicotine is the first step. Seeing the cigarette as the enemy rather than a companion or part of your identity can be more difficult.

Most of the studies into self-quitting show that after six to 12 months, only 3–5 per cent of people have been able to maintain abstinence. But among people with cancer, long-term quit rates often exceed 50 per cent.

If you are making the decision to quit, different methods work for different people. Don't give up if your first attempt at quitting fails. You might need to try a number of different techniques before you find something that works for you in the long term.

NON-PHARMACEUTICAL METHODS

Going 'cold turkey' is, in my opinion, the best way to quit if you can. The reason for this is that pharmacological methods to aid smoking cessation all have significant potential side effects, and nicotine replacement therapy can continue the addiction to nicotine.

If you are due to go into hospital for surgery, this may be a decision that is made for you.

You can expect some short-term discomfort, particularly if you are physically addicted. Some people suffer more withdrawal symptoms than others, with symptoms like impatience, irritability, anger outbursts, anxiety, depression, difficulty concentrating, insomnia and restlessness. This is not inevitable, but if it does happen you can expect it to last for up to four weeks.

It is quite likely that you will need some non-pharmacological techniques to help you cope with the withdrawal from nicotine, especially in the early stages. Cognitive behavioural techniques and hypnotherapy provided by a qualified psychologist will help with this. Additionally, you might like to try acupuncture, herbal medicines, hypnotherapy or cutting down the number of cigarettes you smoke until you are able to quit.

ACUPUNCTURE

Anecdotally, some people say that acupuncture has helped them to overcome cravings and withdrawal from nicotine, but evidence at this stage does not support it.

HERBAL MEDICINES

The herb St John's wort (*Hypericum perforatum*) can help stabilise your mood and is best started two to three weeks before your quit date to prepare for the transition. To minimise herb–drug interactions, choose a high-quality preparation that has a low hyperforin content. You will need to check with your GP or pharmacist for any potential interactions. St John's wort is not recommended during chemotherapy for this reason.

'CUT DOWN TO QUIT'

If stopping suddenly is too difficult for you, then another way to quit is to gradually and consciously reduce the number of cigarettes by stretching out the intervals between one cigarette and the next.

You may have some time in your prehabilitation phase to cut down with the aim of quitting within a few weeks. Set a date and make a plan. Timing will depend on your cancer treatment plan.

Let's say you usually smoke an average of 25 cigarettes a day. From the day you start the cut-down plan, set side 20 cigarettes a day as the maximum number you will smoke for the next four to seven days. The following few days, make it 15 a day. Then cut down to 10 a day. If that speed of reduction is going well, you might then reduce by one or two a day over the next few weeks. When the number per day gets down to about four or five, only light up if you are suffering withdrawal effects and smoke only half that cigarette. Gradually reduce to zero.

As you plan the reduction, think about the routines you might need to change to make it easier for you to avoid your usual smoking triggers or environments once life returns to normal.

PHARMACEUTICAL OPTIONS

There are three main pharmaceutical options for aiding smoking cessation. They are nicotine replacement therapy, bupropion and varenicline.

None of these aids works particularly well without psychological support to change entrenched behaviour patterns associated with smoking, and particularly situations where you are likely to be tempted to take up smoking again. In fact, long-term quitting rates are modest at best using these aids. And bupropion and varenicline have significant side effects and interactions with other drugs that need to be considered.

Remember that the most powerful factor in your decision to quit smoking and to stay away from cigarettes is what is going on in your own head.

If you have a history of depression, you will need to have the support of your GP, psychologist or psychiatrist through the quitting process, as depression might become temporarily worse in the early weeks or months after you quit smoking.

NICOTINE REPLACEMENT THERAPY

Nicotine replacement therapy (NRT) is available in the form of patches, lozenges, gum, inhalers and nasal spray. The idea is to eliminate the cigarettes and replace the cocktail of carcinogenic chemicals with nicotine only.

I have seen a lot of patients who start smoking again or they are still chewing away on nicotine gum years after they stopped smoking, and studies show that the majority of people who try to quit using NRT are back smoking within six months. Adverse effects from using NRT are related to the type of product, and include skin irritation from patches, irritation to the inside of the mouth from gum and tablets, and nausea. There is no evidence that NRT increases the risk of heart attacks.

So the problems are that the nicotine in the NRT is still addictive and has side effects, and quitting needs commitment and some form of behavioural support and monitoring to be successful. Plus we do not know a lot about the health effects of long-term nicotine replacement.

NRT is a transitional aid to weaning off the habit of smoking, so you will need to start the therapy with the intention of gradually reducing the doses to zero. I would advise you to talk to your GP about the right starting dose for you, which will depend on your usual and current level of smoking, and your estimated level of addiction. You can also discuss your need for psychological counselling and support which will increase the likelihood of you successfully quitting.

It is better, if you can, to try methods of helping you quit that don't use nicotine or other pharmaceuticals.

'ELECTRONIC CIGARETTES'

It's a weird experience the first time you walk past someone smoking an 'electronic cigarette'. There they are, sucking on a plastic tube, fumes inhaled and then expelled in a plume of what looks like smoke but has no odour. This is called 'vaping'. The questions I had were 'What are these "electronic cigarettes"?', 'Do they help anyone quit tobacco smoking?' and 'What is the downside?'.

Here is what I found out. 'Electronic cigarettes' are battery-operated devices that dispense nicotine but not the other harmful chemicals in tobacco. So they are a type of NRT delivery system. The plume of 'smoke' that is exhaled is not smoke, but vaporised liquid (hence the term 'vaping'), designed to give the smoker the sensation of blowing out smoke.

The reasons for using them are to be able to smoke without affecting other people around you, as a way of quitting smoking without quitting nicotine, and as an aid to the 'cut down and quit' method of reducing nicotine use as a strategy for quitting the habit.

They were marketed as a quit smoking aid, but the evidence really does not support their effectiveness in helping you to quit smoking, or their safety. In particular, it is not clear whether 'vaping' reduces or in fact increases nicotine addiction. In fact, at this stage they would seem to be just another method for people with a nicotine addiction to inhale nicotine.

VARENICLINE AND BUPROPION

I am highly sceptical about the hype around the pharmaceutical drugs varenicline and bupropion for quitting smoking. They promise to make the quitting process easier, but these medications can have serious side effects such as cardiovascular events and suicidal thoughts. For this reason I would certainly not consider them as first-line treatments.

Varenicline side effects

The common side effects include nausea (usually mild to moderate and fades with time), stomach or bowel problems (for example, constipation, bloating, dry mouth, vomiting, indigestion), headache, dizziness, sleeping problems, unusual dreams, feeling tired, increased appetite, and changes in taste perception.

The more serious side effects include depression, agitation, aggression, thoughts of self-harm, self-harm, thinking about suicide, suicidal behaviour and hallucinations Because of the potential for these more serious side effects, even in people with no prior history of mental illness, you need to let someone close to you know when you start to take the medication, and ask them to tell you if they notice any change in your mood or personality.

Bupropion side effects

The most common side effects include difficulty sleeping, dry mouth, headache, dizziness, anxiety and nausea. The most serious side effect is the risk of seizure, which is estimated to occur in about one in 1000 patients (or 0.1 per cent).

It is possible to have an allergic reaction to bupropion, including itching, hives, or trouble breathing. There have been a few cases of fever, joint and muscle pain, with skin rash occurring 10–20 days after starting treatment. If you think you are having an allergic reaction to bupropion, stop taking it and tell your GP immediately or go to the casualty department at your nearest hospital.

It is also possible to develop mental health problems, such as depression and suicidal or self-harming behaviour. Symptoms are more likely to occur early in the treatment. Bupropion can worsen symptoms in people with certain types of mental illness, so it is important to discuss your history with your GP before you consider taking it.

You also need to consider the potential for any interactions with prescribed medications you are taking as part of your cancer treatment, so it is important to weigh up the risks and benefits in a careful individual discussion with your doctor.

DOES QUITTING MAKE A DIFFERENCE?

According to the American Cancer Society:

5 years after quitting: your risk of cancer of the mouth, throat, oesophagus and bladder are halved. Cervical cancer risk falls to that of a non-smoker.

10 years after quitting: your risk of dying from lung cancer is about half that of a person who is still smoking The risk of cancer of the larynx and pancreas decreases.

To maintain your determination to quit smoking, focus on the reality of smoking: smoking-related cancers, shortened life span, smelly breath, wheezy cough, yellowed teeth, bouts of bronchitis, deep wrinkles across your face, so puffed you can't walk from one room to another without stopping to catch your breath. Look at your children, your partner, your friends and think of them losing you to a smoking-related disease.

If you quit for a while but relapse, it is not a failure. See it as a temporary setback and try again.

Travel Plans

If you are undergoing cancer treatment or you have recently completed your treatment and you are feeling better, you might intend to travel, either for work or for a holiday. Alternatively, travel might be on your bucket list.

This decision to travel is one you need to discuss with your GP and oncologist because travel, even first-class travel, is physically and emotionally challenging. There are many factors to consider, but the first and most important issue is whether you are fit to travel at this stage.

You and your doctor will need to consider:

- your general state of health
- the severity of any current symptoms
- how stable your medical condition is
- whether you need immunisations for your destination countries.

The choice of destinations and itinerary is critical to this last point. There are some immunisations that cannot be given if you are on immunosuppressant drugs.

If you are on medications that suppress your immune system, it would be inadvisable to travel to countries where there is a high risk of diseases such as dengue fever or chikungunya virus. You will need to carefully work out which immunisations are needed for your destination.

The other considerations are fatigue, cabin air pressure, the risk of thromboembolism (deep vein thrombosis [DVT] and pulmonary embolism), and symptom management when you are away from your usual team of healthcare practitioners.

FATIGUE

When you are planning your itinerary you will need to be mindful of your level of fatigue and any other physical limitations. Look at the length of flights or journeys and the number and timing of stopovers and transfers. If you are a seasoned traveller, you will need to turn down the pace of your usual travel, even if you think you could cope with more.

Rather than jumping from one place to another, plan your itinerary so that you can have rest days, as well as controlled activities with rest periods during each day.

If you are flying, some of the international terminals can be very large and require you to walk long distances to the gate or to baggage handling. You can ask airlines in advance to arrange wheelchair transport through air terminals.

BE PREPARED

Take a supply of all of the medications, non-prescription items and supplements that you are likely to need for the entire trip. It is possible to get medication overseas and in regional areas of Australia but the less common medications and supplements may not be easily obtainable in some places you might travel.

Make inquiries about the standard of health services in your destination countries.

Check out the standard of health services and emergency services in the regions where you plan to travel.

Your travel plans may need to be flexible too. If you are planning to visit family and they live in a part of the world that is medically underserviced or where the journey there is difficult, perhaps they could meet you in another destination more suitable to your condition?

MEDICAL DOCUMENTATION

Ask your GP to give you a letter containing a list of all of the medications and supplements you will be carrying, and include the words 'for personal medical use'. This will help you through customs if you are carrying large quantities of medicines. It is an offence in some countries to carry certain drugs such as narcotic analgesics, even if you have a prescription for them. Check the regulations in your destination countries.

Ask your general practitioner and your oncologist to write a medical introduction for you in case you need to seek medical treatment while you are away. Your GP's letter will contain a list of all of your significant medical conditions, past and current treatments and a full list of medications and supplements.

Make sure you have an action plan in case you become unwell. Have a discussion with your doctor about medications you need to take with you in case of emergency. This usually includes regular medications and supplements as well as a first aid kit with topical antiseptic ointment, appropriate antibiotics, medicines for diarrhoea and vomiting and other emergency supplies.

Be alert to the fact that some common medications like anti-malaria medications can interact with some chemotherapy drugs. If your immunity is significantly weakened, I usually advise patients to avoid malaria-prone countries.

Remember you can call your regular doctor from overseas during office hours if you run into trouble and the doctors treating you need more information.

You will need travel insurance suitable to the countries you are visiting, and your travel insurance should include medical evacuation.

ALTITUDE

Flying stresses your body in a number of ways. One is the altitidue and changing air pressures. Planes do not pressurise to sea level, but to 1500–2500 m above sea level. This will effectively reduce the pressure of oxygen available to breathe. Healthy people will compensate for these changes but if you have health problems, particularly with your lungs or circulation, your doctor will have to consider whether you are safe to fly at all. One indication is if you are short of breath when you are at rest or if you become breathless with minimal exertion.

Before you travel is it also wise to have blood tests for anaemia. This is a common consequence of cancer treatment and may be able to be corrected with appropriate supplementation. A low oxygen pressure environment will worsen the effects of anaemia.

If you have had chest surgery within the last month or a pneumothorax you will be advised against flying.

If there is any doubt, there is a test called hypoxic challenge testing to see how you fare.

DVT (DEEP VENOUS THROMBOSIS)

These days you can't miss the messages about long haul flights and the risk of DVT (deep vein thrombosis) and pulmonary embolism (blood clots in the lungs). It is common to see these messages about exercises to reduce the risk of blood clotting as a part of the general safety warnings during takeoff. Most experienced travellers wear compression stockings to help venous blood return.

Malignancy increases your risk of clotting. Over and above this, many people in the population have a genetic predisposition to blood clotting. You can have blood tests to see if you are genetically at increased risk.

There is no evidence that taking aspirin before you fly reduces the risk of DVT.

Discuss with your doctor whether it would be wise for you to use injected anti-clotting medication before you fly. If you are advised to inject blood thinning medications, you will need to check the protocols for carrying hypodermic syringes across borders. This is problematic in some countries, even if you are carrying medical certificates explaining their necessity.

IMMUNISATION

One of the essential preparations for travel is to find out what immunisations are recommended or compulsory before you leave. There are different types of vaccine. Some are in the category of 'live attenuated vaccine' and these are the ones you have to be cautious about if your immunity is compromised. Yellow fever and typhoid are the main travel vaccines in this category. Some countries will not let you in unless you have a current certificate of yellow fever vaccination or a certificate from your doctor explaining why you cannot have it.

Inactivated vaccines are safe for you to have, but they may be less effective if you are immune suppressed. See this website for more information: wwwnc.cdc.gov/travel/destinations/list

DIET

If you have special dietary needs, it is worth doing some homework before you go to make sure your accommodation can either supply the food you are able to eat, or that you stay nearby to a supermarket or grocery store to buy indgredients and that you have facilities to prepare food. Staying in a serviced apartment may be preferable to a hotel for example. Make sure you take a day pack of food as it may be difficult to find suitable foods for you at the times that you need to eat.

· PART SEVEN ·

The most common forms of cancer

Bowel Cancer

Let's get the terminology right to begin with. 'Bowel cancer' is a term usually used to describe cancers of the caecum, large bowel, and rectum. These cancers are also collectively known as 'colorectal cancer'.

I make special mention of colorectal or bowel cancer because it is one of the most common causes of cancer deaths, yet is almost entirely preventable with the right screening, good timing, and a bit of luck. In fact, it is estimated that almost one-half of cases can be prevented by following a healthy lifestyle. I have also focused on bowel cancer because it is one of the conditions that requires special management after treatment to maximise your recovery.

The five-year relative survival for bowel cancer for the period 2006–2010 in Australia was 65.3 per cent for men and 67.1 per cent for women. If bowel cancer is detected and treated early, it can be cured.

BOWEL CANCER TESTING

Bowel cancer most often arises from precancerous lumps in the bowel wall called polyps. This condition can sometimes run in families, or just happen in an individual without a family history. The aim of screening is to detect these polyps at an early and treatable stage.

More than 95 per cent of colorectal cancers are adeno-carcinomas. This means they started in the gland cells in the bowel wall. Other types are rare and they include squamous cell cancers, carcinoid tumours, sarcomas and lymphomas.

FAECAL OCCULT BLOOD TESTING

The most established population screening test is FOBT, or faecal occult blood testing. Australia has a National Bowel Cancer Screening program that offers FOBT, which I fondly refer to as the 'Poo-in-the-Post' test.

'Screening' refers to testing whole populations of people with no symptoms to detect diseases at an early and hopefully treat-able stage. A test kit is sent to individuals at particular ages over 50, a sample of faeces ('poo') is then collected and sent back to a central laboratory to be tested for the presence of blood. This test is notoriously non-specific – meaning that there are many reasons other than a polyp or a cancer for why there might be blood in a faeces sample – and it misses a lot of cancers. But it certainly does detect a large number of cancers at a treatable stage, so that is good news for those people.

If you have a negative test, meaning there is no blood present, it is not a guarantee that you do not have a bowel cancer or a polyp. A polyp or cancer just may not have been bleeding at the time the sample was taken. But the expense to the health system is justified because it is said to be 'better than nothing'. It is also a test we use in some cases where the preparation for a colonoscopy or the colonoscopy itself is judged to be too dangerous for a patient to undertake, or where colonoscopy is inaccessible or too expensive.

FLEXIBLE SIGMOIDOSCOPY

Another test that can be used if colonoscopy is not possible is flexible sigmoidoscopy. Like colonoscopy, this is a direct look at the inside of the colon, but only sees the lower end of the colon (the sigmoid colon) and rectum. This will identify problems in the lower part of the bowel, but would obviously miss any lesions higher up in the large bowel.

COLONOSCOPY

The most accurate screening test for bowel cancer is colonoscopy. This involves a clear fluid fast and cleaning out your bowel by drinking a preparation that causes your gut to flush through until it is empty. A camera on a long fibre-optic scope is then inserted into the rectum and passed up to the end of the large bowel. Any suspicious areas or polyps are removed and examined.

The limitations of this test are the preparation, the small risk of perforation of the bowel during the test, the time involved, the expense of the test for people who do not have medical insurance, and the concern that some people take a while to get their bowels working normally again after the test.

Once you have been diagnosed with cancer, regular colonoscopy becomes a monitoring test, not a screening test. You will also be advised to have a regular blood test for the bowel cancer tumour marker CEA (chorio-embryonic antigen).

Investigating suspicious symptoms

Aside from looking for microscopic amounts of blood in the stool, any symptoms suggesting bowel cancer or its recurrence need to be investigated as a matter of urgency. These symptoms might include:

- visible blood or mucus in the faeces (check the toilet bowl)
- an unexpected and persistent change in bowel habit (for example, diarrhoea or constipation)
- discomfort, bloating, fullness, pain, cramps in your abdomen
- constant tiredness
- low or falling iron or haemoglobin levels on blood testing with no apparent cause (such as a dietary deficiency of iron or heavy periods in a woman).

STAGING SYSTEM

In Australia, the staging system for bowel cancer is the Australian Clinico-Pathological Staging (ACPS) System. The four stages are:

- Stage A – the cancer is confined to the bowel wall.
- Stage B – the cancer has spread to the outer surface of the bowel wall.
- Stage C – cancer is found in lymph nodes near the bowel.
- Stage D – cancer is found at distant sites away from the primary cancer, such as in the liver or lungs.

You may also hear about the 'Dukes' system, which is like the ACPS system. Dukes Stage A equals ACPS Stage A, and so on.

The TNM system records how far the tumour (T) has spread through the bowel wall, if lymph nodes (N) are affected by the cancer, and whether the cancer has spread (metastasised) to other parts of the body (M).

Your oncologist or surgeon will explain your stage and what that means for your prognosis.

Make sure you obtain and keep copies of your original pathology results. This will be important for future treatment planning, particularly once you have completed your initial round of cancer-specific treatments.

Also maintain a record of all of the test results and treatments you have along the way.

TREATMENT

Cancer-specific treatment for bowel cancer usually involves surgery to remove the affected section of bowel. Surgical procedures will vary depending on the type and location of your tumour. You may have a hemicolectomy (removal of part of your large bowel) or a total colectomy (removal of all of your large bowel).

Depending also on the location of the tumour, the end of the bowel will either be opened through the skin on your abdomen, forming a stoma where your bowel contents are collected in a bag temporarily (until the bowel heals) or permanently, or the ends are joined up to form a shorter large bowel.

Chemotherapy or radiotherapy is nearly always recommended in addition to surgery. Your cancer specialists will advise you on the most effective treatment for you.

COLOSTOMY CARE

My grandfather had bowel cancer, which means that I have a family history and something of a memory for his bowel cancer experience.

I remember he emerged from the operating theatre with a colostomy. At the time he was told that it would be permanent because of the technical difficulty in reattaching the two ends of his bowel. Before he left hospital, he had a lot of education from the stoma therapist in how to look after his colostomy and, in his usual manner, he dealt with it with little fuss. That was over 30 years ago. We do not see too many colostomies these days, certainly not permanent ones, because the surgical techniques have improved so much over the years. But it is sometimes still necessary.

If you are having surgery for bowel cancer, the surgeon will discuss the possibility of a stoma with you. Sometimes it is difficult for your surgeon to say for sure whether or not they will be able to reattach the end of bowel until they see what they are dealing with in your lower abdomen. You may find that you have to manage a colostomy temporarily or permanently.

Larger hospitals and cancer units will have a specialist stoma care nurse who will be able to give you any information you need and answer your questions.

If you have a partner, it will be important for him or her to attend these information sessions. You may also have questions about managing sexuality and intimacy after stoma surgery. (See the chapter on intimacy, sexuality and cancer recovery on page 106.)

RISK FACTORS FOR BOWEL CANCER

The risk factors for bowel cancer include some you cannot do anything to change:

- getting older – bowel cancer more commonly affects people aged 50 and over
- inheriting a fairly rare genetic disorder – familial adenomatous polyposis (FAP) or hereditary non-polyposis colorectal cancer (HNPCC)
- a strong family history of bowel cancer
- having ulcerative colitis (inflamed colon lining) for longer than eight to 10 years
- undetected and untreated coeliac disease.

If any of these risks is relevant for you, then your GP will talk to you about a program of close monitoring. It will also mean that throughout your life, and passed on to your children and their children, you will need to be even more mindful of the things you can do to reduce your risk of bowel cancer occurring or recurring. In other words, you may have the gene or the predisposition to bowel cancer, but you do not have to surrender to your genes or to your own bowel cancer history.

Some of the things you *can* change to reduce your bowel cancer risk and help your recovery are:

- Don't smoke. Bowel cancer risk is higher for current smokers.
- Keep your body weight in a healthy range.
- Pay attention to nutrition throughout your life.
- Have a blood test for vitamin D level. If the level is low, increase your skin exposure to sunlight (without risking sunburn) and supplement with vitamin D.
- Exercise regularly as a lifelong habit. (See the chapter on exercise, page 307). You can start gentle walking or other mild exercise soon after surgery, but be mindful it is important to wait for at least six weeks or longer depending on advice from your surgeon, before you do abdominal exercises so that you do not risk incisional hernia. If you experience pain or discomfort during exercise, stop and ask your doctor to check why.

Overall colorectal cancer rates in Australia have been stable or declining, however a 2014 South Australian study has found that the incidence of colorectal cancer among people in their twenties has doubled over the past two decades. Rates have also risen 35 per cent among people in their thirties. People with early onset bowel cancer are around four times more likely to have a family history of bowel cancer compared with other cases, but the majority still have no known predisposition.

The theory is that the increase in incidence is likely to be linked to behavioural changes in children and young adults, such as greater consumption of high-fat processed food, obesity, a sedentary lifestyle, and the increasing rate of early diabetes. The researchers also suggested that binge drinking and recreational drug use among teenagers and young adults could be another factor.

Younger patients tend to present with more advanced cancer, with around 90 per cent of patients having symptoms of cancer at the time they were diagnosed. This is probably because younger patients are not subject to the screening that is offered to people over 50 to detect asymptomatic disease, but may also be due to the more aggressive forms of cancer found in early onset disease.

To my mind the strong message is to continue protective life-style measures throughout life.

AFTER BOWEL CANCER SURGERY
NUTRITION

I have detailed the general elements of healthy nutrition after a cancer diagnosis in the chapter on nutrition (see page 323). There are some special dietary considerations if you have had bowel cancer, however, and particularly if you have had a significant part of your bowel removed.

In my experience of managing the health care of people who have been through standard hospital treatment, nutrition is not given the detailed attention that it deserves and many patients need a lot of nutritional rehabilitation. It is common for patients to tell me that the only advice about nutrition they received was, 'Make sure you eat a healthy diet'.

Here are some more helpful guidelines:

- Prefer organic foods where possible and available.
- Eat small amounts only of lean red meat as part of a mixed diet including carbohydrates (breads and cereals), vegetables and fruit.

- Keep your dietary content of animal fats very low.
- Exclude trans fats, found in some processed and packaged foods.
- Include low-fat dairy foods in your diet as they seem to be protective against bowel cancer. Use lactose-free products if you have lactose intolerance.
- Avoid eating processed meats including ham, bacon, sausages, salami and pâté.
- Avoid alcohol. If you do have a few drinks, the fewer the better but certainly keep it at two or less a day, no more than five days a week. Remember, there is no known safe minimum threshold of alcohol consumption for cancer risk.

DRINK PLENTY OF FLUIDS

Remember to drink plenty of fluids, especially if you have had a total colectomy (removal of all of the large bowel). One of the major roles of the large bowel is to absorb water and electrolytes. After a colectomy you can lose half a litre to a full litre of water a day, plus electrolytes, and end up chronically dehydrated and depleted of electrolytes. Symptoms of this can include fatigue, thirst, muscle cramps and headaches.

You will need to drink a lot more water than before your surgery in order to avoid becoming dehydrated, and also consider taking an electrolyte replacement. This is particularly important when you do aerobic exercise because you will lose additional fluid due to sweating.

FIBRE INTAKE

How much fibre you need can be more difficult to estimate. Some people will need more fibre while others need less than before surgery. You may find that raw vegetables cause some discomfort in the early stages of recovery but you can gradually increase these as you are able to tolerate them. You might need the guidance of a skilled dietitian to help you work out how much fibre is right at various stages of your recovery.

SUPPLEMENTS

Supplements may be prescribed after bowel cancer surgery to account for the possibility of nutritional deficiencies or to reduce the risk of recurrence. In other cases, specific supplements need to be avoided.

Vitamin B_{12} (cyanocobalamin) – If you have had a hemicolectomy (removal of part of your large bowel) or a total colectomy, sometimes the lower part of the ileum (terminal ileum or end of the small bowel) is also removed. The terminal ileum is the part of the bowel where most of the absorption of vitamin B_{12} occurs. If your terminal ileum was removed in surgery you will need to supplement with vitamin B_{12} to avoid deficiency. The symptoms of vitamin B_{12} deficiency include fatigue, anaemia, loss of appetite, weight loss, apathy and depression. You might get a smooth tongue. Eventually vitamin B_{12} deficiency can lead to degeneration of peripheral nerves progressing to paralysis.

Obviously there is no point taking tablets because you can't absorb the vitamin B_{12} through the remaining gut. There are two options here: vitamin B_{12} can be absorbed under your tongue or through the lining of your mouth. You can use an oral spray or sublingual tablets daily. The other option is an injection of vitamin B_{12} once a month with regular monitoring of your blood levels of vitamin B_{12}.

Vitamin B_6 (pyridoxine) – Vitamin B_6 is thought to play a preventive role in the prevention of bowel cancer. It is important to avoid Vitamin B_6 deficiency, before or after a diagnosis of colorectal cancer. Food sources include sunflower seeds, pistachios, tuna, chicken, turkey, bananas, avocado and spinach.

Folate – Studies suggest an approximately 40 per cent reduction in the risk of colorectal cancer in individuals who have the highest dietary folate intake compared with those with the lowest intake. The recommendation is to increase dietary folate from food sources such as whole grains and green leafy vegetables, and definitely *not* take high-dose long-term supplementation. This is because a 2009 meta-analysis found no effect of taking folic acid supplements for less than three years, but showed that taking folic acid supplements for three years or more increased the risk of precancerous bowel adenomas and bowel cancer by 35 per cent.

Selenium – It is not clear from evidence whether selenium is protective against bowel cancer. The simplest form of dietary selenium is to eat two Brazil nuts a day. If your food supply comes from selenium-depleted soil, then supplementation may be warranted, but it is important not to overdose as this can cause side effects.

Calcium – Calcium supplementation, particularly in combination with vitamin D, appears to reduce the risk of bowel cancer.

Vitamin D – Low vitamin D is associated with a higher risk of bowel cancer. An agreed protocol for the optimal dose for prevention has not yet been established. Ask your GP for advice about this, but as a general rule, if your vitamin D level is low, supplement with 2000–5000 IU (depending on how deficient you are) per day for one month, then 1000–2000 IU per day for maintenance. Recheck your vitamin D blood levels after four months. I also recommend increasing outdoor exercise and regular exposure of your skin to sunlight.

Magnesium – Higher magnesium intake is associated with lower risk of colorectal cancer. After colectomy, absorption of magnesium can be decreased and magnesium loss increased. A supplement of magnesium is recommended after a colectomy to avoid magnesium deficiency.

Potassium and sodium are electrolytes that can be lost if you have diarrhoea and may need to be replaced with electrolyte solution, especially with exercise. These levels are easily checked with a standard blood test.

PROBIOTICS

Perhaps the most exciting field of discovery in anything to do with gut health is the field of probiotic research and practice. This is certainly true of bowel cancer. There are two main reasons for using probiotics after bowel cancer surgery. Firstly is the emerging research on cancer prevention. We are still a long way from understanding the exact mechanisms by which probiotics help to prevent bowel cancer, but based on research to date, it seems that the many mechanisms will include:

- altering the balance and mix of the intestinal microflora (bugs inhabiting the intestine)
- inactivation of cancer-causing compounds
- competition with damaging and disease-causing microorganisms
- improvement of your immune response
- anti-cancer effects via regulation of gut cell behaviour
- fermentation of undigested food
- other biochemical activities.

Antibiotic treatment is virtually universal during surgical procedures involving the gut and this can disturb the normal gut flora. But you can't just take any probiotic off the shelf and expect to get the result you want. We do know that different specific probiotic strains have different and specific actions.

I am often asked if the sweetened yoghurt drinks are 'enough'. These usually contain a single strain of lactobacillus. *Lactobacillus acidophilus* and *Bifidobacterium lactis* are commonly used in probiotic supplements but a variety of different types of 'good bugs' is important in the long term for gut health. Some foods contain probiotic bacteria, such as yoghurt and fermented milk drinks with live cultures, sauerkraut, miso, and kim chee. Some commercially available probiotic supplements have between two and 45 or more different probiotic strains, all with slightly different activity.

Research is not yet at a stage where we can recommend a particular strain or combination of probiotics that have been shown to reduce bowel cancer risk or recurrence, but normalising your gut flora is important. Your doctor may be able to arrange a stool analysis at a specialised laboratory to look at the balance of 'good' and 'bad' bacteria in your gut. This can give some guidance.

PREBIOTICS

Beneficial bacteria also need the right environment to thrive in your gut. We achieve this with prebiotics.

Prebiotics are types of fibre that escape digestion to reach the large intestine and selectively stimulate the growth and/or activity of bacteria that are believed to be beneficial to health, such as bifidobacteria and lactobacillus species. Typically, they are oligosaccharides, oligofructose, galacto-ologosaccharides and inulin.

Inulin is a form of partly indigestible starch found in many root vegetables, including onion and garlic. Supplements may be necessary because it can be difficult to obtain enough inulin and other prebiotics in your diet.

Some prebiotic foods are chicory root, raw oats, wholemeal flour, barley, onions (raw and cooked), leeks (raw), Jerusalem artichoke, asparagus, wheat bran and bananas.

RESOURCES

For more information on bowel cancer risk factors see this website: www.cancerresearchuk.org/cancer-info/cancerstats/types/bowel/riskfactors/bowel-cancer-risk-factors

For more information on stoma care, see this website: www.bowelcanceraustralia.org/

Breast Cancer

Breast cancer is the most common cancer in Australian women (excluding non-melanoma skin cancer). In 2010, breast cancer accounted for 28 per cent of all new cancers in women. This means that, at some stage, you are very likely to have to confront a diagnosis of breast cancer in yourself, a family member or a friend.

There has been an enormous international effort to develop screening programs for the early detection of breast cancer and to raise much-need funding for research into the most effective treatments.

THE CAUSE OF BREAST CANCER

Like other cancers, we cannot say for sure what causes breast cancer but we are aware of some significant risk factors. For instance, we know that breast cancer is much more common in women than in men, but it does also occur in men. It is also more common in people with the BRCA1 and BRCA2 gene mutation, although about nine out of 10 women who develop breast cancer do not have a family history of the disease and so are unlikely to have had their genes tested.

Breast cancer is a hormonally dependent cancer, and there seems to be an increased risk of breast cancer in women who have taken combined (oestrogen and progesterone) hormone replacement therapy (HRT) after menopause for more than three years. According to Cancer Australia, evidence suggests that once you stop taking HRT, the risk of breast cancer diminishes to end up being comparable with women who have never-used HRT within five years of ceasing it. The way you use HRT, whether oral, transdermal patches or creams, or implants, does not appear to make a difference to the risk of breast cancer.

Alcohol increases the risk of breast cancer and there is no safe minimum threshold, particularly if you have already had breast cancer. The more you drink, the greater the increase in risk.

You can calculate your risk of breast cancer at this website: http://canceraustralia.gov.au/affected-cancer/cancer-types/breast-cancer/your-risk/calculate

DO BREAST IMPLANTS CAUSE BREAST CANCER?

There is no evidence that implants increase the risk of breast cancer or recurrence after mastectomy.

BRCA1 AND BRCA2

BRCA stands for BReast CAncer susceptibility gene. BRCA1 and BRCA2 are human tumour suppressor genes. A mutation, or gene fault, in either of these genes means that the ability of cells to repair damage is affected, and uncontrolled cell growth leading to cancer is more likely to develop but is not inevitable. Only about one in 20 cases of breast cancer involves a faulty gene. For those women with the gene, the risk is much greater.

GENETIC TESTING

If you have a close family member known to have the BRCA1 or BRCA2 gene mutation, you may be advised to have genetic counselling. You are likely to be at higher risk if you have two or more first-degree relatives (mother, daughter or sister) with breast or ovarian cancer, or three or more second-degree relatives (for instance, grandmother, aunt). Talk to your GP about the need for genetic testing if you have close female relatives who have the genes or, if you don't have that information, several close female relatives with breast cancer. If you have been diagnosed with breast cancer and you want to know the risk for your daughters or sisters, then you need to discuss this with your doctors.

The genetic test is a blood test. Counselling is always recommended first to make sure the test is appropriate, and also so that the implications of a positive or negative result can be discussed.

PREVENTIVE MASTECTOMY

The actor, director and humanitarian Angelina Jolie decided to have her breast tissue removed to drastically lower her risk of breast cancer after losing her mother and aunt to the disease and finding out she had the same BRCA1 gene mutation. This decision caused a worldwide flurry of interest in breast cancer prevention and this seemingly radical surgical procedure. Preventive mastectomy is a major surgical procedure that involves removing breast tissue in a person who does not have breast cancer but who is considered to be at high risk of developing it. In subcutaneous mastectomy the nipple and skin over the breasts is preserved and implants are inserted for reconstruction. The risk of breast cancer doesn't go down to zero if the breast tissue is removed because it is very difficult to remove all breast tissue, but with preventive mastectomy, the risk is reduced by about 90 per cent.

Ovarian cancer risk is also increased in women with BRCA1 or BRCA2 mutations, so at an appropriate time, removal of the ovaries and fallopian tubes will also be considered. Ms Jolie also had her ovaries removed to further reduce her cancer risk.

Men with harmful BRCA1 or BRCA2 mutations have an increased risk of breast cancer and, possibly, of pancreatic cancer, testicular cancer, and early-onset prostate cancer.

WHAT IS THE SURVIVAL TREND FOR WOMEN WITH BREAST CANCER?

In the 10 years from 1994 to 2003, the incidence of breast cancer rose by 7 per cent. The mortality rates fell by 22 per cent over the same period.

Women diagnosed between the ages 50 and 69 have a reasonably positive prognosis, with 72 per cent expected to survive for 20 years.

Improved treatment and population screening have contributed to the fall in mortality from breast cancer and the statistics are improving with time and advances in management.

MEDICAL ADJUVANT THERAPY OR ANTI-HORMONE TREATMENTS

Breast cancer treatment involves initial staging procedures, then usually surgery to remove the primary lump in the breast, before a decision is made about radiotherapy and/or chemotherapy to follow. Most breast cancers are hormone-dependent cancers. Currently, women who have been diagnosed with a breast cancer that is hormone-sensitive will be advised to take a medication to block the action of oestrogen/progesterone and reduce the risk of recurrence. Selective oestrogen receptor modulators (SERMs) bind to oestrogen receptors, preventing oestrogen from binding to oestrogen sensitive tumour tissue. An example of a SERM is tamoxifen.

The known, serious side effects of tamoxifen are blood clots, strokes, uterine cancer and cataracts. Other side effects include menopausal symptoms such as hot flushes, vaginal dryness, joint pain and leg cramps. This has to be weighed against your prospect of increased survival. The benefits of tamoxifen as a treatment for breast cancer are firmly established and are thought to far outweigh the potential risks. But the side effects can be difficult to tolerate.

Aromatase inhibitors such as Arimidex block the production of oestrogen.

Your oncologist will advise you about whether you need to take one of these medications, which one is best for you, and for how long you need to take it.

In my clinical experience some women tolerate the medication well and have little difficulty in taking it long term. Other women suffer terribly from side effects, particularly joint pains, hot flushes and fatigue. In some cases a switch to another type of hormone therapy fixes the problem, and we can use herbal therapies to help. For some women the side effects are intolerable and they decide to rely on lifestyle measures and other therapies to stay in remission. This is always an individual decision made by each woman in consultation with her oncologist. Sometimes women will ask for a second opinion, although in my experience the advice on this issue rarely differs from one oncologist to the next.

If I think a woman's symptoms are being caused by the hormone treatment, I will discuss with her and her oncologist the option of taking a holiday from the medication to see if the side effects go away. You should not do this without medical supervision and support. Once we know whether you feel much better off the medication or not, we can make a more informed decision about whether or not to continue taking it, or whether to try a different medication.

OSTEOPOROSIS

Osteoporosis is a common side effect of the hormone-blocking treatments. For this reason, your bone density will need to be monitored regularly. Weight-bearing and muscle-strengthening exercises will be particularly important, and you will need to make sure you have adequate calcium in your diet and your blood levels of vitamin D are adequate. Your vitamin D levels should be monitored and supplemented as required (see the section on supplements in the herbs and supplements chapter, page 188).

Medications to stop osteoporosis may be necessary if your bone density declines significantly.

There is current debate in the medical community about whether five years, 10 years or some other length of time is ideal for women to take one of these medications to reduce the statistical risk of breast cancer recurrence. In the early days of use of tamoxifen and other hormone therapies, it was thought that about five years was the right time.

The use of aromatase inhibitors such as Arimidex is limited to five years because of the risk of osteoporosis with more extended use. After five years there will be a reassessment. If you had a low-risk cancer that might be the end of it; if you had a higher risk cancer, you may be advised to switch to tamoxifen. As time progresses and new evidence is gathered or new treatments are developed, this protocol is likely to change.

Hormone therapies for breast cancer can result in a significantly increased risk of cardiovascular disease, obesity, type 2 diabetes, osteoporosis, and muscle wasting, so you will need to actively manage your risk factors for other chronic diseases if you are taking one of these drugs.

CHEMOTHERAPY

Once you have had surgery to remove any localised cancer and investigate what sub-type of breast cancer you have, you will be advised on whether to have follow-up radiotherapy and/or chemotherapy. Chemotherapy should only be administered in cases where there is a significant risk of cancer recurrence if it is not given.

It is important for you to ask detailed questions so that you can make an informed decision about whether or not to have chemotherapy. You will need to satisfy yourself that the risk of short-term and long-term side effects is worth the potential for increased survival.

The advice you are given will depend on the type and stage of your breast cancer, any other health issues you have, and the theoretical likelihood that chemotherapy will prolong your remission.

The types of chemotherapy are changing and improving all the time, so the evidence you are provided with may change in future depending on the current state of medical knowledge.

INTEGRATIVE BREAST CANCER CARE

Beyond the stage of active surgical and medical treatment and rehabilitation comes the question of enhancing your wellbeing and, ultimately, your longevity. It is important to discuss any adjunctive therapies you may be considering or taking during treatment, as some interfere with conventional therapies and may cause harm. Other complementary therapies can work effectively and safely alongside your conventional treatment.

WHAT ELSE YOU CAN DO TO RECOVER

The integrative management of breast cancer is a long-term joint effort between you, your health advisers and your support network, with the aim of improving your quality of life and your survival. There are some fundamental questions you need to ask about quality of life such as: 'Do I have ongoing symptoms I need to relieve?' Your symptoms might include pain, anxiety, fatigue, nausea, lymphoedema, insomnia (See part five 'Symptoms and side effects of cancer treatment' on page 245). 'Is my treatment plan sufficient to manage these problems now and into the future?' and 'What additional treatments might give me the results I am looking for?'

Maintaining remission takes a lifelong, whole-of lifestyle plan of action.

AVOID LONG-TERM HORMONE REPLACEMENT THERAPY

After a breast cancer diagnosis you will have to avoid hormone replacement therapy (HRT) for menopause symptoms. We know there is a relationship between HRT and breast cancer because many countries reported significant drops in breast cancer incidence after the sharp reduction in HRT use early this century.

Because breast cancer is a hormone-dependent cancer, you need to make an effort to minimise your exposure to hormones that might encourage the growth of any residual breast cancer. This is the reason why hormone-suppressing medications and, in some cases, surgery to remove your ovaries is recommended.

You will need to try to manage your menopause symptoms with non-HRT options, such as herbal medicines and acupuncture.

WHAT ABOUT VAGINAL OESTROGEN?

The aromatase inhibitors and other anti-hormone treatments aim to reduce your circulating oestrogens to zero. For younger women especially, this can precipitate profound menopausal symptoms such as dry vulva and vagina, and can make sexual intercourse painful or even impossible. If you read the prescribing information about vaginal oestrogen cream, you will see that it comes with strongly worded warnings for women who have had breast cancer. Over the years, prescribing oestrogen cream for women with breast cancer has been a definite no-no, but that stance has softened in recent times.

I recently called a number of oncologists specialising in breast cancer treatment to gauge the current practice. There has not been any scientific studies done to guarantee the safety, but the oncologists I spoke to were confident that only a tiny, insignificant amount of oestrogen is absorbed into the bloodstream from vaginal use of oestrogen so the risk of promoting a recurrence of cancer is minimal. If you are taking tamoxifen, there is 'no risk' from vaginal oestrogen cream. If your cancer was a low-risk cancer and your vaginal symptoms are troublesome, current advice is that you can use oestrogen cream sparingly twice a week with minimal risk. This is a question you need to ask your oncologist who will assess your individual risk and discuss the balance of your realistic level of risk against your quality of life.

GENERAL ADVICE

- Avoid alcohol
- Don't smoke
- Keep your weight in the healthy range
- Exercise
- Practice yoga

STRESS

It is important to eliminate as many stressful elements from your life as possible and make time for yoga, meditation and relaxation. I recommend you consider yoga practice which is supported by scientific evidence. A 2012 University of Texas study, presented at the annual meeting of the American Society of Clinical Oncology, divided 61 women into two groups. All of these women were undergoing radiation treatment for breast cancer. One group took twice-weekly yoga classes, and the other group did not do any yoga. After six weeks, the yoga group reported better physical function (including, for example, the ability to lift groceries with ease and enjoy walking a mile). They also reported fewer sleep problems and felt less depressed and withdrawn.

A German study also found that yoga helped the psychological health of women during breast cancer treatment.

ENVIRONMENT

In the health audit you will see a list of environmental toxins to consider and remove where you can. You can reduce your exposure to environmental toxins and radiation to assist your recovery and your general health into the future.

YOUR EMOTIONAL HEALTH

Finding out you have breast cancer is one of the most stressful days of your life. The diagnosis will set off a cascade of emotions from fear and anxiety to depression. You need to watch out for signs or symptoms of emotional distress, and your GP or oncologist can refer you to a clinical psychologist or psychiatrist for assessment and help if necessary. Psychological therapies help to improve emotional adjustment and social functioning, reduce stress, and improve quality of life for people with breast cancer.

A range of therapies is available to improve your quality of life while you are going through breast cancer treatment. The effectiveness of many of these therapies is influenced by your attitudes, beliefs and personality, and so treatment will need to be tailored specifically for you. Your partner and family members might also need support.

Accurate information about your cancer and any planned

treatments, as well as your response to treatment, is important. Some people feel less anxious and more optimistic about the future after involvement in peer support programs, but the programs may not be universally useful. Cognitive behaviour techniques such as relaxation therapy, guided imagery, systematic desensitisation, and problem-solving can reduce anxiety.

There is more information see part two ' Dealing with cancer emotionally', see page 63.

MINDFULNESS

Mindfulness-based stress reduction (MBSR) and mindfulness-based cognitive therapy (MBCT) taught by a psychologist trained in this technique has been trialled in patients with breast cancer and seems to be helpful in improving psychological health and decreasing depression.

SLEEP

Regular restful sleep is essential to how you cope. See the chapter on sleep (page 360).

HOW MUCH DOES DIET MATTER?

The short answer is: A lot. A large study showed that higher consumption of vegetables and fruit results in a modest reduction in risk of breast cancer. Food sources, rather than supplements, are best for nutrients.

Eat foods high in B vitamins, calcium, and iron, such as almonds, beans, whole grains (if no allergy), dark leafy greens (such as spinach and kale) and sea vegetables.

Cruciferous vegetables (such as broccoli, Brussels sprouts, kale, bok choy, cauliflower and cabbage) contain indole-3-carbinol and this impacts on the body hormonally by helping to break down oestrogen. I recommend eating 2–3 cups per day, raw or lightly steamed, and getting creative in how to get this in – for example, kale in smoothies, cauliflower dipped in hummus for a snack, included in salads.

Eat antioxidant foods, including fruit (such as blueberries, cherries and tomatoes) and vegetables (such as squash and capsicum).

Avoid refined foods, such as white bread, pasta and sugar.

Ensure any red meat you eat is lean.

Include fish, tofu (soy, if no allergy), or beans for protein. If you choose to follow a vegetarian diet you will need to eat quality protein sources. If you are not accustomed to a vegetarian diet, I advise you to see a dietitian to make sure you are getting adequate nutrition and micronutrients. If you do not want to follow a vegetarian diet, you will still need to concentrate on high-quality protein such as organic meat and eggs, whey, and vegetable protein shakes as part of a balanced program aimed at gaining muscle mass and preventing muscle wasting that can sometimes be a side effect of cancer therapies.

You often see questions raised about the safety of eating soy foods after breast cancer. This is a persistent myth. Some studies show that people who ate soy were less likely to get breast cancer. Consumption of soy foods by women with a breast cancer diagnosis has been shown to decrease risk of death by 54 per cent. The current research does not support avoiding whole soy foods, for cancer patients or survivors. The best forms of soy are organic tofu, tempeh, miso soup, edamame beans and soy milk (unsweetened).

Use healthy cooking oils, such as olive oil.

Reduce or eliminate trans-fats, which are found in commercially baked goods such as cookies, crackers, cakes, French fries, onion rings, doughnuts, processed foods and margarine.

And here's some good news. Caffeine does not seem to have any significant effect on increasing breast cancer risk.

Increase your intake of green tea. A plethora of studies has shown the benefit of green tea's polyphenols for prevention of breast cancer. Consuming organic sources of green tea daily is recommended as well as taking additional green tea supplements.

Linseeds are not only a great source of fibre and omega-3 fats, they also help your body to eliminate oestrogen and have been shown to benefit breast cancer. The benefit will come from the seeds (not the oil), when they are ground into a meal. Also, the meal is best kept in the fridge because it goes off quickly.

Eating high-fibre food helps your body flush out oestrogen. Most people don't get nearly enough fibre in their diet. Try increasing the vegetable content and including lentils and beans into your daily diet.

SUPPLEMENTS

If you are considering the use of any herbs or supplements as part of the integrative management of your breast cancer recovery, then I advise you get qualified, personalised professional advice. You need to be clear about your purpose in deciding on a program of supplements. It is also important to have a plan for how long you intend to continue the supplements, and to take advice on reviewing your doses and combinations from time to time.

Supplements may be recommended as adjunctive therapy to support your nutritional intake and the function of your immune system and for reducing the side effects and toxicity of breast cancer treatment (see part five 'Symptoms and side effects of cancer treatment' on page 245, and the chapter on herbs and supplements, page 188).

Your individual requirement for supplements will vary depending on your general state of health, age, stage of cancer treatment, current diet, any specific deficiencies, and your personal preferences.

Antioxidants

Many patients raise the question of antioxidant use (such as high-dose vitamin C infusions or other antioxidant supplements) during chemotherapy. Despite the concerns of some oncologists, no trials have reported evidence of any decrease in the effectiveness of chemotherapy or radiotherapy from antioxidant supplementation during chemotherapy.

Many of the studies indicated that antioxidant supplementation resulted in either increased survival times, increased tumour responses, or both, as well as less toxicity from cancer treatments. I discuss this more in chapter on herbs and supplements (see page 188).

If you are considering using supplements to control the side effects of radiotherapy, then you must abstain from smoking tobacco if you take antioxidants during radiotherapy treatment. Apart from the obvious reason that smoking is damaging to pretty much every part of your health, a study found that patients with head and neck cancer who took synthetic betacarotene had increased recurrence rates and lower survival if they had smoked during the course of their radiation treatment, whereas those who did not smoke during treatment showed no detrimental effects, even if they smoked before the initiation or after the completion of treatment.

Patients receiving antioxidant supplements during radiotherapy in this study had statistically significantly fewer severe acute side effects than those not receiving supplements.

Vitamin C

Vitamin C (ascorbate, or ascorbic acid) is possibly the best known of the antioxidants. Your body cannot make this vitamin so you need to get it from food sources or supplements. The best food sources are citrus fruits, tomatoes, capsicums, strawberries, guava, dark green leafy vegetables, papaya and broccoli.

Many women with breast cancer are deficient in vitamin C. While food sources are preferable to avoid deficiency, if you are not able to eat those foods for any reason, you will need to supplement. You need vitamin C for your tissues to heal and to assist your recovery. Vitamin C supplementation is available as oral pills or powders, or as intravenous infusion.

A meta-analysis published in the *European Journal of Cancer* found that post-diagnosis vitamin C supplement use was associated with a reduced risk of mortality. Dietary vitamin C intake was also significantly associated with a reduced risk of total mortality and breast cancer-specific mortality. This large study would suggest that both dietary vitamin C as well as supplementation could be important.

In the chapter on intravenous vitamin C (page 173), I outline the use of high-dose intravenous vitamin C during the treatment and recovery phase. There are some interesting and convincing studies on the use of IVC as adjunctive breast cancer treatment. A German study found that IVC was well-tolerated and helped to optimise cancer-specific treatments, and reduced quality of life-related side effects of chemotherapy and radiotherapy. No side effects were documented in this study.

Coenzyme Q10

Coenzyme Q10 (ubiquinone) was first identified in 1957 and chemical structure was determined in 1958. Interest in CoQ10 as a possible part of treatment for cancer began in 1961, when it was found that some cancer patients had a lower than normal amount of it in their blood. Low blood levels of CoQ10 have been found in patients with myeloma, lymphoma, and cancers of the breast, lung, prostate, pancreas, colon, kidney, and head and neck.

Because CoQ10 helps the immune system to function and in laboratory tests appears to have some anti-cancer effects, it is used as adjuvant therapy for cancer. It also helps to counter fatigue.

The studies of CoQ10 for cancer thus far have been fairly small and did not have scientifically strong designs. More studies are needed with larger groups of patients to determine what effect, if any, it has on cancer.

The usual dose is 100–300 mg daily.

Vitamin D

Women who have low exposure to sunlight and lower levels of vitamin D as a result are more likely to develop breast cancer and other forms of cancer. A 2014 study looked at the relationship between vitamin D levels and mortality from breast cancer. It found that a high vitamin D level was associated with lower mortality and recommended that serum vitamin D in all patients with breast cancer should be restored to the normal range with appropriate monitoring.

There are also other important reasons to maintain your vitamin D levels, including bone density, quality of life and mood. I strongly recommend you to maintain adequate vitamin D stores throughout your lifetime.

You need to be aware of your vitamin D levels and make sure you maintain them at the high end of the healthy range, now and throughout the rest of your life. You can do this with daily exposure of your skin to sun (without sunburn), but vitamin D deficiency is common and supplementation is often necessary.

Calcium

Calcium is necessary for your bone health, particularly if you are post-menopausal or if you are taking an aromatase inhibitor (hormone) adjunctive therapy. Ensure adequate dietary calcium, mainly from low fat dairy foods and supplement where necessary.

Selenium

Studies show that low levels of selenium are associated with a higher risk of cancer death. We also know that people with cancer often have low selenium levels.

Some countries do not have adequate selenium in their soils, so the food supply lacks selenium. The most reliable food source of selenium is from Brazil nuts (two per day) as well as whole grains, sunflower seeds, shellfish, fish and garlic.

The data on the relationship between selenium supplements and cancer is not conclusive, so at this stage the jury is still out on whether supplementation is of any benefit.

Melatonin

Melatonin is a hormone with antioxidant properties. It is best known for its role in helping to regulate sleep cycles. Some studies have found that women with lower levels of melatonin, such as those who work the night shift or sleep fewer hours, have a higher risk of developing breast cancer. Women with breast cancer tend to have lower levels of melatonin than those without the disease.

Melatonin has virtually no contraindications. It can be used as an adjuvant with the anti-oestrogen and aromatase-inhibiting hormone therapies. It is also helpful in reducing oxidative stress associated with chemotherapy and radiotherapy.

Laboratory studies have shown that melatonin inhibits oestrogen-sensitive human breast cancer cells and can augment the action of the hormone treatment tamoxifen. Whether melatonin supplements can help prevent or even treat breast cancer is yet to be determined, but there is a fair amount of circumstantial evidence around the role of melatonin in the prevention and treatment of breast cancer.

The dose is 2–6 mg at sundown, for immune support and sleep. Higher doses are often used under professional supervision in women after a breast cancer diagnosis.

Probiotics

Probiotic supplements such as lactobacilli are recommended for maintenance of gastrointestinal and immune health. Laboratory and animal studies suggest that probiotics may slow the growth of breast cancer cells, but there are some conflicting results on efficacy and safety at different stages of cancer treatment. You may need to take short courses of probiotics if you are given courses of antibiotics during treatment.

Human studies are needed before we know what role probiotics have in adjunctive breast cancer treatment or in helping to prevent recurrence, and which particular probiotics are most useful in different clinical situations.

Optimal bowel function is crucial for health, especially when it comes to breast cancer. Lactobacillus and other probiotics help to break down oestrogen into a form that is easily eliminated in stools. If you lack healthy levels of these bacteria in your gut, your oestrogen will not get broken down and eliminated.

Traditional Chinese Medicine

Traditional Chinese Medicine (TCM) herbs and acupuncture can help you manage the symptoms of menopause induced by hormone-suppressing treatments. It can also help with the side effects of cancer-specific treatments and recovery after treatment. Check the qualifications and experience of the TCM practitioner, particularly whether they have training and experience in managing people who have had cancer.

Herbs

There are a number of herbs that are useful in minimising the side effects of hormone-reducing medications. I advise you to get personalised professional advice rather than self-medicating.

Black cohosh may help to reduce hot flushes if you are on tamoxifen or aromatase inhibitors. It generally takes about eight weeks to start seeing an effect so be patient!

Astragalus is commonly used by women with breast cancer to enhance the effectiveness and reduce the side effects of chemotherapy. This herb is also used in TCM to reduce fatigue and help recuperation from chemotherapy.

St John's wort is a commonly prescribed and effective herbal medicine for treatment of anxiety and depression. It is also used as a herbal treatment for the symptoms of menopause. Be aware it has many herb–drug interactions so it is generally not recommended until after chemotherapy is completed. Low hyperforin formulas are less likely to cause herb–drug interactions. If you have had depression and you are stabilised on St John's wort, you will need to discuss this with your oncologist. The herb may interfere with the choice of chemotherapy agent, so it is very important that you let your oncologist know. The dose of chemotherapy may need to be adjusted, or there may be a decision to stop the St John's wort, in which case you will need to carefully plan for management of your depression symptoms.

Hot flushes and sleep issues can be particular problems after breast cancer treatment, especially with hormone-blocking drugs, and St John's wort can help to reduce these symptoms. You will need well-informed professional advice on the use of this herb, even though it is available without a prescription.

Green tea (*Camellia sinensis*) is a traditional source of antioxidants which help the liver to detoxify carcinogens. If you are a big coffee drinker, you could replace some of your coffee for green tea to gain this benefit. Green tea does contain caffeine, so all of the usual recommendations about caffeine apply, such as avoiding it at night if you have difficulty with sleeping or anxiety. The dose needs to be high to gain the therapeutic benefit from the phytochemical EGCG (epigallocatechin-3-gallate), and this is difficult to achieve without taking a supplement.

Many laboratory studies have shown green tea has activity against cancer cells in cell cultures. Studies have involved cancer of the stomach, lungs, liver, breast and colon. But it has not been tested in humans so it is not possible to make firm recommendations.

A WARNING ABOUT 'BLACK SALVE'

Also known as red salve, Cansema, or Bloodroot (*Sanguinaria canadensis* with the active caustic ingredient sanguinarine)

It can be frightening to be told you have breast cancer and to then have to face decisions about treatment.

Some women defer cancer-specific treatment so that they have time to do their homework and consider their options. Unfortunately, some of the options are not safe. In recent times I have encountered a number of women who have tried a substance called black salve, because they have been convinced by unregistered practitioners to try this to 'draw the cancer out' through the skin. They describe dramatic and painful eruptions of tissue through the skin of their breast where the black salve is applied. I know of cases where the breast and nipple had been virtually burnt off, making reconstructive surgery far more difficult than it would otherwise have been if she had been treated conventionally in the first place.

In other cases, the black salve caused significant scarring

and the delay in treatment following diagnosis resulted in the cancer growing and spreading.

Here is my warning: please do not touch this substance. It does not work. It will not cure your breast cancer. It will damage you. It may delay you getting effective treatment for your breast cancer at an earlier stage.

If you have started using black salve, stop now and see your doctor for a referral for effective treatment.

Turmeric

Turmeric (curcumin) is thought to have anti-inflammatory, anti-cancer, and antioxidant properties. A 2007 US study in mice showed that curcumin helped to stop the spread of breast cancer cells to other parts of the body. Human studies have also shown potential anti-breast cancer effects but it is early days in terms of evidence.

Turmeric may interfere with some forms of chemotherapy, so talk with your doctor first. You may be advised to wait until after treatment is finished.

Indole-3-carbinol

Indole-3-carbinol is a substance found in cruciferous vegetables. It is also available in supplement form. Studies indicate that I-3-C has potential value as a preventive agent for breast cancer through its oestrogen receptor modulating effect. While studies of populations show that higher levels of cruciferous vegetables in the diet are associated with lower risk of breast cancer, it is not possible to extrapolate that to the use of supplements of indole-3-carbinol. There is evidence to support the fact that I-3-C has a different mechanism of action to tamoxifen and that these two can be used together to support the action of the other.

Multivitamins

Multivitamins, as the name suggests, are combinations of different vitamins and sometimes minerals. If you have had a cancer diagnosis, you need specific advice about whether you need to be taking a multivitamin and if so, which one. Some contain iron and others don't, some are formulated with high levels of B vitamins, some contain selenium.

One example for this need for advice is the copper content of a multivitamin supplement. Copper is needed to form new blood vessels, and cancers need new blood vessels in order to grow. For this reason, if you take a multivitamin, avoid supplements containing copper as there is some suggestion that excessive copper levels may contribute to the development of new blood vessels. Another example is that high levels of B vitamins may make it difficult for you to sleep particularly if taken in higher doses or later in the day.

LYMPHOEDEMA MANAGEMENT

Lymphoedema of the arm is a possible complication of breast cancer treatment, particularly where there has been surgery or radiotherapy affecting the lymph nodes in your armpit. Lymphoedema involves swelling of the soft tissues of the arm, hand, and fingers on the affected side. There may be associated numbness, discomfort, and an increased risk of infection in that limb.

Lymphoedema management needs to be undertaken with a specially qualified lymphoedema therapist who will use specialised massage techniques, exercises and compression bandaging.

Low-level laser therapy may be helpful.

Medications to avoid

The following medications can make lymphoedema worse and should be avoided where possible:

- calcium channel blockers used to treat high blood pressure
- non-steroidal anti-inflammatory agents
- hormone replacement therapy (avoided after breast cancer generally)
- corticosteroids
- some oral hypoglycaemic agents (glitazones) for treatment of diabetes.

Thank you to naturopath Laura Brass ND (Canada) and Teresa Mitchell-Patterson for assistance with review of this chapter.

RESOURCE

Check out this website for more information on hormone therapy and breast cancer: www.cancer.gov/types/breast/breast-hormone-therapy-fact-sheet

Prostate Cancer

Many of the men I see with prostate cancer are motivated to work on their lifestyle for the first time in many years, if ever. We have a lot of evidence that changes to diet, activity levels, and other lifestyle factors make a big difference to recovery and survival from this cancer.

Prostate cancer is the most common cancer in men, and men over 50 years old are at greater risk, although we do see it diagnosed in younger men as well. The current trend is to direct early detection at men from the age of 40, and especially in those men at a higher risk, after appropriate informed consent, particularly about the benefits of early detection versus the risks of overtreatment.

Prostate cancer has been a focus of intensive research activity as new information about the disease, its causes, treatment, and improved technology for diagnosis and treatment emerge at a rapid pace. So let's take a look at some of the big questions you may have since your diagnosis of prostate cancer.

THE CAUSE OF PROSTATE CANCER

There is some inherited risk. It is estimated that up to 40 per cent of prostate cancers may have an inherited or genetic component, according to studies of twins. Men with a family history of prostate cancer have an increased risk of developing prostate cancer. There is a twofold risk if you have one first-degree relative with prostate cancer and a fivefold risk with two first-degree relatives.

Where you live and your ethnic background may have also played a part. There is approximately a 40-fold difference in the reported incidence and a 12-fold difference in death rate from prostate cancer between various geographic and ethnic populations. The highest reported incidence of prostate cancer is in African–Americans.

Studies of men who have migrated from one part of the world to another provide strong evidence that environmental (where you live) and lifestyle factors (how you live) are important in the development of prostate cancer. Age is another factor. The older you get, the more likely you are to be diagnosed with prostate cancer. That said, it does occur in younger men too.

BRCA1 OR BRCA2 GENE MUTATIONS

Men with harmful BRCA1 or BRCA2 mutations have an increased risk of breast cancer and, possibly, of pancreatic, testicular, and early-onset prostate cancer. This has not yet translated into advice for genetic screening for men with a family history of breast or prostate cancer, but this could change in future.

VASECTOMY AND THE RISK OF PROSTATE CANCER

I have wondered if this was a rumour generated by men who did not want to have a vasectomy, but the argument is not settled.

Until recently it was thought that vasectomy was not a factor in the development of prostate cancer, but recent evidence suggests that while vasectomy is not associated with the risk of low-grade or localised disease, it may slightly increase the risk of the most aggressive form of prostate cancer, although this form of cancer is rare.

AFTER THE DIAGNOSIS

When you have been diagnosed with prostate cancer, you will have an initial shock reaction and possibly feel overwhelmed. It is important for you to take the time to gather information so that you can make well-informed decisions about your treatment and how to live your life, regardless of the treatment you decide.

Professor Phillip Stricker from St Vincent's Prostate Cancer Centre in Sydney is one of the pre-eminent experts in the field of prostate cancer management. Like other urologists specialising in this field, he is in the position of doing the biopsies on men suspected of having prostate cancer, and then discussing the results and what they mean in terms of the options for treatment and the prognosis. I asked him what questions patients and their partners have when they are diagnosed with prostate cancer, and what issues they need to consider. The following is a very helpful checklist to make sure you cover all the areas where you will need information from your surgeon or oncologist.

QUESTIONS FOR YOUR PROSTATE CANCER SPECIALIST

- Do I have a curable cancer?
- Do I have a cancer that needs to be treated or is it one that can be monitored?
- If it needs to be treated, what is the least invasive treatment that has a high chance of cure?

- If the treatment has side effects, what are the common side effects, in particular the concern about sexual function and urinary control?
- If I do get sexual problems, how long will these last and what options do I have to treat them?
- If I do get urinary problems, how long will they last, what can I do to speed up their recovery, and what options do I have if they do not recover?
- If I do monitor the tumour, what is the best way of monitoring it and what lifestyle modifications can I make? In particular, can I avoid having multiple biopsies and perhaps rely more on MRI, and what foods should I eat and lifestyle modification should I make to minimise impact?
- Is it possible that I could have only the cancer treated rather than the whole prostate with new focal therapy?
- What actually is nerve-sparing surgery and how effective is it?
- Is robotic surgery better than open surgery?
- What caused my cancer and what should I tell my children?
- If I do not do anything about it, how long have I got to live?
- What are the major factors I should take into consideration in making my decision?
- Does it matter if I delay for a period of time to make it fit in with my time schedule?
- If surgery is undertaken, will I need follow-up radiotherapy?

HOW TO DECIDE ON THE BEST TREATMENT

It is most likely that you will have seen your GP for screening or investigation of symptoms related to prostate cancer. The usual practice is then to be referred to a urologist for further investigation and biopsy, where fine needles are passed into the prostate gland to assess the grade of cancer. Some specialists are now routinely using MRI to assess prostate cancer. The main aim of these investigations is to determine which are the significant cases of prostate cancer needing medical or surgical treatment and which are the insignificant ones that can be safely monitored.

Depending on the microscopic appearance of the cancer, it will be given a grading called a Gleason score and this result along with the MRI appearance guides the decisions about treatment. Possible treatments include active surveillance, open surgery, robotic surgery, focal therapy, brachytherapy (a type of radiation therapy), external beam radiotherapy, and hormonal therapies. The detail of these cancer-specific treatment options is beyond the scope of this book. At the end of this chapter you will see some references for where you can find further information.

The final decision about treatment for a localised prostate cancer needs to be based on your individual preferences, the nature of your cancer, your general wellbeing and other health issues, and your particular priorities (such as the importance of erectile function). You may also need to consider other factors such as where you live, how far you might need to travel for treatment, the cost of the different treatments, and the skill and expertise of the doctors.

The key person to help you make the decision will be a urologist with expertise in multiple treatment options, or multiple specialists with different areas of expertise. Because you may face some choices in the treatment you are offered, and because this will be influenced, at least to some degree, by the preferences of the surgeon or specialists, it would be very reasonable for you to ask for a second opinion. This may be offered to you in the form of a multidisciplinary meeting of several specialists who review your case and make a recommendation, or it may require a referral by your GP to another urologist for a second opinion. You may also need some help with the decision about which treatment to choose, from a clinical psychologist and possibly a sexual health physician.

MEDICATION AND PREVENTION

Your doctor may talk to you about some options for prescribed pharmaceuticals. You will need to weigh up the purported benefits of these medications against the risk of side effects. A few studies have been done to determine whether prostate cancer can be prevented by taking drugs called 5 alpha-reductase inhibitors (finasteride and dutasteride).

The finasteride (Proscar) trial showed a 25 per cent reduction in the prevalence of prostate cancer over a seven-year period. There has been some concern there may be a slight increase in the incidence of more aggressive tumours in the men who use this medication, but subsequent, more careful analyses have not supported this. Currently, finasteride is not recommended by most urologists for the purpose of preventing cancer.

Further major studies that have recently been reported include a prevention study using dutasteride (Avodart). The dutasteride study reported a 20 per cent decrease in the detection of prostate cancer after only four years of follow-up in a slightly higher-risk group of men without any increase in detection of high-grade disease. There was a 4 per cent increased incidence of reduced libido, which was similar to the finasteride study.

The cholesterol-lowering drugs called statins have been implicated in possible prevention. There is currently low-level evidence of a possible risk reduction but this would have to be weighed against the risk of the side effects of these drugs. Side effects such as fatigue, brain fog, liver function abnormalities, and muscle pain can be a problem with the statins. Recently emerging evidence suggests that it is quite possibly the 'bad cholesterol' or LDL-cholesterol that is the cancer factor here.

TREATMENT SIDE EFFECTS

Erectile problems

The incidence of impotence (erectile dysfunction) after prostatectomy or radiotherapy is dependent upon your level of potency before the treatment, the experience of your surgeon, the ability of your surgeon to spare nerves, and the time elapsed after surgery.

The overall incidence of impotence is extremely variable depending upon the expertise of your surgeon. Generally, if you are potent preoperatively and you are under the age of 65 and both nerves are spared, you should expect at least a 70–80 per cent chance of sexual recovery over an 18-month period. This is the result from the best units in the world currently. It is quite common for the erectile recovery to be incomplete but adequate for intercourse, and often requiring medication help with PDE5 inhibitors such as the medications sildenafil, vardenafil and tadanafil (familiar brand names are Viagra, Levitra and Cialis).

It is also mandatory that sexual rehabilitation is part of your recovery process. If sexual recovery after surgery or indeed after any form of therapy such as brachytherapy or radiotherapy is incomplete, then your first option is to try one of the PDE5 inhibitors.

If these medications do not work, then the next options would be a vacuum device and penile injection therapy, and the final option would be a penile implant. Generally, penile implants are reserved for those patients who do not succeed with simpler therapy.

Urinary incontinence

The incidence of incontinence after a radical prostatectomy varies depending on your age, the extent of your cancer, the type of treatment you need, and the skill and experience of your surgeon.

Incontinence is more common after surgery than after radiotherapy. After surgery there is often a period of temporary incontinence, but once again this is largely dictated by the experience of the surgeon. The technique of surgery, be it open, laparoscopic, or robot-assisted laparoscopic surgery is probably less important than the experience of the surgeon; however, some data suggests that early recovery of continence in a very experienced robotic surgeon's hands is marginally better.

The chance of becoming incontinent after surgery in the short term is 20–30 per cent and in the long term should be less than 5 per cent. In the best series in the world, it is only 1 or 2 per cent. The definition of continence should be no requirement for any continence pads at all.

The most important factor is the experience of the surgeon, but it has been strongly shown that the use of pelvic floor exercises prior to surgery, particularly supervised by an experienced pelvic floor physiotherapist, is key to the early recovery of urinary control.

PELVIC FLOOR PHYSIOTHERAPY

It is important to arrange to see a pelvic floor physiotherapist soon after surgery to help with muscle exercises to build the strength of your pelvic floor muscles, which support your bladder. This will help to reduce the incidence of urinary incontinence. Most cases of incontinence will resolve after six to 12 months. If they do not resolve, treatments include injections with collagen and Macroplastique, urethral slings or, for the more severe types of incontinence, an artificial urinary sphincter. You can discuss these options with your urologist.

ACTIVE SURVEILLANCE

Men with lower grade, small volume prostate cancers will be given the option of 'active surveillance' – 'active' because you are doing a lot to optimise your health to keep the prostate cancer under control, and 'surveillance' because your cancer is monitored with regular blood tests, MRI scans and biopsies. This means there are no cancer-specific measures such as surgery, radiotherapy, chemotherapy, or hormone therapies, but an intense focus on lifestyle factors that have been shown to slow the progression of prostate cancer. The course of the disease can be monitored and different lifestyle interventions assessed over time.

Active surveillance includes:

- PSA tests every three to six months
- periodic biopsy (at between 12 and 48 months from the start of the program until life expectancy is less than 15 years)
- multiparametric MRI at entry and potentially again at 12 to 24 months to reduce the need for repeat biopsies
- progression to active treatment if the cancer significantly progresses
- adoption of intensive lifestyle measures.

We have loads of information about the effect of lifestyle measures on the progression of prostate cancer and survival rates after it has been diagnosed.

If you are recommended to take the active surveillance path, then you will need to gather a team of advisers, which might include your GP, a dietitian, an exercise physiologist, a meditation/mindfulness teacher, a qualified naturopath and others.

While you may be given comprehensive lifestyle advice, it is up to you whether or not you actually take the advice and incorporate that strategy into your life in the long term.

LIFESTYLE AND PROSTATE CANCER MANAGEMENT

You may be diagnosed with a low-grade prostate cancer and depending on the pathology, your age, and general state of health, your doctors may advise you to manage this conservatively. More severe grades of prostate cancer or a cancer diagnosed in a younger man will most likely need less conservative treatments such as surgery.

Regardless of the grade of your prostate cancer, there is evidence that comprehensive lifestyle measures and dietary habits will reduce the rate of progression of the disease and increase your survival time.

HEALTHY DIET

Obesity, high saturated-fat intake, and high-calorie intake may increase the risk of developing prostate cancer, so these are areas where you can concentrate your attention. You may need to work with a dietitian to help you adjust your eating plan.

Diets that can reduce prostate cancer risk

The Mediterranean diet and the traditional Japanese diet are both considered protective against prostate cancer. In particular, both are very low in animal fats. The Japanese diet is low in calories and animal fat, and high in green tea, soy foods, vegetables and fish. The Mediterranean diet is high in fresh fruit, vegetables and fish; excludes red meat; and includes garlic, tomatoes, and olive oil.

We do know some other specific dietary elements that give some protection against prostate cancer.

Lycopene

Lycopene is a potent antioxidant that gives some foods their red colour. It is found in tomatoes, tomato-based products, watermelon and strawberries, and may help lower your risk of prostate cancer. Cooked tomato products are better than raw for lycopene content. (See the chapter on nutrition page 323 for more information.)

Cruciferous vegetables
Cruciferous vegetables include broccoli, cauliflower, cabbage and kale. They have been shown to have an anti-cancer effect.

Soy foods
If you live in Japan, it is likely that soy foods will be a regular part of your diet. But if soy foods are new or just an occasional food for you, consider including them regularly because they contain an isoflavone called genistein which has been associated with a lower risk of prostate cancer.

Pomegranate
Pomegranate juice is known to have anti-inflammatory effects and high levels of antioxidants. It also contains polyphenols and isoflavones, which are believed to have an anti-cancer effect.

Pomegranate juice helps stop prostate cancer from spreading – scientists from the University of California identified components in pomegranate juice that help slow the progression of prostate cancer. In a study of men with recurrent prostate cancer and rising prostate-specific antigen (PSA) levels, researchers found that taking pomegranate juice extract significantly slowed the rate at which PSA was rising.

Pomegranate juice may affect some medications including the blood thinner warfarin (Coumadin) and some medications for treating high blood pressure and high cholesterol. You also may need to be careful about drinking juice if you have diabetes. In this case, the extract in tablet form may be preferable.

Selenium and Vitamin E

Studies show that low levels of selenium are associated with a higher risk of cancer death. We also know that people with cancer often have low selenium levels.

A trial using selenium and vitamin E reported no benefit in taking selenium and vitamin E in the prevention of prostate cancer. The trial was, however, performed in a country where the soil was not deficient in selenium.

Some countries do not have adequate selenium in their soils, so the food supply lacks selenium. In countries where the soil is deficient in selenium, such as in Australia, taking a supplement of 100–200 µg of selenium daily is considered safe and does appear to reduce the incidence of prostate cancer. The data on the relationship between selenium supplements and cancer is not conclusive, so at this stage the jury is still out on whether supplementation is of any benefit.

The most reliable food source of selenium is from Brazil nuts (two per day) as well as whole grains, sunflower seeds, shellfish, fish and garlic.

Green tea

If you only drink coffee and black tea, switch some of these over to green tea. Green tea has an antioxidant action and helps the liver to detoxify carcinogens. Many laboratory studies have shown green tea acts against cancer cells in cell cultures.

Vitamin D

Adequate vitamin D intake is to be encouraged, usually by natural means for exposure of your skin to sunshine without sunburn, but possibly by supplementation.

Probiotics

Optimal bowel function is crucial for health. Probiotic supplements such as lactobacilli are recommended for maintenance of gastrointestinal and immune health. You may need to take short courses of probiotics if you are given courses of antibiotics during treatment, for example after a prostate biopsy.

Human studies are needed before we know what role probiotics have in adjunctive prostate cancer treatment or in helping to prevent recurrence and which particular probiotics are most useful in different clinical situations.

Turmeric

Turmeric (curcumin) is a member of the ginger family and is thought to have anti-inflammatory, anti-cancer, and antioxidant properties. Curcumin has been shown in laboratory tests to interfere with prostate cancer proliferation and metastasis (spread to other organs). It is thought to be a non-toxic herbal treatment for prostate cancer prevention, or adjunctive treatment.

If you are considering using herbal medicines, you will need to seek professional advice on correct forms and dosages.

DIETARY FACTORS TO AVOID

Flaxseed oil can stimulate prostate cancer to grow. You can get the omega-3 fatty acids you need through fresh fish, fish oil supplements and nuts.

Also avoid **high-calcium** diets or supplements, as they have been shown to stimulate prostate cancer growth. If you supplement with calcium, or with a product that contains calcium, keep your total intake of calcium from all diet or supplement sources below 700 mg a day.

Alcohol

We know that alcohol is a carcinogen, so it follows that the more alcohol you drink, the higher the risk of cancer. Prostate cancer is one of the cancers associated with alcohol consumption. Men who drink four or five standard drinks or more of alcohol per day, five or more days a week, are at an increased risk of developing high-grade, more aggressive prostate cancer.

I find that men who are dependent on alcohol in any way will try to negotiate a 'safe' level of drinking, or try to minimise the risk so that they can continue to drink as they did before. If you want to eliminate as many risk factors as possible, then you will reduce your alcohol consumption, preferably to zero. The decision is entirely up to you.

Eliminating alcohol will also help you to avoid osteoporosis, which is a side effect of long-term hormone therapy for prostate cancer.

NUTRITION AND LIFESTYLE ADVICE FOR PROSTATE CANCER

In a nutshell, the advice for men who have been diagnosed with prostate cancer is:

- healthy heart diet (Mediterranean or traditional Japanese
- daily aerobic exercise and regular resistance training
- low animal fats and eat little or no red meat
- avoid trans-fats found in many processed and packaged foods
- maintain a low calorie/kilojoule intake to keep body weight in the healthy range
- avoid obesity
- reduce alcohol consumption (preferably to zero)
- selenium (100–200 µg of selenium daily)

- high lycopene foods with natural red colour (such as tomatoes)
- vitamin D – ensure sufficient sun exposure or adequate supplement dosage to correct deficiency
- fish oil/omega-3 fatty acids are considered to provide a protective role and can be taken as 4000 mg/day or > 3 serves of fish a week
- soy foods included regularly in your diet
- pomegranate juice or tablets
- antioxidants (green tea, soy protein, red clover; all have a low-level evidence)
- increase foods containing natural vitamin C (citrus, berries, capsicums)
- vitamin E supplementation may help some men if the dose is limited to less than 400 IU per day
- avoid a high-calcium diet
- curcumin supplement.

ADVANCED PROSTATE CANCER

Generally, if the PSA is higher than 50 or there is evidence of metastatic disease, the cancer is regarded as advanced. Hormone therapy, either continuous or intermittent, remains the mainstay for this stage of the disease.

Hormone therapy medications include goserelin, leuprorelin or Eligard. These may be combined with anti-androgens drugs, including bicalutamide, flutamide, nilutamide or cyproterone.

If you have advanced prostate cancer, lifestyle measures are every bit as important as they are with the less aggressive, lower grades of cancer. Apart from helping to slow the progression of the disease, lifestyle measures can help to combat some of the side effects of the hormone therapies.

The side effects of hormone therapies include weight gain,

tiredness, decreased muscle mass, depression, mood swings, decreased libido, hot flushes and osteoporosis. You will need to avoid or manage any weigh gain with careful attention to your dietary calorie/kilojoule intake.

Regular resistance exercises, as well as a carefully planned diet, can prevent many of the side effects of hormone therapy. Both aerobic and resistance exercise are important. See the chapter on exercise for further detail on this (page 307).

There is some evidence that soy isoflavones may have a role in treating hot flushes. If this approach is not successful, hot flushes can be treated with cyproterone or oestrogen patches.

Depression and mood swings may be treated with St John's wort.

OSTEOPOROSIS

Long-term hormone therapy for prostate cancer can lead to osteoporosis. You can reduce your risk by making sure you do regular aerobic and resistance exercise, keeping your vitamin D in the normal to high range, and having adequate calcium in your diet.

The risk of osteoporosis can also be reduced by keeping alcohol intake to a minimum, increasing weight-bearing and resistance exercise, and increasing isoflavone intake.

If you are on long-term hormone therapy, you will need regular bone mineral density (BMD) tests and, if your BMD significantly deteriorates to the osteoporotic range, you may also be advised to have specific osteoporosis medication along with continuing diet, supplements and lifestyle measures.

WHAT DOES THE FUTURE HOLD?

There is a large amount of research and development in the pipeline aimed at investigation of prostate cancer to more accurately predict how a particular cancer will behave in a particular man, and more refined treatment techniques.

In the next five to 10 years we are likely to see the development of:

- biomarkers predicting the natural history of the cancer
- focal treatments aimed at treating the initial cancer
- better imaging (including MRI and PET/CT scanning)
- improved delivery of radiation therapy
- increased use of high-tech surgical treatments using modalities such as intensity-modulated radiotherapy, the CyberKnife system and robot-assisted surgery.

Thanks to Professor Phillip Stricker, Urologist and director of St Vincents Prostate Cancer Centre Sydney Australia.

Thanks to dietician Jaime Rose Chambers for review of nutritional advice.

RESOURCES

See these three website for information for men and their families about prostate cancer:

http://www.prostate.com.au

http://cancer.org.au

http://cancercouncil.com.au

See these two online resources:

Rashid P, *Prostate cancer: your guide to the disease, treatment options and outcomes*, 3rd edn, http://prostate.org.au

Stricker P, Phelps K, *Prostate cancer for the general practitioner*, 2nd edn, Churchill Livingstone, Elsevier, http://prostate.com.au

Cancer of the Cervix

The most common cervical cancer is squamous cell carcinoma, which accounts for 80 per cent of cases. Adenocarcinoma is less common and more difficult to diagnose because it starts higher in the cervix. The risk of a woman being diagnosed by age 85 is one in 155.

In Australia there were 818 new cases of cervical cancer diagnosed in 2010, and in 2011 there were 229 deaths caused by cervical cancer. Cervical cancer death rates have halved since the National Cervical Screening Program began in 1991. Although these are relatively low numbers, abnormal Pap smears are common and they are a cause of concern.

Abnormal Pap test results are graded in increasing order of severity: minor atypia, CIN 1 (for cervical intraepithelial neoplasia), CIN 2, CIN 3 and cervical cancer. Mild abnormalities may revert to normal or progress to higher grades of CIN and eventually to cancer of the cervix. Higher grade abnormalities will need to be treated, usually with laser surgery.

Cervical abnormalities detected by Pap smears are completely treatable in the early stages before they develop into cervical cancer. Your GP or gynaecologist will advise you on how often you need to be tested and how to respond to an abnormal test.

Almost all cases of cervical cancer are caused by persistent infection with some high-risk types of the human papillomavirus (HPV); this is the biggest risk factor for cervical cancer. The other main risk factor for cervical cancer is smoking.

Through the national immunisation program, most girls in Australia will receive the HPV vaccine around the age of 12. Since 2013, boys have also been included in the immunisation program because the vaccine also helps prevent some HPV-related cancers and diseases that affect men.

The HPV vaccine was introduced with great fanfare back in 2007. Could this new Australian-developed vaccine mean the end of cervical cancer and other diseases caused by some types of HPV? It was greeted more cautiously by GPs. Although we generally welcomed the introduction of a vaccine which had the potential to reduce the impact of wart virus (HPV), and particularly the incidence of abnormal Pap smears and cervical cancer, we feared that young women would think they were protected from cervical cancer and so they could forget about having regular Pap smears.

That concern was vindicated when it emerged that many women who have had the HPV vaccine are wrongly assuming that it makes them immune to cervical cancer and are avoiding having Pap smears, creating the potential for a spike in cervical cancer in years to come. The study, by the Victorian Cytology Service, showed 'alarmingly lower' rates of Pap smears for cervical cancer screening in young women who have been vaccinated against HPV compared with women who have not been vaccinated. Unvaccinated women had Pap smears screening rates of 61.3 per cent compared with women who chose to get vaccinated (27.5 per cent).

There is still a lot of misunderstanding about what the HPV vaccine can and cannot do. The vaccines available in Australia have been shown to prevent infection and cervical abnormalities from two sexually transmissible cancer-causing types of HPV, specifically type 16 and type 18. The vaccine prevents infection only if it is given before infection with the virus and does not prevent persistent infection or cervical abnormalities if you have already been infected with the HPV type before you had the vaccination. Another issue is that the vaccine does not cover all types of HPV that can cause cancer, so if you have been vaccinated you should continue to have Pap smears.

Whether or not you have been vaccinated, you need to be screened for cervical cancer with a regular Pap smear every two years, or more frequently if your doctor recommends it. If you have had an abnormal smear in the past or you have had HPV show up on previous testing, then you will be advised to have the test more often. You will be sent a reminder, either from the Pap test register in your state, or from your doctor, or both. Please don't ignore it.

IMPORTANT ADVICE

If you are under 26 years old, ask your GP about HPV vaccination for men and women. Continue with regular Pap smears, whether or not you are vaccinated against HPV.

Take precautions against sexually transmissible infections. Use barrier methods of contraception and STI prevention. Ask any new sexual partner to have STI testing.

Symptoms of cervical cancer include irregular vaginal bleeding between periods or after intercourse, vaginal bleeding after menopause, pain during intercourse, and unusual vaginal discharge. These symptoms should be reported to your GP for investigation with Pap test, colposcopy, and biopsy.

If you have been told you have an abnormal Pap smear and you have to wait for a follow-up test, use the opportunity to strengthen your body's own healing potential. This is akin to the active surveillance recommended for men with suspected low-grade prostate cancer.

WAYS TO HELP YOUR IMMUNE SYSTEM TO COUNTER HPV

Don't smoke. Chemicals in tobacco concentrate in the cervix and damage cervical cells and increase cancer risk.

Minimise (by this I mean stop) alcohol consumption.

Reduce sources of stress in your life.

Eat a healthy diet with a variety of colours of plant-based foods and minimise processed foods. Increase your intake of cruciferous vegetables and consider a supplement of indole-3-carbinol. And avoid animal fats.

Check for and correct nutritional deficiencies such as vitamin C, iron, vitamin B_6, Vitamin B_{12}, folate, betacarotene, zinc and selenium. There are blood tests for most of these nutrients:

- increase your dietary intake of vitamin C as inadequate vitamin C intake is a risk factor for the development of precancerous abnormalities and cancer
- low dietary iron levels and low iron stores (shown as low ferritin) are associated with a higher cervical cancer risk
- low serum betacarotene rates have been associated with a greater risk of cervical dysplasia
- vitamin B_6 levels are decreased in one-third of patients with cervical cancer
- blood and dietary levels of the trace mineral selenium have been found to be significantly lower in women with cervical dysplasia, particularly where levels of selenium in the soil are deficient, as they are in Australia.

Stomach Cancer

Stomach cancer is also known as gastric cancer. This cancer tends to affect people over the age of 50, men more so than women. There is no routine screening test for gastric cancer, so we rely on the investigation of any suspicious symptoms.

Signs of early stomach cancer include heartburn or indigestion, a sense of fullness even after a small meal, loss of appetite, weight loss, nausea and/or vomiting, unexplained tiredness or weakness, bloodstained vomit or black-coloured bowel motions.

If you present to your doctor with indigestion, initial investigations will include a blood test and a breath test for a bacterial infection with *Helicobacter pylori*. Presence of this bug is associated with the development of stomach cancer. Investigation is by direct vision with a gastroscopy (also called an endoscopy) with biopsy of any suspicious areas.

The risk factors for stomach cancer include:

- smoking
- aged over 50 years
- chronic untreated *Helicobacter pylori* infection

- a diet low in fruit and vegetables
- eating a lot of smoked, pickled or salted foods
- partial gastrectomy (removal of part of the stomach) for peptic ulcer disease 20 years in the past
- a family history of stomach cancer, familial adenomatous polyposis (FAP), or hereditary non-polyposis colorectal cancer (HNPCC).

There are wide cultural differences. For example, stomach cancer accounts for 2 per cent of cancers in the US but 20.8 per cent of cancers in South Korea.

PREHABILITATION

After staging, a treatment plan is devised. Cancer prehabilitation involves planning for the treatment ahead and also for the consequences of treatment.

Your stomach plays an important role in digestion. It acts as a reservoir where food is mixed with stomach acid as part of the digestion process. Prehabilitation involves anticipating the impact the removal of your stomach will have on your health and wellbeing.

NUTRITION

If you have been experiencing symptoms for some time, such as loss of appetite, nausea and weight loss, and you were not supplementing for inadequacies in your diet, it is likely that you will already have nutritional deficiencies. These need to be corrected as much as possible before you undergo surgery.

You will need a nutritional assessment, and an assessment about whether you are currently experiencing a degree of malnutrition. A dietitian will help you with an eating plan for now and also for the post-operative period.

SUPPLEMENTS

Protein, vitamin, and mineral supplementation will need to be professionally assessed and prescribed. Vitamin B_{12}, folate, and iron deficiency are common in people who have had a gastrectomy. Vitamins D and C, and protein are also commonly deficient preoperatively. All these nutrients can be supplemented.

Rapid replenishment of some nutrients can be done by injection or infusion. For example, vitamin D is available by injection, high-dose B vitamins can by given by injection or intravenous infusion, and high-dose vitamin C and iron are available by infusion.

EXERCISE

If you have become physically weakened by your condition, you will need help to improve your strength and fitness. An exercise physiologist or specialised physiotherapist can help you with a program.

STRESS MANAGEMENT

As with any cancer prehabilitation program, having counselling or participating in group sessions to learn relaxation and stress management techniques will improve your emotional health and coping strategies.

POST-GASTRECTOMY SYNDROME

A gastrectomy is the surgical removal of the stomach. If you have been diagnosed with stomach cancer, this the main treatment you will be offered. Nutritional deficiencies are common at the time of diagnosis in people with gastric cancer, and surgery makes the problem of deficiencies worse, so careful attention needs to be paid to diet and supplementation for the rest of your life.

Because of the removal of the stomach and therefore its role in digestion, you will not be able to get all the nutrients your body needs from food. The main deficiencies to consider are vitamin C, vitamin D, vitamin B_{12}, calcium, magnesium, protein, thiamine and iron.

Long-term problems of uncorrected deficiencies include anaemia, poor healing, infection and osteoporosis. Get your bone density level checked pre-operatively as this will need to be monitored over time.

The primary function of the stomach is to act as a reservoir, initiate the digestive process, and release its contents gradually into the duodenum for digestion in the small bowel. When your stomach is removed, food travels rapidly into the small intestine. A condition called 'dumping syndrome' is common after gastrectomy. It involves intolerance for large meals, where two to four hours after eating you may experience cramping abdominal pain, diarrhoea, light-headedness, and a sudden drop in blood pressure accompanied by a rise in your heart rate.

After gastrectomy you will have a specially designed diet that is high in protein, low in carbohydrates, and low in sugars. You will be advised to gradually increase your fibre intake, and eat five or six small meals a day, with limited fluid intake during meals.

You can take vitamin B_{12} as a sublingual spray or as regular injections. Oral iron, magnesium and calcium supplements, vitamin C, D and other B vitamins are often needed to prevent deficiencies in these vitamins and minerals.

What the Future Holds

Over my career I have been privileged to see first hand the incredible advances in cancer treatment. People diagnosed with previously lethal cancers are now surviving. Yet the 'cure for cancer' remains elusive. Research around the world is focused on prevention, treatment and cure. We are learning more and more about the complex and detailed biology of cancer and over the coming years the progress that is being made will help to reduce the fear of cancer into the future.

There are many things about a cancer diagnosis that you cannot control. But there are many things that have a significant impact on cancer recovery that you can control.

The process of cancer treatment can be gruelling and exhausting. By taking control of your lifestyle and health habits, you can improve your chances of recovery.

You can get your life back.

I hope with the information and advice provided in this book you will be able to navigate your cancer journey and regain your health and confidence.

Acknowledgements

The Cancer Recovery Guide represents my own evolution over several decades of clinical practice, personal experiences and careful thought about what people diagnosed with cancer want and need.

From my earliest experiences as a junior doctor on the oncology wards through many years of general practice, I have developed a sense of what 'best practice' should look like, and my patients have guided me in exploring territories beyond the boundaries of my conventional medical training.

I cannot thank them all by name, but I have dedicated this book to them collectively. I can specifically mention my mother-in-law, Jutta, who sadly lost her battle with bowel cancer despite the best medical and palliative care available at the time.

Thanks go to my wife, Jackie Stricker-Phelps, for constantly challenging me to dig deeper in finding solutions for the most complicated clinical problems.

His Royal Highness The Prince of Wales has for decades been a thought leader in integrative medicine, environmental protection, and concepts of sustainability. I had the privilege of meeting him in India, along with Prof Dean Ornish, Dr Woodson Merrell, Dr Michael Dixon OBE and Dr Isaac Mathai where we discussed the future of global healthcare. I am profoundly honoured that HRH Prince Charles has written the foreword to the book. My gratitude goes to Dr Michael Dixon OBE, Chair of the College of Medicine UK and Chair of the NHS Alliance, for reviewing the manuscript.

I would like to thank several valued colleagues for their advice and chapter reviews:

- Prof Phillip Stricker AO for his input and review of the chapter on prostate cancer. Phillip is a rare type of cancer surgeon who encourages all of his patients to take an integrative approach to their cancer treatment and their overall lifestyle. Our many early conversations about how we could improve the treatment process and the future lives of our patients through a blend of conventional and adjunctive therapies were pivotal in my thinking.
- Integrative GP Dr Claudia Lee at Sydney Integrative Medicine for her review of the chapter on vitamin C and other intravenous nutriceuticals.
- Dietician Jaime Rose Chambers for sharing her professional experience of managing the nutrition of patients diagnosed with cancer. This book is obviously something of a family event as Jaime is my oldest daughter and our dietician at Cooper Street Clinic and Sydney Integrative Medicine. She is also a member of Prof Stricker's multidisciplinary prostate cancer treatment team.
- Naturopaths Laura Brass from Canada and Teresa Mitchell-Paterson of Sydney Integrative Medicine for their detailed advice on aspects of herbal medicines and nutritional supplements.
- Psychologists Lissy Abrahams and Jace Cannon-Brooks of the Heath Group Practice in Sydney for their review of the chapter on emotional health.

I must express my appreciation to my marvellous publishing team at Pan Macmillan: publisher Ingrid Ohlsson, editor Samantha Sainsbury and copy editor Glenda Downing.

Endnotes

PART ONE – DIAGNOSIS
HEARING THE WORD 'CANCER' IS SCARY

Page

11.   According to the Cancer Council . . .: Cancer Council Australia, 'Facts and figures', 5 April 2015, www.cancer.org.au

11.   Cancer remains the second most . . .: The American Cancer Society, 'Cancer facts and statistics', www.cancer.org/research/cancerfactsstatistics/index American Cancer Society.

13.   A group from the National Cancer Institute . . .: Esserman LJ, Thompson IM, Reid B 'Overdiagnosis and Overtreatment in Cancer. An Opportunity for Improvement', *The Journal of the American Medical Association*, vol. 310, no. 8, 2013, pp. 797–798, doi:10.1001/jama.2013.108415.

SPEAKING THE LANGUAGE

Page

21.   In a 2012 study of older disabled adults . . .: Ahalt C, Walter LC, Yourman L, Eng C, Pérez-Stable EJ, Smith AK, ' "Knowing is better": preferences of diverse older adults for discussing prognosis', *Journal of General Internal Medicine*, vol. 27. no. 5, 2012, pp. 568-75, doi: 10.1007/s11606-011-1933-0. Epub 2011 Nov 30.

PART TWO – DEALING WITH CANCER EMOTIONALLY
MENTAL HEALTH

Page

75. You need to be able to recognise . . .: American Psychiatric Assocation, *Diagnostic and stastical manual of mental disorders*, 5th ed (DSM-V), Washington, DC, APA.

82. The *Medical Journal of Australia* reviewed . . .: Lombard CB, 'What is the role of food in preventing depression and improving mood, performance and cognitive function?', *Medical Journal of Australia*, 2000 Nov 6;173 Suppl:S104–5.

84. St John's wort has also been shown. . .: Medina MA, Martinez-Poveda B, Amores-Sanchez M et al., 'Hyperforin: more than an antidepressant bioactive compound?', *Life Science*, vol. 79, no. 2, 2006, pp. 105–111.

85. Scientific reviews have shown that . . .: Fournier J, DeRubeis R, Hollon S et al., 'Antidepressant Drug Effects and Depression Severity A Patient-Level Meta-analysis', *Journal of the Americal Medical Association*, vol. 303, no. 1, 2013, pp. 47–53.

86. One study looked at . . .: Carlson LE, Doll R, Stephen J, 'Randomized controlled trial of Mindfulness-based cancer recovery versus supportive expressive group therapy for distressed survivors of breast cancer', *Journal of Clinical Oncology*, vol. 3, no. 25, 2013, pp. 3119–26, doi: 10.1200/JCO.2012.47.5210.

88. Studies have shown that yoga . . .: Buffart LM, van Uffelen JG, Riphagen II, 'Physical and psychosocial benefits of yoga in cancer patients and survivors, a systematic review and meta-analysis of randomized controlled trials', *BMC Cancer*, 2012, 12:559, doi: 10.1186/1471–2407-12-559.

89. Relaxation therapy with breathing . . .: Song QH, Xu RM, Zhang QH et al., 'Relaxation training during chemotherapy for breast cancer improves mental health and lessens adverse events', *Integrative Journal of Clinical Experimental Medicine*, vol. 6, no. 10, 2013, pp. 979–84.

91. The level of stress at the time . . .: Andersen BL, Shapiro CL, Farrar WB et al., 'Psychological responses to cancer recurrence', *Cancer*, vol. 104, no. 7, 2005, pp. 1540–7.

92. A study by the Ohio State University . . .: Yang HC, Thornton LM, Shapiro CL, Andersen BL, 'Surviving recurrence: psychological and quality-of-life recovery', vol. 112, no. 5, 2008, pp. 1178–87.

CONNECTEDNESS

Page

95. The Harvard Nurses' Study . . .: The Nurses' Health Study, Harvard University, http://www.channing.harvard.edu/nhs/

95. According to a study . . .: Waxler-Morrison N, Gregory T, Mears B, Kan L, 'Effects of social relationships on survival for women with breast cancer: A prospective study', *Social Science Medicine*, vol. 33, no. 2, 1991, pp. 117–83.

SPIRITUALITY AND CANCER

Page

102. Spiritual beliefs will influence . . .: Peteet JR, Balboni MJ, 'Spirituality and religion in oncology', *CA: A Cancer Journal for Clinicians*, 63, pp. 280–289.

INTIMACY, SEXUALITY AND CANCER RECOVERY

Page

113. This is thought to be due . . .: Macmillan UK, www.macmillan.org.uk

PART THREE – CANCER-SPECIFIC TREATMENTS
PREHILBILTATION

Page

119. There is a growing body of . . .: Silver JK, Baima J, 'Cancer prehabilitation: an opportunity to decrease treatment-related morbidity, increase cancer treatment options, and improve physical and psychological health outcomes', *American Journal of Physical Medicine & Rehabilitation*, vol. 92, no. 8, 2013, pp. 715–27, doi: 10.1097/ PHM.0b013e31829b4afe.

126. It is estimated to happen to 30–50 per cent . . .: Monk TG et al., 'Predictors of Cognitive Dysfunction after Major Non-Cardiac Surgery', *Anaesthesiology*, 2008, 108:18-30, www.anesthesiaweb. org/images/pocd/Monk-2008.pdf

CHEMOTHERAPY

Page

131. It has been shown to ameliorate fatigue . . .: Graziano F et al., 'Potential role of levocarnitine supplementation for the treatment

of chemotherapy-induced fatigue in non-anaemic cancer patients', *British Journal Cancer*, vol. 86, no. 12, 2002, pp. 1854–7.

131. No severe adverse events were . . .: Wang YM et al., 'The efficacy and safety of melatonin in concurrent chemotherapy or radiotherapy for solid tumors: a meta-analysis of randomized controlled trials', *Cancer, Chemotherapy and Pharmacology*, vol. 69, no. 5, 2012.

136. Glutamine increases regeneration . . .: Daniele B, Perrone F et al., 'Oral glutamine in the prevention of fluorouracil induced intestinal toxicity: a double blind, placebo controlled, randomised trial', *Gut*, vol. 48, no. 1, 2001, pp. 28–33.

136. A Mayo Clinic study showed. . .: Anderson PM, Schroeder G, Skubitz KM, 'Oral glutamine reduces the duration and severity of stomatitis after cytotoxic cancer chemotherapy', *Cancer*, vol. 83, no. 7, 1998, pp. 1433–9.

136. A randomised human study . . .: Savarese DM, Savy G, Vahdat L, Wischmeyer PE, Corey B, 'Prevention of chemotherapy and radiation toxicity with glutamine', *Cancer Treatment Review*, vol. 29, no. 6, 2003, pp. 501–13.

139. A Cochrane review of Chinese herbs . . .: Taixiang W, Munro AJ, Guanjian L, 'Chinese medical herbs for chemotherapy side effects in colorectal cancer patients', Cochrane Database System Review 2005; 1: CD 04540.

139. There is potential for role . . .: Davis L, Kuttan G, 'Immunomodulatory activity of *Withania somnifera* extract in mice', *Journal of Ethnopharmacology*, 71(1/2), 2000, pp. 193–200.

140. Neuropathy, or nerve damage, is estimated . . .: Forman A, 'Peripheral neuropathy in cancer patients: incidence, features and pathophysiology', *Oncology*, vol. 4, no. 1, 1990, pp. 57–62.

141. One double-blind trial . . .: Cascinu S et al., 'Neuroprotective effect of reduced glutathione on cisplatin-based chemotherapy in advanced gastric cancer: a randomized double-blind placebo-controlled trial', *Journal of Clinical Oncology*, vol. 13, no. 1, 1995, pp. 26–32, www.ncbi.nlm.nih.gov/pubmed/7799029

142. A second randomised, placebo-controlled trial . . .: Cascinu S et al., 'Neuroprotective effect of reduced glutathione on oxaliplatin-based chemotherapy in advanced colorectal cancer: a randomized, double-blind, placebo-controlled trial', *Journal of Clinical Oncology*, vol. 15, no. 16, 2002, pp. 3478–83.

142. Vitamin E has been studied . . .: Pace A, Carpano S, Galié E et al., 'Vitamin E in the neuroprotection of cisplatin-induced peripheral neurotoxicity and ototoxicity', *Journal of Clinical Oncology*, vol. 25 (18S), 2007, p. 9114.

142. It was also found to help . . .: Argyriou AA, Chroni E, Koutras A et al., 'Preventing paclitaxelinduced peripheral neuropathy: a phase II trial of vitamin E supplementation', *Journal of Pain Symptom Management*, vol. 32, no. 3, 2006, pp. 237–244.

142. A study in 2008 . . .: Nikcevich DA, Grothey A, Sloan JA et al., 'Effect of intravenous calcium and magnesium (IV CaMg) on oxaliplatin-induced sensory neurotoxicity in adjuvant colon cancer: Results of the phase III placebo-controlled, double-blind NCCTG trial N04C7', *Journal of Clinical Oncology*, vol. 26 (15S), 2002, p. 4009.

143. A series of 15 patients . . .: Gedlicka C et al., 'Effective treatment of oxaliplatin-induced cumulative polyneuropathy with alpha-lipoic acid', *Journal of Clinical Oncology*, 2002, pp. 3359–3361.

143. Alpha-lipoic acid . . .: Gedlicka C et al., 'Amelioration of docetaxel/cisplatin induced polyneuropathy by alphalipoic acid', *Annals of Oncology*, vol. 14, 2003, pp. 339–340.

143. A recent review of these studies . . .: Schröder S et al., 'Can medical herbs stimulate regeneration or neuroprotection and treat neuropathic pain in chemotherapy-induced peripheral neuropathy?', *Evidence-Based Complementary Alternative Medicine*, 423713, doi:10.1155/2013/423713. Epub 2013 Jul 31.

144. 'While CIPN has multiple . . .: ibid.

144. According to the Mayo Clinic, acupuncture . . .: Wong R, Sagar S, 'Acupuncture treatment for chemotherapy-Induced peripheral neuropathy', *Acupuncture in Medicine*, vol. 24, no. 2, 2006, pp. 87–91.

146. Milk thistle, which is used to prevent and treat . . .: Gholamreza Karimi, Mohammad Ramezani and Zahra Tahoonian, 'Cisplatin Nephrotoxicity and Protection by Milk Thistle Extract in Rats', *Evidenced-Based Complementary Alternative Medicine*, vol. 2, no. 3, 2005, pp. 383–386, www.ncbi.nlm.nih.gov/pubmedhealth/PMH0032607/

146. There are many studies reporting . . .: Herschmann DL, 'Randomised double blind placebo-controlled trial of acetyl-L-carnitine for the prevention of taxane-induced neuropathy in

women undergoing adjuvant breast cancer therapy', *Journal of Clinical Oncology*, vol. 31, no. 202627-2633, 2013.

147. Late reactions can sometimes . . .: Pai VB, Nahata MC, 'Cardiotoxicity of chemotherapeutic agents: incidence, treatment and prevention', *Drug Safety*, vol. 22, no. 4, 2000, pp. 263–302.

147. The dose of anti-cancer drug . . .: Yeh ET, Tong AT, Lenihan DJ et al., 'Cardiovascular complications of cancer therapy: diagnosis, pathogenesis, and management', *Circulation*, vol. 109, no. 25, 2004, pp. 3122–3131.

148. Long-term L-carnitine . . .: Mijares A, Lopez JR, 'L-carnitine prevents increase in diastolic Ca^{2+} induced by doxorubicin in cardiac cells', *European Journal of Pharmacology*, vol. 425, no. 2, 2001, pp. 117–120.

148. Coenzyme Q10 provides . . .: Bryant J, Picot J, Baxter L et al., 'Clinical and cost-effectiveness of cardioprotection against the toxic effects of anthracyclines given to children with cancer: a systematic review', *British Journal of Cancer*, no. 96, vol. 2, 2007, pp. 226–230 and Roffe L, Schmidt K, Ernst E, 'Efficacy of coenzyme Q10 for improved tolerability of cancer treatments: a systematic review', *Journal Clinical Oncology*, vol. 22, no. 21, 2004, pp. 4418–4424.

148. Studies suggest that coenzyme Q10 . . .: Conklin KA, 'Coenzyme q10 for prevention of anthracycline-induced cardiotoxicity', *Integrative Cancer Therapy*, vol. 4, no. 2, 2005, pp. 110–30.

152. There are some preliminary studies . . .: Huang X, Whitworth CA, Rybak LP, 'Ginkgo biloba extract (EGb 761) protects against cisplatin-induced ototoxicity in rats', *Otology & Neurotology*, vol. 28, no. 6, 2007, pp. 828–33.

152. El-Boghdady NA, 'Increased cardiac endothelin-1 and nitric oxide in adriamycin-induced acute cardiotoxicity: protective effect of Ginkgo biloba extract', *Indian Journal of Biochemistry and Biophysics*, vol. 50, no. 3, 2013, pp. 202–9.

153. It has also been shown to be effective . . .: Raghav S, Singh H, Dalal PK et al., 'Randomized controlled trial of standardized Bacopa monniera extract in age-associated memory', *Indian Journal of Psychiatry*, vol. 48, no. 4, 2006, pp. 238–42.

153. While there are studies to show that brahmi . . .: Kongkeaw C, Dilokthornsakul P, Thanarangsarit P, Limpeanchob N, Norman Scholfield C, 'Meta-analysis of randomized controlled trials on cognitive effects of Bacopa monnieri extract', *Journal of*

Ethnopharmacology, vol. 151 no. 1, 2014, pp. 528–35, doi: 10.1016/j.jep.2013.11.008.

RADIOTHERAPY

Page

159. Supplements which may be helpful . . .: Thomas G, Asher G, Mounsey A, 'PURLs: Finally, a way to relieve cancer-related fatigue', Journal of Family Practice, vol. 63, no. 5, 2014, 270–272. PMCID: PMC4043102.

159. It may be useful in supporting . . .: Pittler MH, Ernst E, 'Horse chestnut seed extract for long-term or chronic venous insufficiency', Cochran review, 2012, www.cochrane.org/CD003230/PVD_horse-chestnut-seed-extract-for-long-term-or-chronic-venous-insufficiency.

160. A clinical trial involving . . .: Ryan J, Heckler C, Ling M et al., 'Curcumin for radiation dermatitis: A randomized, double-blind, placebo-controlled clinical trial of thirty breast cancer patients', *Radiation Research,* vol. 180, 2013, pp. 34–43.

161. Calendual ointment . . .: Pommier P, Gomez F, Sunyach M et al., 'Calendula ointment and radiation dermatitis during breast cancer treatment', *Journal of Clinical Oncology*, vol. 22, no. 8, 2004, pp. 1447–1453.

161. Topical aloe vera . . .: Haddad P et al., 'Aloe vera for prevention of radiation-induced dermatitis: a self-controlled clinical trial', *Current Oncology*, vol. 20, no. 4:e345–8, 2013, doi: 10.3747/co.20.1356. www.ncbi.nlm.nih.gov/pubmed/23904773

164. Herbs used with radiotherapy: Phelps K, Hassed C, *General Practice: The Integrative Approach*, Elsevier, 2010.

164. Milk thistle . . .: Greenlee H, Abascal K, Yarnell E, Ladas E, 'Clinical applications of Silybum marianum in oncology', *Integrative Cancer Therapy*, vol. 6, no. 2, 2007, pp. 158–65.

165. Green tea: Pajonk F, Reidisser A, Henke M et al., 'The effects of tea extracts on proinflammatory signaling', *BMC Medicine*, vol. 4, no. 28, 2006.

165. Panax ginseng: Kim SH, Cho CK, Yoo SY et al., 'In vivo radioprotective activity of *Panax* ginseng and diethyl ldithiocarbamate', *In Vivo*, vol. 7, 1993, pp. 467–470.

165. Reishi mushroom: Wang D, Weng X, 'Antitumor activity of extracts of Ganoderma lucidum and their protective effects on damaged HL-7702 cells induced by radiotherapy and chemotherapy',

Zhongguo Zhong Yao Za Zhi, vol. 31, no. 19, 2006, pp. 1618–1622.

165. Holy basil: Ganasoundari A, Zare SM, Uma Devi P, 'Modification of bone marrow radiosensitivity by medicinal plant extracts', *British Journal of Radiology*, vol. 70, 1997, pp. 599–602.

165. Calendaul: Pommier P, Gomez F, Sunyach MP et al., 'Phase III randomized trial of Calendula officinalis compared with trolamine for the prevention of acute dermatitis during irradiation for breast cancer', *Journal of Clinical Oncology*, vol. 22, no. 8, 2004, pp. 1447–1453.

PART FOUR – ADJUNCTIVE THERAPIES
INTRAVENOUS VITAMIN C AND OTHER NUTRIENTS

Page

174. There is some evidence that intravenous vitamin C . . .: Fritz H et al., 'Intravenous Vitamin C and Cancer: A Systematic Review', *Integrative Cancer Therapy*, vol. 13, no. 4, 2014, pp. 280–300.

174. In some cases there is evidence that it makes chemotherapy . . .: ibid.

175. High dose vitamin C therapy in cancer patients has been studied . . .: Cameron E, Pauling L, 'Supplemental ascorbate in the supportive treatment of cancer: Prolongation of survival times in terminal human cancer', *Proceedings of the National Academy of Science USA*, 1976, 73:3685–3689 and Cameron E, Pauling L, 'Supplemental ascorbate in the supportive treatment of cancer: Reevaluation of prolongation of survival times in terminal human cancer', *Proceedings of the National Academy of Science*, 5:4538–4542, 37, http://www.kumc.edu/school-of-medicine/integrative-medicine/patientservices/infusion-clinic.html

176. Other clinics such as the University of Kansas . . .: University of Kansas, Patient services at Integratve Medicine, 'Infusion clinic', www.kumc.edu/school-of-medicine/integrative-medicine/patient-services/infusion-clinic.html

176. The H_2O_2 preferentially kills . . .: Chen Q, Espey MG, Krishna MC, et al., 'Pharmacologic ascorbic acid concentrations selectively kill cancer cells: Action as a pro-drug to deliver hydrogen peroxide to tissues', *Proceedings of the National Academy of Science*, 2005.

177. Ascorbic acid with arsenic . . .: National Cancer Institute, 'High-dose Vitamin C (PDQ)', 2015, www.cancer.gov/cancertopics/pdq/cam/highdosevitaminc/patient/page2

177. Ascorbic acid with gemcitabine . . .: ibid.

177. Ascrobic acid with gemcitabine and . . .: ibid.

177. A variety of animal studies . . .: Qi Chen, 'Pharmacologic doses of ascorbate act as a prooxidant and decrease growth of aggressive tumor xenografts in mice', Proceedings of The National Academy of Sciences of the USA, www.pnas.org/content/105/32/11105

177. Researches at the University of Kansas . . .: Ma Y, Chapman J, Levine M et al., 'High-dose parenteral ascorbate enhanced chemosensitivity of ovarian cancer and reduced toxicity of chemotherapy', Science Translational Medicine, 2014, 5;6(222):222ra18, doi:10.1126/scitranslmed.3007154.

178. A 2011 study . . .: Vollbracht C1, Schneider B, Leendert V et al., 'Intravenous vitamin C administration improves quality of life in breast cancer patients during chemo-/radiotherapy and aftercare: results of a retrospective, multicentre, epidemiological cohort study in Germany', In Vivo, vol. 25, no. 6, 2011, pp. 983–90.

178. A series of case reports . . .: Padayatty SJ, Riordan HD, Hewitt SM, Katz A, Hoffer LJ, Levine M, 'Intravenously administered vitamin C as cancer therapy: three cases', Canadian Medical Association Journal, vol. 174, no. 7, 2006, pp. 937–42.

178. A study at the Riordan Clinic . . .: Mikirova N, Casciari J, Rogers A, 'Effect of high-dose intravenous vitamin C on inflammation in cancer patients', Journal of Translational Medicine, vol. 11, no. 10, 2012, p. 189.

178. High dose IVC has also recently . . .: Fowler AA, Syed AA, Natarajan R, 'Phase 1 safety trial of intravenous ascorbic acid in patients with severe sepsis', Journal of Translational Medicine, vol. 12, no. 32, 2014.

179. Studies have also shown that Vitamin C levels in . . .: National Cancer Institute, 'Questions and Answers About High Dose Vitamin C', http://www.cancer.gov, Accessed 23 March 2014.

181. One of the concerns surrounding . . .: Lawenda BD, Kelly KM, Ladas EJ et al., 'Should supplemental antioxidant administration be avoided during chemotherapy and radiation therapy?', Journal of the National Cancer Institute, vol. 100, no. 11, 2008, pp. 773–783.

181. One clinical study, however, showed . . .: Pathak AK, Bhutani M, Guleria R et al., 'Chemotherapy alone vs. chemotherapy plus high dose multiple antioxidants in patients with advanced non small cell lung cancer', Journal of the American College of Nutrition, vol. 24, no. 1, 2005, pp. 16–21.

181. Another study found an increase . . .: Kennedy DD, Tucker KL, Ladas ED et al., 'Low antioxidant vitamin intakes are associated with increases in adverse effects of chemotherapy in children with acute lymphoblastic leukaemia', *The American Journal of Clinical Nutrition,* vol. 79, no. 6, 2004, pp. 1029–1036.

181. The University of Kansas advises . . .: The University of Kansas Medical Centre, www.kumc.edu/school-of-medicine/integrative-medicine, 2015, Accessed 24 March 2014.

181. A German study showed that high dose . . .: Vollbracht C, Schneider B, Leendert V, Weiss G, Auerbach L, Beuth J, 'Intravenous vitamin C administration improves quality of life in breast cancer patients during chemo-/radiotherapy and aftercare: results of a retrospective, multicentre, epidemiological cohort study in Germany', *In Vivo,* vol. 25, no. 6, 2011, pp. 983–90.

182. The Riordan Clinic in the USA . . .: The Riordan IVC Protocol for Adjunctive Cancer Care, 'Intravenous Ascorbate as a Chemotherapeutic and Biological Response Modifying Agent', 2015, www.riordanclinic.org/research/research-studies/vitaminc/protocol

182. 'A variety of laboratory . . .: Fromberg A et al., 'Ascorbate exerts anti-proliferative effects through cell cycle inhibition and sensitizes tumor cells toward cytostatic drugs', *Cancer Chemotherapy Pharmacology,* vol. 67, 2011, pp. 1157–66 and Shinozaki K et al. 'Ascorbic acid enhances radiation-induced apoptosis in an HL60 human leukemia cell line', *Journal of Radiation Research,* vol. 52, 2011, pp. 229–37.

182. The protocol at the University of Kansas . . .: The University of Kansas Medical Centre, www.kumc.edu/school-of-medicine/integrative-medicine, 2015.

185. One double-blind trial . . .: Cascinu S, Cordella L, Del Ferro E, Fronzoni M, Catalano G, 'Neuroprotective effect of reduced glutathione on cisplatin-based chemotherapy in advanced gastric cancer: a randomized double-blind placebo-controlled trial', *Journal of Clinical Oncology,* vol. 1, no. 1, 1995, pp. 26–32, www.ncbi.nlm.nih.gov/pubmed/7799029

186. This study was followed by . . .: Cascinu S, Catalano V, Cordella L, 'Neuroprotective effect of reduced glutathione on oxaliplatin-based chemotherapy in advanced colorectal cancer: a randomized, double-blind, placebo-controlled trial', *Journal of Clinical Oncology,* vol. 20, no. 16, 2002, pp. 3478–83.

HERBS AND SUPPLEMENTS

Page

189. A review of 32 studies . . .: Velicer CM, Ulrich CM, 'Vitamin and Mineral Supplement Use Among US Adults After Cancer Diagnosis: A Systematic Review', *Journal of Clinical Oncology*, 2008, pp. 665–673.

190. Reasons for using herbal medicines include . . .: Damery S, Gratus C, Grieve R, 'The use of herbal medicines by people with cancer: a cross-sectional survey', *British Journal of Cancer*, vol. 104, no. 6, 2011, pp. 927–933.

191. Most of the concerns about . . .: Cheng CW, Fan W, Ko SG et al., 'Evidence-based management of herb-drug interaction in cancer chemotherapy', *Explore* (NY) vol. 6, no. 5, 2010, pp. 324–9.

198. Additionally, preliminary research . . .: Rajagopal S et al., 'Andrographolide, a potential cancer therapeutic agent isolated from Andrographis paniculata', *Therapeutic Oncology*, vol. 3, no. 3, 2003, pp. 147–58.

199. Two of the components of . . .: Willoughby JA Sr, Sundar SN, Cheung M, et al., 'Artemisinin blocks prostate cancer growth and cell cycle progression by disrupting Sp1 interactions with the cyclin-dependent kinase-4 (CDK4) promoter and inhibiting CDK4 gene expression', Journal of Biology and Chemistry, vol. 284, no. 4, pp. 2203-13.3;284 and Singh NP, Lai HC, 'Artemisinin induces apoptosis in human cancer cells', Anticancer Research, vol. 24 no. 4, 2004, pp. 2277–80.(4):2203–13.

200. A 2005 Cochrane review . . .: Taixiang W, Munro AJ, Guanjian L, 'Chinese medical herbs for chemotherapy side effects in colorectal cancer patients', Cochrane Database System Review 2005; 1:CD04540.

200. Astragalus extracts . . .: Cho WC, Leung KN, 'In vitro and in vivo anti-tumor effects of Astragalus membranaceus', *Cancer Letters*, vol. 25, no. 1, 2007, pp. 43–54.

200. Delay chemical-induced liver . . .: Rajagopal S, Kumar RA, Deevi DS, Satyanarayana C, Rajagopalan R, 'J Exp Andrographolide, a potential cancer therapeutic agent isolated from Andrographis paniculata', *Therapeutic Oncology*, vol. 3, no. 3, 2003, pp. 147–58.

200. Have anti-angiogenic property . . .: Mijares A, Lopez JR, 'L carnitine prevents increase in diastolic Ca^{2+} induced by doxorubicin in cardiac cells', *European Journal of Pharmacology*, vol. 425, no. 2, 2001, pp. 117–120.

200. In vitro, animal . . .: Velicer CM, Ulrich CM, 'Vitamin and Mineral Supplement Use Among US Adults After Cancer Diagnosis: A Systematic Review', *Journal of Clinical Oncology*, February 1, 2008:665-673 and Damery S, Gratus C, Grieve R, 'The use of herbal medicines by people with cancer: a cross-sectional survey', *British Journal of Cancer*, vol. 104, no. 6, 2011, pp. 927–933.

200. May also enhance the effects . . .: Cheng CW, Fan W, Ko SG et al., 'Evidence-based management of herb-drug interaction in cancer chemotherapy', *Explore (NY)* 2010, vol. 6, no. 5, pp. 324–9.

201. Baical skullcap . . .: Sagar S, Yance MN, Wong RK, 'Natural health products that inhibit angiogenesis: a potential source for investigational new agents to treat cancer Part 1', *Current Oncology*, vol. 13, no. 1, 2006, pp. 14–26.

201. A 2014 review found that . . .: Fritz H, Seely D, McGowan J et al., 'Black cohosh and breast cancer: a systematic review', *Integrative Cancer Therapy,* vol. 13, no. 1, 2014, pp. 12–29, doi:10.1177/1534735413477191.

202. Apply calendula . . .: Pommier P, Gomez F, Sunyach MP et al., 'Phase III randomised trial of Calendula officinalis compared with trolamine for the prevention of acute dermatitis during irradiation for breast cancer', *Journal of Clinical Oncology*, vol. 22, no. 8, 2004, pp. 1447–1453.

203. Diabetics should use the tablet . . .: *American Journal of Obstetrics and Gynaecology*, 2015.

204. Ginger: Bode AM, Dong Z, 'The amazing and mighty ginger', *Herbal Medicine: Biomolecular and Clinical Aspects*, CRC Press, 2011, www.ncbi.nlm.nih.gov/books/NBK92775/

204. High doses of pure American . . . .: Barton DL, Heshan L, Shaker DR et al., 'Wisconsin Ginseng (*Panax quinquefolius*) to Improve Cancer-Related Fatigue: A Randomized, Double-Blind Trial', N07C2 JNCI, *Journal of the National Cancer Institute*, 2013, djt181 doi: 10.1093/jnci/djt181.

205. Green tea . . .: Pajonk F, Reidisser A, Henke M et al., 'The effects of tea extracts on proinflammatory signaling', *BMC Medicine*, vol. 4, no. 28, 2006.

206. Licorice is often . . .: Madisch A, Holtmann G, Mayr G, et al., 'Treatment of functional dyspepsia with a herbal preparation. A double-blind, randomized, placebo-controlled, multicenter trial', *Digestion*. vol. 69, no. 1, 2004, pp. 45-52.

208. Reishi mushroom . . .: Wang D, Weng X, 'Antitumor activity of extracts of Ganoderma lucidum and their protective effects on damaged HL-7702 cells induced by radiotherapy and chemotherapy', 2006, *Zhongguo Zhong Yao Za Zhi*, vol. 31, no. 19, pp. 1618–1622.

208. A few studies have shown it to have . . .: Jin X, 'G. lucidum (Reishi mushroom) for cancer treatment', *Cochrane Review*, 2012, www.ncbi.nlm.nih.gov/pubmedhealth/PMH0046740/

208. Meta-analysis results showed . . .: Chan GC, 'Ganoderma lucidum (Reishi mushroom) for cancer treatment', *Cochrane Database System Review*, 2012 Jun 13;6:CD007731, doi: 10.1002/14651858. CD007731.pub2.

208. From animal studies it is thought . . .: Zhang C, Feng Y, Qu S et al., 'Resveratrol attenuates doxorubicininduced cardiomyocyte apoptosis in mice through SIRT1-mediated deacetylation of p53,' *Cardiovascular research,* vol. 90, no. 3, 2011, pp. 538–545.

209. Extensive scientific testing . . .: Linde K, Berner MM, Kriston L, 'St. John's wort for treating depression', *Cochrane Review*, 2009, www.cochrane.org/CD000448/DEPRESSN_st.-johns-wort-for-treating-depression.

209. Laboratory studies . . .: National Cancer Institute, 'Mary's thistle – for health professionals', 2015, www.cancer.gov/cancertopics/pdq/cam/milkthistle/HealthProfessional/page1

277. One animal study compared the protective . . .: Yakup Yürekli et al., 'L-Carnitine Protection Against Cisplatin Nephrotoxicity In Rats: Comparison with Amifostin Using Quantitative Renal Tc 99m DMSA Uptake', *Molecular Imaging and Radionuclide Therapy*, vol. 20, no. 1, 2001, pp. 1–6.

212. It has been shown to improve . . .: Baliga MS, Joseph N, Venkataranganna MV, Saxena A, Ponemone V, Fayad R, 'Curcumin, an active component of turmeric in the prevention and treatment of ulcerative colitis: preclinical and clinical observations', *Food & Function*, vol. 3 no. 11, 2012, pp. 1109-17, doi: 10.1039/c2fo30097d.

212. Laboratory studies have shown that curcumin . . .: López-Lázaro M, 'Anticancer and carcinogenic properties of curcumin: considerations for its clinical development as a cancer chemopreventive and chemotherapeutic agent', *Molecular Nutrition and Food Research*, 2008, 52 Suppl 1:S103-27, doi: 10.1002/mnfr.200700238 and Johnson JJ, Mukhtar H, 'Curcumin for chemoprevention of colon cancer', *Cancer Letters*, vol. 255, no. 2, 2007, pp 170-81.

212. Some studies have shown it is as effective . . .: Donath F, Quispe S, Diefenbach K, Maurer A, Fietze I, Roots I, 'Critical evaluation of the effect of valerian extract on sleep structure and sleep quality', *Pharmacopsychiatry.* 2000, 33, pp. 47–53.

213. There is a potential role for withania . . .: Davis L, Kuttan G, 'Immunomodulatory activity of *Withania somnifera* extract in mice', *Journal of Ethnopharmacology*, vol. 71(1/2), 2000, pp. 193–200.

213. It has been shown to improve . . .: Biswal BM, 'Effect of Withania somnifera (Ashwagandha) on the development of chemotherapy-induced fatigue and quality of life in breast cancer patients', *Integrative Cancer Therapy*, vol. 12, no. 4, 2013, pp. 312–22, doi:10.1177/1534735412464551.

214. A 2015 survey of North American Cancer . . .: Hong G, White J, Zhong L, Carlson LE, 'Survey of Policies and Guidelines on Antioxidant Use for Cancer Prevention, Treatment, and Survivorship in North American Cancer Centers: What Do Institutions Perceive as Evidence?' *Integrative Cancer Therapy*, 2015, pii: 1534735415572884.

215. Researches have begun to look at whether . . .: Aparna Areti, Veera Ganesh Yerra, VGM Naidu, Ashutosh Kumar, 'Oxidative stress and nerve damage: Role in chemotherapy induced peripheral neuropathy', *Redox Biology*, vol, 2, 2014, pp. 289–295

216. Low folate is linked to . . .: Pelucchi C, Talamini R, Negri E, Levi F, Conti E, Franceschi S, La Vecchia C, 'Folate intake and risk of oral and pharyngeal cancer', *Annals of Oncology*, vol. 14, no. 11, 2003, pp. 1677-81.

216. Low vitamin B_6 intake has been . . .: Larsson SC1, Orsini N, Wolk A, 'Vitamin B6 and risk of colorectal cancer: a meta-analysis of prospective studies' *Journal of American Medical Association*, vol. 303, no. 11, 2010, pp. 1077–83, doi: 10.1001/jama.2010.263.

217. A randomised clinical trial . . . .: Lappe JM, Travers-Gustafson D, Davies KM, 'Vitamin D and calcium supplementation reduces cancer risk: results of a randomized trial', *American Journal of Clinical Nutrition,* vol. 85, no. 6, 2007, pp. 1586–91.

218. It supports the body's immune . . .: Rajiv S, 'Coenzyme Q10: The essential nutrient', *Journal of Pharmacy and Bioallied Sciences*, vol. 3, no. 3, 2011, pp. 466–467, doi: 10.4103/0975-7406.84471 PMCID: PMC3178961.

219. It has been shown to help prevent . . .: Langsjoen PH, Langsjoen AM, 'Overview of the use of CoQ10 in cardiovascular disease', *Biofactors*, 9(2-4),1999, pp. 273-84.

219. According to the National Cancer Institute . . .: National Cancer Institute, 'Coenzyme Q10 (PDQ), http://www.cancer.gov/about-cancer/treatment/cam/patient/coenzyme-q10-pdq

220. CoQ10 provides some protection against . . .: Bryant J, Picot J, Baxter L et al., 'Clinical and cost-effectiveness of cardioprotection against the toxic effects of anthracyclines given to children with cancer: a systematic review', *British Journal of Cancer*, vol. 96, no. 2, 2007, pp. 226–230 and Roffe L, Schmidt K, Ernst E, 'Efficacy of coenzyme Q10 for improved tolerability of cancer treatments: a systematic review', *Journal of Clinical Oncology*, vol. 22, no. 21, 2004, pp. 4418–4424.

220. According to the Cancer Council NSW, there is . . .: Cancer Council NSW, Position Statement on Fish Oil, Omega-3 Fatty Acids and Cancer www.cancercouncil.com.au/682/reduce-risks/diet-exercise/nutritionadvice/meat-fish/fish-omega-3-and-cancer/

221. This leads to increased tolerance . . .: Gaurav K et al., 'Glutamine: A novel approach to chemotherapyinduced toxicity', *Indian Journal of Medical and Paediatric Oncology*, www.ncbi.nlm.nih.gov/pmc/articles/PMC3385273/

221. Glutamine: Kumar G, Goel RK, Shukla M, Pandey M, 'Glutamine: A novel approach to chemotherapy-induced toxicity', *Indian Journal of Paediatric Oncology*, vol. 33, no. 1, 2012, pp. 13–20.

221. It may also protect . . .: Savarese DM, Savy G, Vahdat L, Wischmeyer PE, Corey B, 'Prevention of chemotherapy and radiation toxicity with glutamine', *Cancer Treatment Review*, vol. 29, no. 6, 2003, pp. 501-13.

222. Glutathione intravenous infusions . . .: Di Re F, Bohm S, Oriana S, Spatti GB, Pirovano C, Tedeschi M, Zunino F, 'High-dose cisplatin and cyclophosphamide with glutathione in the treatment of advanced ovarian cancer', *Annals of Oncology*, vol. 4 no. 1, 2003, pp. 55-61.

222. Human clinical trials showed that . . .: Bell MC et al., 'Placebo-controlled trial of indole-3-carbinol in the treatment of CIN', *Gynecological Oncology*, vol. 78, 2000, pp. 123–9.

222. Shown on abnormal Pap smears . . .: Naik R, Nixon S, Lopes A et al., 'A randomized phase II trials of indole-3-carbinol in the treatment of vulvar intraepithelial neoplasia', *International Journal of Gynaecology Cancer*, vol. 16, no. 2, 2006, pp. 786–90.

222. Long-term L-carnitine administration . . .: Mijares A, Lopez JR, 'L carnitine prevents increase in diastolic Ca^{2+} induced by doxorubicin in cardiac cells', *European Journal of Pharmacology*, vol. 425, no. 2, 2001, pp. 117–120.

223. Some studies have found that people . . .: Giovannucci E, 'Tomatoes, tomato-based products, lycopene, and cancer: review of the epidemiologic literature', *Journal of the National Cancer Institute*, vol. 91 no. 4, 1999, pp. 317-31.

223. A study published in the *European* . . .: Chen GC, Pang Z, Liu QF, 'Magnesium intake and risk of colorectal cancer: a meta-analysis of prospective studies', *European Journal of Clinical Nutrition*, vol. 66, no. 11, 2012, pp. 1182-6, doi: 10.1038/ejcn.2012.135.

224. Melatonin has been used alone and combined . . .: Wang YM, Jin BZ, Ai F, Duan CH, Lu YZ, Dong TF, Fu QL, 'The efficacy and safety of melatonin in concurrent chemotherapy or radiotherapy for solid tumors: a meta-analysis of randomized controlled trials', *Cancer Chemotherapy Pharmacology*, vol. 69 no. 5, 2012, pp. 1213-20, doi: 10.1007/s00280-012-1828-8.

224. Melatonin may decrease surgery-associated . . .: Caumo W, Levandovski R, Hidalgo MP, 'Preoperative Anxiolytic Effect of Melatonin and Clonidine on Postoperative Pain and Morphine Consumption in Patients Undergoing Abdominal Hysterectomy: A Double-Blind, Randomized, Placebo-Controlled Study', *Journal of Pain*, 2008.

225. They may increase the body's . . .: Poutahidis T, Kleinewietfeld M, and Erdman S, 'Gut Microbiota and the Paradox of Cancer Immunotherapy', *Frontiers in Immunology*, 2014; 5: 157, www.ncbi.nlm.nih.gov/pubmed/24778636

226. Selenium deficiency . . .: Beck M, Orville LA, Handy J, 'Selenium Deficiency and Viral Infection' , *Journal of Nutrition*, vol. 133, no. 5, 2003, 1463S-1467S http://jn.nutrition.org/content/133/5/1463S. full and National Institutes of Health, Selenium Dietary Supplement Fact Sheet, 2013, http://ods.od.nih.gov/factsheets/Selenium-HealthProfessional and Dennert G et al., 'Selenium for preventing cancer', Cochrane Database System Review, 2011:CD005195 and Flores-Mateo G et al., 'Selenium and coronary heart disease: a meta-analysis', *American Journal Clinical Nutrition*, 84 2006, pp. 762-73.

226. It also appears that selenium . . .: Chen YC, Prabhu KS, Mastro AM, 'Is selenium a potential treatment for cancer metastasis?', *Nutrients*, vol. 5, no. 4, pp. 1149-68, doi: 10.3390/nu5041149.

226. Selenium has been shown to . . .: Ohkawa K et al., 'The effects
of coadministration of selenium and cisplatin (CDDP) on CDDP
induced toxicity and anti-yumour activity', *British Journal of
Cancer*, 58.1, 1998, pp. 123–7.

227. Overall evidence from research has shown . . .: Heart Foundation
Position Statement, 'Antioxidants in food, drinks and supplements
for cardiovascular health', 2010, www.heartfoundation.org.au/
SiteCollectionDocuments/Antioxidants-Position-Statement.pdf

229. Evidence suggests that it may be of particular importance . . .:
Ho E, 'Zinc deficiency, DNA damage and cancer risk', *Journal of
Nutritional and Biochemistry*, vol. 15, no. 10, 2004, pp. 572–8.

229. Zinc supplementation . . .: Yarom N, Ariyawardana A, Hovan A
et al., 'Systematic review of natural agents for the management of oral
mucositis in cancer patients', *Support Care Cancer*, June 14, 2013.

229. Zinc sulfate has also been shown . . .: Ripamonti C, Zecca E,
Brunelli C et al., 'A randomized, controlled clinical trial to evaluate
the effects of zinc sulfate on cancer patients with taste alterations
caused by head and neck irradiation', *Cancer*, vol. 82, no. 10, 1998,
pp. 1938–45.

OTHER THERAPIES

Page

231. The Dutch government's . . .: Office of Medicinal Cannabis, The
Netherlands Ministry of Health Welfare and Sports. 'Medicinal
Cannabis, Information for Health Care Professionals', 2008.

232. A growing number of clinical trials . . .: Lynch M and Campbell
F, 'Cannabinoids for treatment of chronic non-cancer pain; a
systematic review of randomized trials', *British Journal of Clinical
Pharmacology*, vol. 72 no. 5, 2011, pp. 735–744, doi: 10.1111/
j.1365-2125.2011.03970.xPMCID: PMC3243008.

232. There is evidence for cannabis . . .: Machado Rocha FD et. al.,
'Therapeutic use of Cannabis sativa on chemotherapy-induced
nausea and vomiting among cancer patients: systematic review
and meta-analysis', 2008, Blackwell Publishing Ltd.,
www.researchgate.net/

232. It has been shown to be effective . . .: Rahn E and Hohmann
A, 'Cannabinoids as Pharmacotherapies for Neuropathic Pain:
From the Bench to the Bedside', *Neurotherapeutics* , vol. 6 no. 4,
2009, pp. 713–737, doi: 10.1016/j.nurt.2009.08.002PMCID:
PMC2755639NIHMSID: NIHMS141302.

233. According to the patient information . . .: www.cannabisbureau.nl

233. Maximum euphoria . . .: Ashton C, 'Pharmacology and effects of cannabis: a brief review', *British Journal of Psychiatry*, 178, pp. 101–106.

233. A New Zealand study involving people under . . .: Aldington S, Harwood M, Cox B et al., 'Cannabis use and risk of lung cancer: a case–control study', *European Repertory Journal*, vol. 31, no. 2, 2008, pp. 280–286.

234. Evidence of a link with cancer . . .: Trabert B, Sigurdson AJ, Sweeney AM, 'Marijuana use and testicular germ cell tumors', *Cancer*, 2011, vol. 117, no. 4, pp. 848–53.

23. Prostate cancer: Sidney S, Quesenberry CP Jr, Friedman GD et al., 'Marijuana use and cancer incidence', *Cancer Causes Control*, vol. 8, no. 5, 1997, pp. 722–8.

234. But a large review by Health Canada . . .: Health Canada, 'M'arihuana (Marijuana, Cannabis): Dried Plant for Administration by Ingestion or Other Means', Ottawa, Canada: Health Canada, 20104.

235. The largest published report on therapeutic . . .: Cassileth BR, Vickers AJ, 'Massage therapy for symptom control: outcome study at a major cancer center', *Journal of Pain Symptom Management*, vol. 28, 2004, pp. 244–9.

238. There is no evidence to suggest that massage . . .: Sagar SM, Dryden T, Wong RK, 'Massage therapy for cancer patients: a reciprocal relationship between body and mind', *Current Oncology*, vol. 14, no. 2, 2007, pp. 45–56, www.ncbi.nlm.nih.gov/pmc/articles/

238. The use of pets in clinical situations . . .: Marcus D, 'Complementary medicine in cancer care: adding a therapy dog to the team', *Current Pain and Headache Report*, vol. 16, no. 4, 2012, pp. 289–91.

241. A 2014 study at the Universtiy of Texas . . .: Chandwani KD, Perkins G, Nagendra HR et al., 'Randomized, Controlled Trial of yoga in Women With Breast Cancer Undergoing Radiotherapy', *Journal of Clinical Oncology*, 2014, doi:10.1200/JCO.2012.48.2752.

241. A 2013 study in the US looked at . . .: Mustian KM, Sprod LK, Janelsins M et al., 'Multicenter, Randomized Controlled Trial of Yoga for Sleep Quality Among Cancer Survivors', *Journal of Clinical Oncology*, 2013, pp. 3233–3241.

241. According to research studies . . .: Kiecolt-Glaser JK, Bennett JM, Andridge R, 'Yoga's Impact on Inflammation, Mood, and Fatigue in Breast Cancer Survivors: A Randomized Controlled Trial Journal of Clinical Oncology', *Journal of Clinical Oncology*, 2012, pp. 1280–1287.

243. Aromatherapy massage is the . . .: Fellowes D, Barnes K, Wilkinson S, 'Aromatherapy and massage for symptom relief in patients with cancer', Cochrane Database System Review 2004; 3:CD002287.

243. Some studies have suggested that . . .: Richardson MM, Babiak-Vazquez AE, Frenkel MA, 'Music therapy in a comprehensive cancer center', *Journal of the Society for Integrative Oncology*, vol. 6, no. 2, 2008, pp. 76–81.

PART FIVE – SYMPTOMS AND SIDE EFFECTS OF CANCER TREATMENT
SYMPTOM MANAGEMENT

Page

255. Acupuncture: Lu W, Dean-Clower E, Rosenthal DS, 'The Value of Acupuncture in Cancer Care', *Hematology/Oncology Clinics of North America*, vol. 22, no. 4, 2008, pp. 831–viii.

255. At this stage, the formal research . . .: Paley CA, Johnson MI, Tashani OA, Bagnali A-M, 'Acupuncture for cancer- related pain in adults', Cochrane Database Review System 2011, CD007753, doi: 10.1002/14651858.CD007753.pub2.

255. But research studies are suggesting . . .: Lu W et al., 'Acupuncture for cancer pain and related symptoms', *Current Pain Headache Report*, vol. 17, no. 3, 2003, pp. 321 and Alimi D, Rubino C, Pichard-Leandri E et al., 'Analgesic effect of auricular acupuncture for cancer pain: a randomized, blinded, controlled trial', *Journal of Clinical Oncology*, vol. 15, no. 21(22), pp. 4120–4126.

255. Massage appears to be of benefit . . .: Cassileth BR, Vickers AJ, 'Massage therapy for symptom control: outcome study at a major cancer center', *Journal of Pain Symptom Management*, vol. 28, no. 3, 2003, pp. 244–249.

256. Very effective and safe . . .: : National Cancer Institute, US National Institutes of Health, 'Effect of acupuncture on chemotherapy-induced nausea and vomiting', 2015, www.cancer.gov/cancertopics/pdq/cam/acupuncture/HealthProfessional/page6#Section_58

259. Ginger (*Zingiber officinale*) . . .: Ryan JL, Heckler C, Dakhil SR et al., 'Ginger for chemotherapyrelated nausea in cancer patients: A URCC CCOP randomized, double-blind, placebo-controlled clinical trial of 644 cancer patients', *Journal of Clinical Oncology*, vol. 27 (Suppl abstr 9511):15S. 2009.

260. Baical skullcap . . .: Aung HH, Dey L, Mehendale S et al., '*Scutellaria baicalensis* extract decreases cisplatin-induced pica in rats', *Cancer Chemotherapy Pharmacology*, vol. 52, no. 6, 2003, pp. 453–458.

260. A Cochrane review of Chinese herbs . . .: Taixiang W, Munro AJ, Guanjian L, 'Chinese medical herbs for chemotherapy side effects in colorectal cancer patients', Cochrane Database System Review 2005; 1:CD04540.

260. One study showed benefit . . .: You Q, Yu H, Wu D et al., 'Vitamin B$_6$ points PC6 injection during acupuncture can relieve nausea and vomiting in patients with ovarian cancer', *International Journal of Gynecological Cancer*, vol. 19, no. 4, 2009, pp. 567–571.

261. Research shows that 20–35 per cent . . .: Beyond Blue, 'Cancer and depression/anxiety', www.beyondblue.org.au

265. American gingseng . . .: Barton DL, Liu H, Dakhil SR et al., 'Wisconsin ginseng (*Panax quinquefolius*) to improve cancer-related fatigue: a randomized, double-blind trial', N07C2, 2013, *Journal National Cancer Institute*, doi:10.1093/jnci/djt181.

265. In a recent study the spores . . .: Zhao H1, Zhang Q, Zhao L, Huang X, Wang J, Kang X., 'Spore Powder of Ganoderma lucidum Improves Cancer-Related Fatigue in Breast Cancer Patients Undergoing Endocrine Therapy: A Pilot Clinical Trial', Evidence Based Complement Alternative Medicine, 2012:809614, doi: 10.1155/2012/809614.

265. A study in China . . .: Zhao H, Zhang Q, Zhao L et al., 'Spore Powder of Ganoderma lucidum Improves Cancer-Related Fatigue in Breast Cancer Patients Undergoing Endocrine Therapy: A Pilot Clinical Trial, *Evidence-Based Complementary and Alternative Medicine*, vol. 2012, article ID 809614, doi:10.1155/2012/809614.

265. A special preparation . . .: Chen HW, Lin IH, Chen YJ et al., 'A novel infusible botanically derived drug, PG2, for cancer-related fatigue: a phase II double-blind, randomized placebo-controlled study', *Clinical & Investigative Medicine*, vol. 35, no. 1, 2013, E1–11.

266. L-carnitine (taken orally, 6 g per day for four weeks) . . .: Gramignano G, Lusso MR, Madeddu C et al., 'Efficacy of

L-carnitine administration on fatigue, nutritional status, oxidative stress, an related quality of life in 12 advanced cancer patients undergoing anticancer therapy', *Nutrition*, 22, 2006, pp. 136–145 and Graziano F et al., 'Potential role of levocarnitine supplementation the treatment of chemotherapy-induced fatigue in non-anaemic cancer patients', *British Journal of Cancer*, vol. 86, no. 12, 2002, pp. 1854–7.

266. Acupuncture does seem to help . . .: Zeng Y, Luo T, Finnegan-John J, Cheng AS, 'Meta-Analysis of Randomized Controlled Trials of Acupuncture for Cancer-Related Fatigue', *Integrative Cancer Therapy*, 2013, PubMed Health, The University of York Centre for Reviews and Dissemination.

268. Bulk-forming laxatives include . . .: Mills S, Bone K, 'Principles and practice of phytotherapy', *Modern Herbal Medicine*, 2000, London, Churchill Livingstone, pp. 168–173.

268. Rhubarb root . . .: Kemper, K, 'Rhubarb root (*Rheum officinale* or *R. palmatum*)', The Center for Holistic Pediatric Education and Research and The Longwood Herbal Task Force, http://m. longwoodherbal.org/rhubarbroot/rhubarb.pdf

270. You will need to see a specially . . .: Vignes S, Porcher R, Champagne A et al., 'Predictive factors of response to intensive decongestive physiotherapy in upper limb Lymphedema after breast cancer treatment: a cohort study', *Breast Cancer Research and Treatment*, no. 98, vol. 1, 2006, pp. 1–6.

271. Studies on women after breast . . .: McKenzie DC, Kalda AL, 'Effect of upper extremity exercise on secondary lymphedema in breast cancer patients: a pilot study', Journal of Clinical Oncology, vol. 21, no. 3, 2003, pp. 463-6.

271. Weight training . . .: Schmitz KH, Ahmed RL, Troxel A et al., 'Weight lifting in women with breast-cancer-related lymphedema', *New England Journal of Medicine*, vol. 361, no. 7, 2009, pp. 664–73.

271. There is some evidence . . .: Shaw C, Mortimer P, Judd PA, 'Randomized controlled trial comparing a low-fat diet with a weight-reduction diet in breast cancer-related lymphedema', *Cancer*, vol. 109, no. 10, 2007, pp. 1949–56.

271. Low-level laser therapy: Carati CJ, Anderson SN, Gannon BJ et al., 'Treatment of postmastectomy lymphedema with low-level laser therapy: a double blind, placebo-controlled trial', *Cancer*, vol. 98, no. 6, 2003, pp. 1114–22.

272. Horse chestnut . . .: Pittler M, Ernst E, 'Horse chestnut seed extract for chronic venous insufficiency', Cochrane Database System Review, 25(1):CD003230.

272. Citrus bioflavonoids . . .: Cluzan RV, Alliot F, Ghabboun S et al., 'Treatment of secondary lymphedema of the upper limb with CYCLO 3 FORT', *Lymphology*, 29, 1996, pp. 29–35.

273. Low-dose glutamine . . .: Anderson PM, Schroeder G, Skubitz KM, 'Oral glutamine reduces the duration and severity of stomatitis after cytotoxic cancer chemotherapy', *Cancer*, vol. 83, no. 7, 1998, pp. 1433–1439.

274. Acupuncture has been shown . . .: Blom M, Dawidson I, Fernberg JO, Johnson G, Angmar-Mansson B, 'Acupuncture treatment of patients with radiation-induced xerostomia', *European Journal of Cancer Part B Oral Oncology*, 1996, 32B(3), pp. 182–190.

274. A clinical trial . . .: Ryan J, Heckler C, Ling M et al., 'Curcumin for radiation dermatitis: A randomized, double-blind, placebo-controlled clinical trial of thirty breast cancer patients', *Radiation Research*, 180, 2013, pp. 34–43.

275. Calendula ointment . . .: Pommier P, Gomez F, Sunyach M et al., 'Calendula ointment and radiation dermatitis during breast cancer treatment', *Journal of Clinical Oncology*, vol. 22, no. 8, 2004, pp. 1447–1453.

275. Also topical aloe vera . . .: Haddad P et al., 'Aloe vera for prevention of radiation-induced dermatitis: a self-controlled clinical trial', *Current Oncology*, vol. 20, no. 4,:e345-8, doi: 10.3747/co.20.1356, 2013.

276. A Cochrane review of Chinese herbs . . .: Taixiang W, Munro AJ, Guanjian L, 'Chinese medical herbs for chemotherapy side effects in colorectal cancer patients', Cochrane Database System Review 2005; 1:CD04540.

276. Milk thistle has a . . .: Ladas EJ, Kroll DJ, Oberlies NH et al., 'A randomized, controlled, double-blind, pilot study of milk thistle for the treatment of hepatotoxicity in childhood acute lymphoblastic leukaemia (ALL)', *Cancer*, vol. 116, no. 2, 2010, pp. 506–513 and Ramasamy K, Agarwal R, 'Multitargeted therapy of cancer by silymarin', *Cancer Letters*, no. 269, vol. 2, 2008, pp. 352–362.

276. Milk thistle has been shown . . .: Memorial Sloan Kettering Cancer Centre, 'Milk Thistle', Gerstner Sloan Kettering Graduate School of Biomedical Science, 2014, http://www.mskcc.org/cancer-care/herb/milk-thistle

278. Oral complications occur in . . .: National Institute of Dental and Craniofacial Research, 'Oral Complications of Cancer Treatment: what the dental team can do', NIH Publication No. 09-4372, www.nidcr.nih.gov/OralHealth/Topics/CancerTreatment/OralComplicationsCancerOral.htm

281. Experimental studies have shown . . .: Skubitz KM, Anderson PM, 'Oral glutamine to prevent chemotherapy induced stomatitis: a pilot study', *Journal of Laboratory Clinical Medicine*, vol. 127, no. 2, 1996, pp. 223–8.

PART SIX – LIFESTYLE ADJUSTMENTS TO SUPPORT RECOVERY

WHY YOUR ENVIRONMENT AND LIFESTYLE MATTER

Page

288. Professor Dean Ornish from . . .: Ornish D et al., 'Intensive lifestyle changes may affect the progression of prostate cancer', *Journal of Urology*, 2005 vol. 174, no. 3, pp. 1065-9, discussion 1069-70.

CANCER AND YOUR ENVIRONMENT

Page

290. There are various ways in which your . . .: Kune G, *Reducing the odds: a manual for the prevention of cancer*, 1999, Allen & Unwin, Sydney.

290. Regular and long-standing exposure . . .: US Department of Health and Human Services, 'The health consequences of involuntary exposure to tobacco smoke: a report of the Surgeon General. Atlanta, Georgia: US Deptartment of Health and Human Services', Centers for Disease Control and Prevention, Coordinating Center for Health Promotion, National Center for Chronic Disease Prevention and Health Promotion, Office on Smoking and Health, 2006, www.cdc.gov/tobacco/data_statistics/sgr/sgr_2006/index.htm

290. For those with heavy exposure . . .: Taylor R, Najafi F, Dobson A, 'Meta-analysis of studies of passive smoking and lung cancer: effects of study type and continent', *International Journal of Epidemiology*, vol. 36, no. 5, 2007, pp. 1048–1059.

291. The International Agency for Reseach . . .: 'IARC: Outdoor air pollution a leading environmental cause of cancer deaths', United Nations Association of Australia, Victorian Division, 2013.

291. A study of 12,000 . . .: Silverman D, Samanic C, Lubin J, 'The Diesel Exhaust in Miners Study: A Nested Case–Control Study of Lung Cancer and Diesel Exhaust', *Journal of National Cancer Institute*, vol. 104, no. 11, 2012, pp. 855–868.

293. Having a simple . . .: US Department of Health and Human Services, Twelfth Report on Carcinogens, 2011, Public Health Services, National Toxicology Program.

293. However, X-rays are classified . . .: International Agency for Research on Cancer (ARC), *Volume 75: Ionizing Radiation, Part 1: X- and Gamma (g)-Radiation and Neutrons, IARC Monographs on the Evaluation of Carcinogenic Risks to Humans*, 2000, IARC, Lyon, France.

293. The story may not . . .: Hutchinson L, 'Breast cancer: Radiation risk in BRCA carriers', *National Review of Clinical Oncology*, vol. 9, no. 11, 2012, p. 611.

293. For example, women with . . .: Andrieu N, Easton DF, Chang-Claude J et al., 'Epidemiological Study of BRCA1 and BRCA2 Mutation Carriers (EMBRACE); Gene Etude Prospective Sein Ovaire (GENEPSO); Gen en Omgeving studie van de werkgroep Hereditiair Borstkanker Onderzoek Nederland (GEO-HEBON); International BRCA1/2 Carrier Cohort Study (IBCCS), Effect of chest X-rays on the risk of breast cancer among BRCA1/2 mutation carriers in the international BRCA1/2 carrier cohort study: a report from the EMBRACE, GENEPSO, GEO-HEBON, and IBCCS Collaborators' Group', *Journal of Clinical Oncology*, vol. 24, no. 21, 2006, pp. 3361–3366.

ALCOHOL

Page

293. The International Agency for . . .: World Health Organization, 'IARC Monograph Evaluation of Carcinogenic Risks to Humans: Alcohol Drinking', Monograph 44, http://monographs.iarc.fr/ENG/Monographs/vol44/volume44.pdf

296. According to the World Cancer Research Fund . . .: Marmot M, *Food, Nutrition, Physical Activity and the Prevention of Cancer: a global Perspective*, World Cancer Research Fund and American Institute for Cancer Research, p. 157, http://eprints.ucl.ac.uk/4841/1/4841.pdf

296. A convincing link: . . .: Boffetta P, Hashibe M, 'Alcohol and cancer', *Lancet Oncology*, vol. 7, no. 2, 2006, pp. 149–56.

296. The Million Women Study . . .: Beral NE et al., 'Moderate Alcohol Intake and Cancer Incidence in Women', The Million Women Study, The University of Oxford, *Journal of National Cancer Institute*, 101, 2009, pp. 296–305.

297. The experts have looked . . .: Winstanley MH et al., 'Alcohol and Cancer: a position statement from Cancer Council Australia', 2011, *Medical Journal of Australia*, 194, pp. 479–482.

298. For example, tobacco smoking . . .: Hashibe M, Brennan P, Benhamou S et al., 'Alcohol drinking in never users of tobacco, cigarette smoking in never drinkers, and the risk of head and neck cancer: pooled analysis in the International Head and Neck Cancer Epidemiology Consortium', *Journal of the National Cancer Institute*, vol. 99, no. 10, 2007, pp. 777-89.

306. Cancer has been found to be . . .: Chen WY, Rosner B, Hankinson SE, Colditz GA, Willett WC, 'Moderate alcohol consumption during adult life, drinking patterns, and breast cancer risk', *Journal of the Amercian Medical Association*, vol. 306, no. 17, pp.188490, doi: 10.1001/jama.2011.1590.

306. The Cancer Council Australia . . .: Winstanley MH et al., 'Alcohol and Cancer: a position statement from Cancer Council Australia', *Medical Journal of Australia*, 194, 2011, pp. 479–482.

EXERCISE

Page

307. It helps to reduce . . .: Galvao DA, Newton RU, 'Review of exercise intervention studies in cancer patients', *Journal of Clinical Oncology*, vol. 23, no. 4, 2005, pp. 899–909.

307. A review of the role . . .: Borjesson M, Karlsson J, Mannheimer C, 'Relief of pain by exercise! Increased physical activity can be a part of the therapeutic program in both acute and chronic pain', *Lakartidningen*, vol. 98, no. 15, 2001, pp. 1786–1791.

308. A review . . .: Lemanne D1, Cassileth B, Gubili J, 'The role of physical activity in cancer prevention, treatment, recovery, and survivorship', *Oncology*, vol. 27, no. 6, 2013, pp. 580–5.

308. A major review of research . . .: Mishra SI, Scherer RW, Geigle PM et al., 'Exercise interventions on health-related quality of life for cancer survivors', 2012, Cochrane Database System Review, 8:CD007566, doi:10.1002/14651858.CD007566.pub2.

309. John Hopkins Hospital . . .: Mock V, Dow KH, Meares CJ et al., 'Effects of exercise on fatigue, physical functoning, and emotional

distress during radiation therapy for breast cancer', *Oncology Nursing Forum*, vol. 24, no. 6, 1997, pp. 991–1000.

309. They found that women . . .: Schwartz AL, Mori M, Gao R, Nail LM, King ME, 'Exercise reduces daily fatigue in women with breast cancer receiving chemotherapy', *Medicine and Science in Sports and Exercise*, vol. 32, no. 5, 2001, pp. 718–723.

309. A recent meta-analysis . . .: Tomlinson D, Diorio C, Beyene J, Sung L, 'Effect of exercise on cancer-related fatigue: a meta-analysis', *American Journal of Physical Medicine and Rehabilitation*, vol. 93, no. 8, 2014, pp. 675-86.

310. A Canadian Study . . .: Courneya KS, Segal RJ, Mackey JR, 'Effects of exercise dose and type on sleep quality in breast cancer patients receiving chemotherapy: a multicenter randomized trial', *Breast Cancer Research and Treatment*, vol. 144, no. 2, 2014, pp. 361–9.

312. The World Cancer Research Fund . . .: Segal JR, Reid RD, Courneya KS, 'Randomized controlled trial of resistance or aerobic exercise in men receiving radiation therapy for prostate cancer', *Journal of Clinical Oncology*, vol. 27, no. 3, 2009, pp. 344–51.

312. Over 30 studies . . .: Slattery M, Potter J, Caan B et al., 'Energy balance and colon cancer – beyond physical activity', *Cancer Research*, vol. 57, 1997, pp. 75–80 and Colditz G, Cannuscio C, Grazier A, 'Physical activity and reduced risk of colon cancer', *Cancer Causes Control*, 1997, 8, pp. 649–667.

313. Large-scale Norwegian studies . . .: Thune I, Brenn T, Lund E, Gaard M, 'Physical activity and the risk of breast cancer', *New England Journal of Medicine*, vol. 336 no. 18, 1997, pp. 1269-75.

313. In those who were lean . . .: Thune I, Lund E, 'The influence of physical activity on lung cancer risk', *International Journal of Cancer*, 70, 1997, pp. 57–62.

313. In post-menopausal women . . .: Eliassen AH, Hankinson SE, Rosner B, Holmes MD, Willett WC, 'Physical activity and risk of breast cancer among postmenopausal women', *Archive of Internal Medicine*, vol. 170, no. 19, 2010, pp. 1758-64, doi: 10.1001/archinternmed.2010.363, www.ncbi.nlm.nih.gov/pubmed/20975025

313. For example, a study of 2987 . . .: Holmes MD, Chen WY, Feskanich D et al., 'Physical activity and survival after breast cancer diagnosis', *Journal of the American Medical Association*, vol. 293, no. 20, 2005, pp. 2479–2486.

313. This was confirmed . . .: Pierce JP, Stefanick ML, Flatt SW et al., 'Greater survival after breast cancer in physically active women

with high vegetable–fruit intake regardless of obesity', *Journal of Clinical Oncology*, vol. 25, no. 17, 2007, pp. 2345–2351.

318. Most research on exercise and . . .: Focht BC, Clinton SK, Devor ST, 'Resistance exercise interventions during and following cancer treatment: a systematic review', *Journal of Community and Supportive Oncology*, vol. 11, no. 2, 2013, pp. 45–60.

NUTRITION

Page

324. Diet-related factors . . .: Doll R, Peto R, 'The causes of cancer: quantitative estimates of avoidable risks of cancer in the United States today', *Journal of National Cancer Institute*, 66, 1981, pp. 1196–1265 and Key TJ, Allen NE, Spencer EA et al., 'The effect of diet on risk of cancer', *Lancet*, 360, 2002, pp. 861–868.

331. The World Health Organization estimates . . .: World Health Organisation, 'Overweight and Obesity', 2015, www.who.int/mediacentre/factsheets/fs311/en/

331. Being overweight or obese . . .: American Cancer Society, 'Body Weight and Cancer Risk', 2015, www.cancer.org/acs/groups/cid/documents/webcontent/002578-pdf.pdf

332. If you are a man . . .: Cancer Council Victoria, 'How does the risk vary?', 2013, www.cancervic.org.au/preventingcancer/weight/obesity-risk

338. Cancer survivors wanting . . .: Dana-Faber Cancer Institute, http://www.dana-farber.org/

339. Two studies . . .: Solon-Biet SM, McMahon AC, Ballard JW et al., 'The Ratio of Macronutrients, Not Caloric Intake, Dictates Cardiometabolic Health, Aging, and Longevity in Ad Libitum-Fed Mice', *Cell Metabolism 19*, 2014, pp. 418–430 and Levine ME, Suarez JA, Brandhorst S et al., 'Low Protein Intake is Associated with a Major Reduction in IGF-1 Cancer, and overall Mortality in the 65 and Younger but not older population', 2014, *Cell Metabolism*, vol. 19, no. 4, pp. 407–417.

341. Seasonings and herbs . . .: Meeran S, Kativar S, 'Cell cycle control as a basis for cancer chemoprevention through dietary agents', *Frontiers in Bioscience*, 2008, 13:2191–2202 and Krishnaswamy K, 'Traditional Indian spices and their health significance', *Asia Pacific Journal of Clinical Nutrition*, 17(Suppl 1), 2008, pp. 265–268.

341. Good-quality dark chocolate . . .: Maskarinec G, 'Cancer protective properties of cocoa: a review of the epidemiologic evidence', *Nutrition and Cancer*, vol. 61, no. 5, 2009, pp. 573–579.

341. Studies have shown that consuming . . .: Larsson SC, Kumlin M, Ingelman-Sundberg M et al., 'Dietary long chain n-3 fatty acids for the prevention of cancer: a review of potential mechanisms', *American Journal of Clinical Nutrition*, 79, 2004, pp. 935–945.

342. Recent US studies . . .: Lu C, Toepel K, Irish R, Fenske RA, Barr DB, Bravo R, 'Organic diets signifi cantly lower children's dietary exposure to organophosphorus pesticides', *Environmental Health Perspective*, vol. 114, no. 22, 2006, pp. 60–3.

342. Organic varieties . . .: Crinnion WJ, 'Organic foods contain higher levels of certain nutrients, lower levels of pesticides, and may provide health benefits for the consumer', *Alternative Medicine Review*, vol. 15, no. 1, 2010, pp. 4–12, www.ncbi.nlm.nih.gov/pubmed/20359265

343. The American Institute of Cancer . . .: Norat T, Aune D, Chan D, Fruits and vegetables: updating the epidemiologic evidence for the WCRF/AICR lifestyle recommendations for cancer prevention. *Cancer Treatment Research*, 2014, 159, pp. 35-50, doi: 10.1007/978-3-642-38007-5_3.

343. According to the Australian . . .: Australian Bureau of Statistics, Profiles of Health, Australia 2011–2013, 'Daily intake of fruits and vegetables', 2013, Accessed 18 May 2014, http://www.abs.gov.au

344. They may not be your . . .: Verhoeven DTH, Goldbohm RA, van Poppel G et al., 'Epidemiological studies on *Brassica* vegetables and cancer risk', *Cancer Epidemiology Biomarkers Prevention*, 5, 1996, pp. 733–748 and Herr I, Büchler MW, 'Dietary constituents of broccoli and other cruciferous vegetables: implications for prevention and therapy of cancer', *Cancer Treatment Review*, 2010.

344. In a study involving . . .: Wiseman, M, 'The second World Cancer Research Fund/American Institute for Cancer Research expert report. Food, nutrition, physical activity, and the prevention of cancer: a global perspective', *Proceedings of the Nutrition Society*, 2008, vol. 67, no. 3, 2008, p. 253-6.

344. Research is looking . . .: National Cancer Institute, 'Cruciferous vegetables and cancer prevention', 2012, http://www.cancer.gov/about-cancer/causes-prevention/risk/diet/cruciferous-vegetables-fact-sheet#q2

345. For example, the cancer-protective . . .: Conway C, Getahun S, Liebes L et al., 'Disposition of glucosinolates and sulforaphane in humans after ingestion of steamed and fresh broccoli', *Nutrition and Cancer*, vol. 38, no. 2, 2000, pp. 168–178.

344. Garlic and onions . . .: Fleischauer AT, Arab L, 'Garlic and cancer: a critical review of the epidemoiological literature', *Journal of Nutrition*, 2011, 131:1032S–1040S.

344. According to the US National Cancer Institute . . .: National Cancer Institute, http://www.cancer.gov/

345. Women with breast cancer . . .: Pierce JP, Stefanick ML, Flatt SW et al., 'Greater survival after breast cancer in physically active women with high vegetable–fruit intake regardless of obesity', *Journal of Clinical Oncology*, vol. 25, no. 17, 2007, pp. 2345–2351.

345. A study found that women . . .: Rock CL, Flatt SW, Natarajan L, 'Plasma carotenoids and recurrence-free survival in women with a history of breast cancer', *Journal of Clinical Oncology*, vol. 23, no. 27, 2005, pp. 6631–6638.

345. For example, while cartenoid . . .: Druesne-Pecollo N, Latino-Martel P, Norat T et al., 'Betacarotene supplementation and cancer risk: a systematic review and metaanalysis of randomized controlled', *International Journal of Cancer*, vol. 127, no. 1, 2010, pp. 172–84, doi: 10.1002/ijc.25008.

346. Several population studies . . .: Kavanaugh, C, Trumbo P, and Ellwood K, 'The U.S. Food and Drug Administration's evidence-based review for qualified health claims: tomatoes, lycopene, and cancer', *Journal of the National Cancer Institute*, vol. 99, no. 4, 2007.

346. There are great differences . . .: Madgee PJ, Rowland IR, 'Phyto-oestrogens, their mechanism of action: current evidence for a role in breast and prostate cancer', *British Journal of Nutrition*, 91, 2004, pp. 513–531.

346. Soy foods have also been . . .: Cotterchio M, Boucher BA, Manno M et al., 'Dietary phytoestrogen intake is associated with reduced colorectal cancer risk 1', *Journal of Nutrition*, vol. 136, no. 12, 2006, pp. 3046–3053.

346. Gastric cancer: Ko KP, Park SK, Yang JJ et al., 'Intake of Soy Products and Other Foods and Gastric Cancer Risk: A Prospective Study', *Journal of Epidemiology*, vol. 23, no. 5, 2013, pp. 337–343.

346. Strawberries . . .: Neto C, 'Cranberry and blueberry: evidence for protective effects against cancer and vascular diseases', *Molecular Nutrition and Food Research*, vol. 51, no. 6, 2007, pp. 652–664.

346. With the potential to . . .: Duthie S, 'Berry phytochemicals, genomic stability and cancer: evidence for chemoprotection at several stages in the carcinogenic process', *Molecular Nutrition and Food Research*, vol. 51, no. 6, 2007, pp. 665–674.

347. There are many mechanisms . . .: Neto CC, 'Cranberry and blueberry: evidence for protective effects against cancer and vascular diseases', *Molecular Nutrition and Food Research*, vol. 51, no. 6, 2007, pp. 652–64.

347. It has shown in vitro . . .: Sliva D, 'Ganoderma lucidum (Reishi) in cancer treatment', *Integrative Cancer Therapy*, vol. 2, no. 4, 2003, pp. 358–64.

347. To stimulate . . .: Weng CJ, Yen GC, 'The in vitro and in vivo experimental evidences disclose the chemopreventive effects of Ganoderma lucidum on cancer invasion and metastasis', *Clinical and Experimental Metastasis*, vol. 27, no. 5, 2010, pp. 361–9.

347. According to the US National Cancer Institute . . .: National Cancer Institute, www.cancer.gov/

347. One recent study found . . .: Alonso EN, Orozco M, Eloy Nieto A, Balogh GA, 'Genes related to suppression of malignant phenotype induced by Maitake D-Fraction in breast cancer cells', *Journal of Medicinal Food*, vol. 16, no. 7, 2013, pp. 602–17.

347. It has been shown to have . . .: Ng ML, Yap AT, 'Inhibition of human colon carcinoma development by lentinan from shiitake mushrooms (Lentinus edodes)', *Journal of Alternative and Complementary Medicine*, vol. 8, no. 5, 2002, pp. 581–589.

348. Green tea contains . . .: Shankar S, Ganapathy S, Srivastava RK et al., 'Green tea polyphenols: biology and therapeutic implications in cancer', *Frontiers in Bioscience*, 2007, 12:4881–4899.

349. There are multiple protective . . .: Divisi D, Di Tommaso S, Salvemini S et al., 'Diet and cancer', *Acta Biomed*, vol. 77, no. 2, 2006, pp. 118–123.

349. This point is illustrated . . .: Ahn J, Gammon MD, Santella RM et al., 'Associations between breast cancer risk and the catalase genotype, fruit and vegetable consumption, and supplement use', *American Journal of Epidemiology*, vol. 162, no. 10, 2005, pp. 943–952.

349. An example is in providing . . .: Moss RW, 'Do antioxidants interfere with radiation therapy for cancer?', *Integrative Cancer Therapy*, vol. 6, no. 3, 2007, pp. 281–292.

350. A trial on nearly 2500 . . .: Chlebowski RT, Blackburn G, Thomson C et al., 'Dietary fat reduction and breast cancer outcome: interim efficacy results from the Women's Intervention Nutrition Study', *Journal of National Cancer Institute*, vol. 98, no. 24, 2006, pp. 1767–1776.

350. There is also a possible . . .: Slattery ML, Benson J, Ma KN et al., 'Trans-fatty acids and colon cancer', *Nutrition and Cancer*, vol. 39, no. 2, 2001, pp. 170–5.

350. The World Cancer Research Fund recommendation . . .: World Cancer Research Fund, http://www.wcrf.org/

351. The official view from the US National Cancer Institute . . .: National Cancer Institute, 'Artificial Sweeteners and Cancer', 2008, http://www.cancer.gov

352. The 5-2 diet . . .: Barnosky AR, Hoddy KK, Unterman TG, Varady KA, 'Intermittent fasting vs daily calorie restriction for type 2 diabetes prevention: a review of human findings', *Translational Research*, vol. 164. no. 4, 2014, pp. 302-11, doi: 10.1016/j. trsl.2014.05.013.

SLEEP

Page

360. Sleep problems such as . . .: Theobald DE, 'Cancer pain, fatigue, distress, and insomnia in cancer patients', Clinical Cornerstone, 2004;6 Suppl 1D:S15-21.

360. Including biochemical . . .: Roscoe JA, Kaufman ME, Matterson-Rusby SE et al., 'Cancer-Related Fatigue and Sleep Disorders', *The Oncologist*, 12(suppl 1), 2007, pp. 35–42.

369. These people not only . . .: Davis S, Mirick DK, 'Circadian disruption, shift work and the risk of cancer: a summary of the evidence and studies in Seattle', *Cancer Causes Control*, vol. 17, no. 4, 2006, pp. 539–45.

369. In particular, research has shown . . .: Davis S, Mirick DK, Stevens RG, 'Night shift work, light at night, and risk of breast cancer', *Journal of National Cancer Institute*, vol. 93, no. 20, 2001, pp. 1557–62.

369. Melatonin secretion is . . .: Srinivasan V, Spence DW, Pandi-Perumal SR, Trakht I, Cardinali DP, 'Therapeutic actions of melatonin in cancer: possible Mechanisms',

Integrative Cancer Therapy, vol. 7, no. 3, 2008, pp. 189–203, doi: 10.1177/1534735408322846.

SMOKING

Page

385. According to the World Health Organization . . .: World Health Organization, 'Tobacco Free Initiative', www.who.int/tobacco/research/cancer/en/

389. But among people . . .: Cancer.net, American Society of Clinical Oncology, 2015, www.cancer.net

390. Anecdotally, some people say . . .: White AR, Rampes H, Liu JP, Stead LF, Campbell J, 'Acupuncture and related interventions for smoking cessation', Cochrane Database System Review, 2011 Jan 19;(1):CD000009, doi: 10.1002/14651858.CD000009.pub3.

390. 'Cut down to quit': I Can Quit, 'How to cut down to quit smoking', Cancer Institute NSW, www.icanquit.com.au/quit-guide/methods-to-quit/cut-down-to-quit

392. There is no evidence . . .: Stead LF, Perera R, Bullen C, Mant D et al., 'Nicotine replacement therapy for smoking cessation', Cochrane Database System Review, 2012 Nov 14;11:CD000146, doi: 10.1002/14651858.CD000146.pub4.

393. In particular, it is not . . .: Palazzolo DL, 'Electronic Cigarettes and Vaping: A New Challenge in Clinical Medicine and Public Health: A Literature Review', *Front Public Health*, 2013 Nov 18;1:56.

393. Varenicline side effects . . .: Quit, 'Side effects of champix', www.quit.org.au/about/frequently-asked-questions/faq-champix-varenicline/faq-varenicline-side-effects.html

394. According to the American Cancer Society . . .: American Cancer Society, 'When smokers quit – what are the benefits over time?', 2014, www.cancer.org/healthy/stayawayfromtobacco/guidetoquittingsmoking/guide-to-quitting-smoking-benefits

PART SEVEN – THE MOST COMMON FORMS OF CANCER
BOWEL CANCER

Page

405. The five-year relative . . .: Australian Institute of Health and Welfare 2012, 'Cancer survival and prevalence in Australia: period estimates from 1982 to 2010', Cancer Series no. 69, Cat. no. CAN 65. Canberra: AIHW.

406. More than 95 per cent . . .: Cancer Research UK, 'Types of Bowel
Cancer', 2013, www.cancerresearchuk.org/about-cancer/type/bowel-
cancer/about/types-of-bowel-cancer

412. Younger patients tend to present . . .: Young JP, Won AK, Rosty C
et al., 'Rising Incidence of early onset colorectal cancer in Australia
over two decades: Report and Review', Journal of Gastroenterology
and Heptatology, vol. 30, no. 1, 2015, pp. 6-13, doi: 10.1111/
jgh.12792.

413. Include low-fat dairy . . .: World Cancer Research Fund/American
Institute for Cancer Research, 'Continuous Update Project:
Colorectal Cancer Report 2010 Summary. Food, Nutrition, Physical
Activity, and the Prevention of Colorectal Cancer', (PDF 1.11MB),
2011.

414. Vitamin B_6 is thought . . .: Larsson SC1, Orsini N, Wolk A,
'Vitamin B6 and risk of colorectal cancer: a meta-analysis of
prospective studies', Journal of the American Medical Association,
vol. 303, no. 11, 2010, pp. 1077–83, doi: 10.1001/jama.2010.263.

415. This is because a 2009 meta-analysis . . .: Kim Yi, 'Role of folate in
colon cancer development and progression', Journal of Nutrition,
2003, 133 (11 Suppl 1):3731S730S).

415. It is not clear from . . .: Pericleous M, Mandair D, Caplin ME, 'Diet
and supplements and their impact on colorectal cancer', Journal of
Gastrointestinal Oncology, vol. 4, no. 4, 2013, pp. 409–23.

415. Calcium supplementation . . .: Wactawski-Wende J, Kotchen JM,
Anderson GL et al., 'Calcium plus vitamin D supplementation
and the risk of colorectal cancer', The New England Journal of
Medicine, vol. 354, no. 7, 2006, pp. 684–96.

416. We are still a long way . . .: Unccello M et al., 'Potential role of
probiotics on colorectal cancer prevention', BMC Surgery, 2012,
12(Suppl 1):S35) and Wollowksi I, Rechkemmer G, 'Protective role
of probiotics and prebiotics in colon cancer', American Journal of
Clinical Nutrition, vol. 73, no. 2, 2001, 451s-455s.

BREAST CANCER

Page
419. In 2010 . . .: Australian Cancer Incidence and Mortality (ACIM)
Books, Breast cancer for Australia (ICD10 C50), www.aihw.gov.au/
acim-books, Accessed March 2014.

420. According to Cancer Australia . . .: Cancer Australia,
canceraustralia.gov.au

420. Only about one in 20 . . .: Breast Cancer Campaign, 'BRCA gene mutations and familial breast cancer', 2015, www.breastcancer campaign.org/about-breast-cancer/breast-cancer-risk-factors/family-history-and-genetics/brca-gene-mutations-and-breast-cancer

422. The incidence of breast cancer . . .: Australian Cancer Incidence and Mortality (ACIM) Books - Breast cancer for Australia (ICD10 C50). http://www.aihw.gov.au/acim-books and Australian Government, 'Breast cancer statistics', 2015, http://canceraustralia.gov.au/affected-cancer/cancer-types/breast-cancer/breast-cancer-statistics

426. We know there is a relationship . . .: Lambe M, Wigertz A, Holmqvist M, 'Reductions in use of hormone replacement therapy: effects on Swedish breast cancer incidence trends only seen after several years', *Breast Cancer Research Treatment*, vol. 121, no. 3, 2010, pp. 679–83 and Katalinic A, Rawal R, 'Decline in breast cancer incidence after decrease in utilisation of hormone replacement therapy', *Breast Cancer Research Treatment*, vol. 107, no. 3, 2008, pp. 427–30.

427. A 2012 University of Texas . . .: Chandwani KD, Perkins G, Nagendra HR, 'A review of yoga research found that yoga improved quality of llfe in women having radiotheapy for breast cancer', *Journal of Clinical Oncology*, vol. 32 no. 10, 2014, pp. 1058-65, doi: 10.1200/JCO.2012.48.2752.

428. A German Study also found . . .: Cramer H1, Lange S, Klose P, Paul A, Dobos G, 'Yoga for breast cancer patients and survivors: a systematic review and meta-analysis', *BMC Cancer*, 2012, 12:412, doi: 10.1186/1471–2407–12–412.

429. Mindfullness-based stress . . .: Cramer H, Lauche R, Paul A, Dobos G, 'Mindfulnessbased stress reduction for breast cancer – a systematic review and meta-analysis', *Current Oncology*, 2012, vol. 19, no. 5, e343–52, doi: 10.3747/co.19.1016.

430. A large study showed . . .: Gandini S1, Merzenich H, Robertson C et al., 'Meta-analysis of studies on breast cancer risk and diet: the role of fruit and vegetable consumption and the intake of associated micronutrients', *European Journal of Cancer*, 2000, vol. 36, no. 5, pp. 636–46.

432. Consumption of soy foods . . .: Caan B, Natarajan L, Parker B et al., 'Soy food consumption and breast cancer prognosis', *Cancer Epidemiology Biomarkers Preview*, vol. 20, no. 5, 2011, pp. 854–858.

432. Despite the concerns . . .: Block KI, Koch AC, Mead MN et al., 'Impact of antioxidant supplementation on chemotherapeutic efficacy: a systematic review of the evidence from randomized controlled trials', *Cancer Treatment Review*, vol. 33, no. 5, 2007, pp. 407–418.

433. A meta-analysis published . . .: Harris H, Orsini N, Wolk A, 'Vitamin C and survival among women with breast cancer: A Meta-analysis', *European Journal of Cancer*, vol. 50, Issue 7, 2014, pp. 1223–1231.

433. A German study . . .: Vollbracht C1, Schneider B, Leendert V, 'Intravenous vitamin C administration improves quality of life in breast cancer patients during chemo-/radiotherapy and aftercare: results of a retrospective, multicentre, epidemiological cohort study in Germany', 2011, 25(6):983–90.

434. A 2014 study looked . . .: Mohr SB1, Gorham ED, Kim J, Meta-analysis of vitamin D sufficiency for improving survival of patients with breast cancer', *Anticancer Research*, vol. 34, no. 3, 2014, pp. 1163–6.

434. There are also other . . .: Hines SL, Jorn HK, Thompson KM et al., 'Breast cancer survivors and vitamin D: a review', *Nutrition*, vol. 26, no. 3, 2010, pp. 255–262.

434. Calcium is necessary . . .: Nogues X, Servitja S, Peña MJ, 'Vitamin D deficiency and bone mineral density in postmenopausal women receiving aromatase inhibitors for early breast cancer', *Maturitas*, 2010.

435. Studies show that low . . .: Bleys J, Navas-Acien A, Guallar E, 'Serum selenium levels and all-cause, cancer, and cardiovascular mortality among US adults', *Archive of Internal Medicine*, vol. 168, no. 4, 2008, pp. 404-10.

435. It is also helpful . . .: Sanchez-Barcelo EJ, Mediavilla MD, Alonso-Gonzalez C, Reiter RJ, 'Melatonin uses in oncology: breast cancer prevention and reduction of the side effects of chemotherapy and radiation', *Expert Opinion on Investigative Drugs*, vol. 21, no. 6, 2012, pp. 819–31.

435. Whether melatonin . . .: Stevens RG, 'Circadian disruption and breast cancer: from melatonin to clock genes', *Epidemiology*, vol. 16, no. 2, 2005, pp. 254–8.

437. Hot flushes and sleep . . .: Al-Akoum M, Maunsell E, Verreault R, 'Effects of Hypericum perforatum (St. John's wort) on hot flashes and quality of life in perimenopausal women: a randomized pilot

trial', *Menopause*, vol. 16, no. 2, 2009, pp. 307–14, doi: 10.1097/gme.0b013e31818572a0.

438. Studies have involved . . .: National Cancer Institute, 'Tea and Cancer Prevention: Strengths and Limits of the Evidence', 2010, www.cancer.gov/about-cancer/causes-prevention/risk/diet/tea-fact-sheet#q5

439. Tumeric (curcumin) . . .: Bachmeier B, Nerlich AG, Iancu CM et al., 'The chemopreventive polyphenol Curcumin prevents hematogenous breast cancer metastases in immunodeficient mice', *Cellular Physiology Biochemistry*, 2009, 19(1–4):137–52.

439. Studies indicate 1-3-C . . .: Meng Q, Yuan F, Goldberg ID, 'Indole-3-carbinol is a negative regulator of estrogen receptor-alpha signaling in human tumor cells', *Journal of Nutrition*, vol. 130, no. 12, pp. 2927–31.

439. While studies of population . . .: Smith-Warner SA, Spiegelman D, Yaun SS et al., 'Intake of fruits and vegetables and risk of breast cancer: a pooled analysis of cohort studies', *Journal of the American Medical Association*, vol. 285, no. 6, 2001, pp. 769-776.

440. Low-level laser . . .: Carati CJ, Anderson SN, Gannon BJ, Piller NB, 'Treatment of postmastectomy lymphedema with low-level laser therapy: a double blind, placebo-controlled trial', *Cancer*, vol. 98, no. 6, 2003, pp. 1114–22.

PROSTATE CANCER

Page

443. It is estimated that . . .: Page WF, Braun MM, Partin AW et al., 'Heredity and prostate cancer: a study of World War II veteran twins', *Prostate*, vol. 33, no. 4, 1997, pp. 240–245.

443. Men with a family history . . .: Bratt O, 'Hereditary prostate cancer: clinical aspects', *Journal of Urology*, vol. 168, no. 3, 2002, pp. 906–913.

443. There is a twofold . . .: Jemal A, Siegel R, Ward E et al., 'Cancer statistics 2007', *CA A Journal for Cancer Clinicians*, vol. 57, no. 1, 2007, pp. 43–66.

443. There is approximately . . .: Kenfield SA, Chang ST, Chan JM, 'Diet and lifestyle interventions in active surveillance patients with favorable-risk prostate cancer', *Current Treatment Options Oncology*, vol. 8, no. 3, 2007, pp. 173–196.

443. The highest reported . . .: Cox B, Sneyd MJ, Paul C et al., 'Vasectomy and risk of prostate cancer', *Journal of the American Medical Association*, vol. 87, no. 23, 2002, pp. 3110–3115.

444. Until recently it was . . .: Yair L et al., 'Implications of the Prostate Cancer Prevention Trial: A Decision Analysis Model of Survival Outcomes', *Journal of Clinical Oncology*, vol. 23, no. 9, 2005.

444. But recent evidence . . .: Siddiqui MM, Wilson KM, Epstein MM et al., 'Vasectomy and Risk of Aggressive Prostate Cancer: A 24-Year Follow-Up Study', JCO.2013.54.8446.

447. A few studies have been . . .: Lucia MS, Epstein JI, Goodman PJ et al., 'Finasteride and high-grade prostate cancer in the Prostate Cancer Prevention Trial', *Journal of the National Caner Institute*, vol. 99, no. 18, 2007, pp. 1375–1383 and Thompson IM, Goodman PJ, Tangen CM et al., 'The influence of finasteride on the development of prostate cancer', *New England Journal of Medicine*, vol. 349, no. 3, 2003, pp. 215–224 and Rubin MA, Kantoff PW, 'Effect of finasteride on risk of prostate cancer: how little we really know', *Journal of Cellular Biochemisty*, vol. 91, no. 3, 2004, pp. 478–482.

447. There has been some concern . . .: Andriole GL, Roehrborn C, Schulman C et al., 'Effect of dutasteride on the detection of prostate cancer in men with benign prostatic hyperplasia', *Urology*, vol. 64, no. 3, 2004, pp. 537–541; discussion 42–43.

447. The dustasteride study . . .: Moyad MA, Merrick GS, Butler WM et al., 'Statins, especially atorvastatin, may favorably influence clinical presentation and biochemical progression-free survival after brachytherapy for clinically localized prostate cancer', *Urology*, vol. 66, no. 6, 2005, pp. 1150–1154.

449. The chance of becoming . . .: Ficarra V, Novara G, Rosen RC et al., 'Systematic review and meta-analysis of studies reporting urinary continence recovery after robot-assisted radical prostatectomy', European Urology, vol. 62 no. 3, 2012 pp. 405-17 doi: 10.1016/j. eururo.2012.05.045. Epub 2012 Jun 1.

449. It is important to arrange . . .: Cornel EB, de Wit R, Witjes JA, 'Evaluation of early pelvic floor physiotherapy on the duration and degree of urinary incontinence after radical retropubic prostatectomy in a non-teaching hospital', *World Journal of Urology*, vol. 23, no. 5, 2005, pp. 353–355 and Tarcia Kahihara C, Ferreira U, Nardi Pedro R et al., 'Early versus delayed physiotherapy in the treatment of post-prostatectomy male urinary incontinence', *Archivos Espanoles Urologia*, vol. 59, no. 8, pp. 773–778.

450. We now have loads of information . . .: Morton MS, Turkes A, Denis L et al., 'Can dietary factors influence prostatic disease?' *British Journal of Urology*, vol. 84, no. 5, 2005, pp. 549–554.

451. Obesity, high saturated-fat. . .: Efstathiou JA, Bae K, Shipley WU et al., 'Obesity and mortality in men with locally advanced prostate cancer: analysis of RTOG 85-31', *Cancer*, vol. 110, no. 12, 2007, pp. 2691–2699 and Gong Z, Agalliu I, Lin DW et al., 'Obesity is associated with increased risks of prostate cancer metastasis and death after initial cancer diagnosis in middle-aged men', *Cancer*, vol. 109, no. 6, 2007, pp. 1192–1202.

453. A trial using selenium . . .: Lippman SM, Klein EA, Goodman PJ et al., 'Effect of selenium and vitamin E on risk of prostate cancer and other cancers. The Selenium and Vitamin E Cancer Prevention Trial (SELECT)', *Journal of American Medical Association*, vol. 301, no. 1, 2009, pp. 39–51.

453. In countries where the soil . . .: Etminan M, FitzGerald JM, Gleave M et al., 'Intake of selenium in the prevention of prostate cancer: a systematic review and meta-analysis', *Cancer Causes Control*, vol. 16, no. 9, 2005, pp. 1125–1131.

453. Adequate vitamin D . . .: Autier P, Gandini S, 'Vitamin D supplementation and total mortality: a meta-analysis of randomized controlled trials', *Archives of International Medicine*, no. 167, vol. 16, 2007, pp. 1730–1737.

454. It is thought to be . . .: Teiten MH, Gaascht F, Eifes S, 'Chemopreventive potential of curcumin in prostate cancer', *Genes and Nutrition*, vol. 5, no. 1, 2010, pp. 61–74.

455. Daily aerobic exercise . . .: Torti DC, Matheson GO, 'Exercise and prostate cancer', *Sports Medicine*, vol. 34, no. 6, 2007, pp. 363–9 and Galvao DA, Taaffe DR, Spry N et al. Exercise can prevent and even reverse adverse effects of androgen suppression treatment in men with prostate cancer', Prostate cancer and prostatic diseases vol. 10, no. 4, 2007, pp. 340–346.

455. Regular resistance exercises . . .: Torti DC, Matheson GO, 'Exercise and prostate cancer'.

455. Long-term hormone therapy . . .: Galvao DA, Taaffe DR, Spry N et al., 'Exercise can prevent and even reverse adverse effects of androgen suppression treatment in men with prostate cancer', *Prostate Cancer Prostatic Diseases*, vol. 10, no. 4, 2007, pp. 340–346 and Vanoni C, 'Treatment of depression with St. Johns wort in general practice', *Praxis* (Bern 1994) 2000; 89(51/52),

pp. 2163–2167 and Morote J, Morin JP, Orsola A et al., 'Prevalence
of osteoporosis during long-term androgen deprivation therapy
in patients with prostate cancer', *Urology*, vol. 69, no. 3, 2007,
pp. 500–504.

457. The risk of osteoporosis can . . .: Yee EF, White RE, Murata GH
et al., 'Osteoporosis management in prostate cancer patients treated
with androgen deprivation therapy', *Journal of General Internal
Medicine*, vol. 22, no. 9, 2007, pp. 1305–1310.

457. Resistance exercise, and increasing . . .: Diamond TH, Higano CS,
Smith MR et al., 'Osteoporosis in men with prostate carcinoma
receiving androgen-deprivation therapy: recommendations
for diagnosis and therapies', *Cancer*, vol. 100, no. 5, 2004,
pp. 892–899 and Kogawa M, Wada S, 'Osteoporosis and alcohol
intake', *Clinical Calcium*, vol. 15, no. 1, 2005, pp. 102–105.

457. Depression and mood . . .: Vanoni C, 'Treatment of depression
with St. Johns wort in general practice', *Praxis* (Bern 1994) 2000;
89(51/52), pp. 2163–2167.

CANCER OF THE CERVIX

Page

459. The most common cervical . . .: Cancer Council Australia, 'Cervical
Cancer', 2015, www.cancer.org.au/about-cancer/types-of-cancer/
cervical-cancer.html

459. Adenocarcinoma is less common . . .: Cancer Research UK, 'Types
of Cervical Cancer', www.cancerresearchuk.org/about-cancer/type/
cervical-cancer/about/types-of-cervical-cancer

459. In Australia there were . . .: Australian Government, 'Cervical
cancer', 2014, http://canceraustralia.gov.au/affected-cancer/cancer-
types/gynaecological-cancers/cervical-cancer/cervical-cancer-statistics

459. Cervical cancer death rates . . .: ibid.

462. Increase your intake of . . .: Bell MC, et al., 'Placebo-controlled
trial of indole-3-carbinol in the treatment of CIN', *Gynecological
Oncology*, 2000;78:123–9.

462. Check for and correct . . .: Yüksel H, Odabasi AR, Cetin G et al.,
'Folate and vitamin B_{12} levels in abnormal pap smears: a case
control study', *European Journal of Gynaecological Oncology*,
2007, vol. 28, no. 6, pp. 526–30.

STOMACH CANCER

Page

464. For example, stomach cancer . . .: World Cancer Research Fund International, 'Stomach Cancer Statistics', 2015, http://www.wcrf. org/int/cancer-facts-figures/data-specific-cancers/stomach-cancer-statistics

464. Cancer prehabilitation . . .: Mayo NE1, Feldman L, Scott S, 'Impact of preoperative change in physical function on postoperative recovery: argument supporting prehabilitation for colorectal surgery', *Surgery*, vol. 150, no. 3, 2011, pp. 505-14, doi: 10.1016/j. surg.2011.07.045.

464. Prehabilitation involves anticipating . . .: Juul JW Tegels et al., 'Improving the outcomes in gastric cancer surgery', *World Journal of Gastroenterology*, vol. 20, no. 38, 2004, pp. 13692-13704, http://www.wjgnet.com/1007-9327/full/v20/i38/13692.htm

Index

Australian Clinico-Pathological Staging (ACPS) System 408

B

herbs and seasonings 341
holistic approach 6
holy basil (*Ocimum sanctum*) 165,
   205–6
hormonal therapy
   breast cancer 12, 110, 135, 422–4
   chemo brain and 151
   fatigue 263
   hair thinning 135
   osteoporosis 217
   prostate cancer 446, 456
   sexual function and 106, 110–13
   side effects 456–7
   sleep problems 362
hormone replacement therapy (HRT)
   207, 420, 426, 441
hormones
   immunity and 95
horse chestnut standardised extract
   159
hospital admissions 30
hot flushes
   self-assessment 32
household cleaners 293
huang-qi *see* astragalus
human papillomavirus (HPV) 460–1
   risk factors, reducing 462
   vaccine 167, 460–1
hydrogen peroxide (H2O2)
   176
Hypericum perforatum see St John's
   wort
hysterectomy 110
   sexual function and 110

I

immune function 355–6
   chemotherapy and 137–40
   diet 356–7
   digestive system, role of 356
   environment 358
   exercise and 317–18
   herbal medications 275–6

inflammatory response 355–6
innate immunity 355
intravenous nutrient therapy 174
   managing 137–40, 275–6, 356–9
   rehabilitation of immune system
     138
   stress management 138, 275
   supplements 139–40, 229, 358–9
immunisation 25, 39–40
   chemotherapy and 137
   travel plans 400
immunotherapy 2, 166–8, 224
   cancer vaccines 167
   fatigue 263
   monoclonal antibodies 166
   questions to ask 168
   targeted immune therapies 167
incontinence 33
   faecal 113
   urinary 34, 279, 449
indole-3-carbinol 222, 439
infections
   avoiding infectious people 137
   chemo brain and 151
   self-assessment 32
   signs, reporting 138
infertility
   chemotherapy and 145
inflammation
   mucous membranes 136, 221
   radiotherapy, caused by 158, 274–5
   yoga and 241–2
information
   collecting 13–14, 69, 91–2
   preparation for surgery 123
   warnings about public 15
insecticides 292–3
insomnia 75, 131, 151, 158, 212,
     223, 261, 263, 360–2, 389, 426
   managing 364–72, 364–71
   medication 370–1
   quitting smoking 389
integrative medicine 4–6, 55–6

malnutrition 334
mealtimes 328–30
mindful eating 327–8, 330
mouth problems and 161, 280, 282–3
mushrooms see mushrooms
nausea and vomiting, treating 260–1
obesity 331–6, 451
oils, healthy 341
omega-3 fatty acids 341
organic foods 342–3
pain management 251
phytonutrients 336–7
plant-based food 336
prehabilitation 119, 120
preparation for surgery 123–4, 126
processed foods 349–52
prostate cancer 451–6
protective elements 324–5
protein see protein
'rainbow diet' 336–7
self-assessment 36–7
sleep and 366
snacking 330
soy 346, 430, 452, 457
stomach cancer 464
superfoods 324
supplements 83, 135–6, 325–6, 335–6
travel plans 401
vegetables see vegetables
water 343

O
obesity 331–6
cancer, links to 331, 451
statistics 331
weight loss see weight loss
occupational therapist 51
Ocimum sanctum see holy basil
oestrogen 420
blocking 201, 224, 265, 422–4
vaginal creams 111, 426–7

oils, healthy 341
olive leaf 207
omega-3 fatty acids 341
oncologist 2, 20, 22, 46, 48, 121, 134
role of 49–50
oncology massage 235–8
chemotherapy and 130
contraindications 236–7
information for therapist 237–8
purpose 236
therapist 53, 56, 237
oncology nurse 50, 56
oncology social worker 51
opioids
pain management 257–8
oral health 121, 273–4 *see also* dental
health
candida 283
checklist 283–4
chemotherapy and 278–80
dentist, role of 280–1
diet and 282–3
flossing 282
fluoride gel 282
glutamine wash 281
jaw exercises 282
medications 283
mouthwash 281–2
neurotoxicity 280
nutrition and 280
radiotherapy and 157, 161–2
riboflavin (vitamin B2*) 281
taste alterations 280
toothbrush, choice of 281
trismus 279
organic foods 342–3
osteopath 51
osteopenia 217–18
osteoporosis 93, 217, 424, 457, 466
ovarian cancer 26, 68, 331
genetic risk factors 422
intravenous vitamin C 177, 178
ovaries, removal of 122

sexuality and recovery 106
'overall survival' 18
overexercising 321–2, 357
oxaliplatin 140, 142, 143, 186
oxytocin 95

P
paclitaxel (Pacific yew) 140, 142, 146,
    177, 181, 188
pain
    associated features 250
    cannabis use and 232–3
    causes 248, 249
    diary 249–50
    duration 250
    exercise and management of 252–3,
        307
    integrative management 251
    intensity 250
    investigations 250–1
    location 249
    management 248–59
    meditation and 87
    neuropathy and 140
    non-pharmalogical therapies 252–6
    onset 249
    pharmalogical therapies 256–9
    quality 250
    relieving factors 250
    self-assessment 32
    sleep problems 362
    supplements and 213, 224
    timing 249
    treatment and 249, 250
Palifermin (Kepivance) 283
palliative care 7, 19
    resources 7
Panax ginseng see ginseng
Panax quinquefolius see ginseng,
    American
pancreatic cancer 19
    supplements and 220
Pap smear 26, 39, 47, 459–61

paracetamol
    pain management 257
passionflower (*Passiflora incarnata*) 84
passive smoking 290–1
PDE5 inhibitors 112, 448
pelvic floor
    exercise 320–1
    physiotherapy 449–50
peppermint (*Mentha piperita*) 207
    precautions 207
personal hygiene 138
personal trainers 315
pesticides 292–3, 342
PET scans 31, 155
pet therapy 238–9
pharmaceutical treatment
    fatigue management 266
    lymphoedema 272
    pain management 256–9
pharmacist 51
phosphatidyl serine 153
phosphatidylcholine 153
physical therapy
    neuropathy, treating 144–5
physiotherapist 51, 315, 320
phytonutrients 336–7
Piper methysticum see kava kava
plant-based food 336
podiatrist 51
pollution
    air 291
    chemical 292–3, 342, 374–6
pomegranate (*Punica granatum l.*)
    347, 452
post-gastrectomy syndrome 465–6
post-operative cognitive dysfunction
    126
potassium 416
prebiotics 224–5
    bowel cancer 417
prehabilitation 119–21, 123, 304,
    322, 390, 464, 465
pressure garments 271

antioxidants and 181, 214–15
bowel cancer 409
breast cancer 12
debulking tumours and 122
dental and oral health 157, 278–84
emotional difficulties 162
fatigue 157–8, 263
fertility and 156
hair loss 162
herbal treatments 164–5
intravenous nutrient therapy and
174
loss of appetite 162
lymphoedema 159–60
methods of radiation delivery 156
mouth problems 161–2,
278–84
nature and purpose 154–5
nausea 162
osteoporosis 217
precautions for support people
162–4
preparation for 155–6
radiation dermatitis 160–1, 274–5
radioactive secretions 163
seed implants 163–4
sexual function and 110–11, 112
side effects 157–62
skin problems related to
32
yoga and 241
rectal cancer 66, 331
sexuality and 113
'recurrence-free survival' 18
red clover 207–8
precautions 208
red grapes 344
red meat 350
red salve (*Sanguinaria canadensis*)
438–9
reishi mushroom (*Ganoderma
lucidum*) 132, 165, 208, 265,
347–8

relapse or recurrence 21–2
mental health and 91–2
relationships 95–100 *see also* support
structures
counselling 100
ending 100
mending 100
post-cancer sexuality and 113–15
'relative survival' 18
relaxation 90, 358
chemotherapy and 130
preparation for surgery 124
therapy 89
remission 14, 21–2
complete 22
partial 22
resilience 65, 70, 88, 92, 102, 123,
287
resistance training 318, 335, 457
resveratrol 148, 208–9, 344–5
rhubarb root (*Rheum officinale* or *R.
palmatum*) 268
riboflavin (vitamin B2*) 281

S
Saccharomyces boulardii 225
safety
exercise, during 319–20
saw palmetto (*Serenoa repens*) 210–11
interactions 210–11
precautions 210
scarring
sexuality and body image 108–10
screening 25–7
bowel cancer 405–8
cervical cancer 26, 459–60
cost 26
following up results 66–7
government subsidy 26
GP, role of 47
mental health issues related to 66–9
purpose 25–6
Scutellaria spp.

allium 344
cancer-protective diet 343–5
cruciferous 344, 452
juicing 348
vegetarian diet 339–40
breast cancer 430
vincristine (Madagascar periwinkle)
140, 188, 280
Viscum album L. see mistletoe
Vitamin A 214–15, 359
Vitamin B group 186, 216, 260, 359,
429
alcohol, withdrawal from
304–6
B1* (thiamine) 142–3, 216, 466
B2* (riboflavin) 281
B6* (pyridoxine) 133, 142–3, 216,
260, 414, 462
B12* (cyancobalamin, cobalamin)
143, 216, 414, 462, 465, 466
intravenous therapy 186
nausea and vomiting, treating 260
vitamin C (ascorbic acid) 179, 226–7,
306, 342, 344, 359, 462, 465, 466
antioxidant, as 176, 214–15
breast cancer and 432–3
intravenous see intravenous vitamin
C
pro-oxidant, as 176–7
vitamin D 357, 359, 411, 415, 434,
453
Vitamin E (*alpha-tocopherol*) 142,
148, 214, 227–8, 359, 453
deficiency 227–8
precautions 228
volatile organic compounds (VOCs)
379
vomiting 207, 229
chemotherapy and 132–3, 272
management of symptoms 259–61
self-assessment 32
vulval cancer 222
sexuality and recovery 106

W

waist measurement 34–5, 332
warfarin 152, 195, 198, 203, 205,
211, 220, 452
water 343, 356
bowel cancer and intake of 413
websites
warnings regarding 15
weedkillers 292–3
weight 34, 356
cancer risk and 332
increasing 334–6
lymphoedema treatment 271
obesity 331–6, 412, 451
quitting smoking 388
underweight 333–6
weight loss 332–3
chemotherapy and 333
depression and 74
preparation for surgery 123
self-assessment 32
unplanned 333–6
wigs 134
withania (*Withania somnifera*,
Ashwagandha, Indian ginseng)
84, 139, 213

X

x-rays 31, 250, 293–4
xerostomia 161–2

Y

yoga 88, 239–43, 358, 427–8
Ashtanga 240
benefits 240–1, 427–8
Bikram 240
chemotherapy and 130, 152
detox process 382
fatigue, and 241–2
inflammation, and 241–2
Iyengar 240
Kundalini 240
pain management 253